*Disordered Thinking
and Schizophrenic
Psychopathology*

Disordered Thinking and Schizophrenic Psychopathology

MARTIN HARROW, Ph.D.
and
DONALD M. QUINLAN, Ph.D.

Foreword by Roy R. Grinker, Sr., M.D.

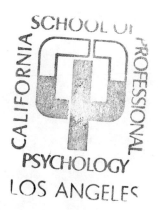

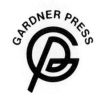

GARDNER PRESS, INC.
New York & London

GARDNER PRESS, INC.
19 Union Square West
New York 10003

Harrow, Martin.
    Disordered thinking and schizophrenic
psychopathology / by Martin Harrow and Donald
Quinlan. Gardner Press, c1985.
ISBN: 0-89876-099-2
                        78-13649

Book Design by Sidney Solomon
PRINTED IN THE UNITED STATES OF AMERICA

CONTENTS

PART II
BIZARRE-IDIOSYNCRATIC THINKING

Drive-Dominated Thinking and Impairment in Perspective
    and Monitoring

PART IV
BOUNDARY-RELATED PHENOMENA

PART V
OTHER IMPORTANT ASPECTS OF
DISORDERED THINKING AND OVERVIEW

PART IV
APPENDIX

Foreword

Whenen a Michael Reese group first began to study schizophrenia in the early 1950s, I was asked, as the Clinical Director, to write the clinical introduction to Samuel J. Beck's book, *The Six Schizophrenias*. I found that the area of schizophrenia contained a large number of diverse theories, most of which paid little attention to data and empirical facts. The field was confusing, and I commented on this to several of my colleagues. Indeed, over the last thirty years advances from my own research program, and from many other research programs, have brought some clarity to the field. When I step back and take another look at the area after many years, I find there are still large gaps in knowledge, and now almost thirty years later, the field is still in confusion. There are diverse facts that have not been put together in coherent fashion to form a strong theory of schizophrenia. The years have moved by, but the sense of confusion and lack of knowledge in schizophrenia continues.

Throughout this period I have attempted to encourage promising mental health professionals in the direction of empirical research. Drs. Harrow and Quinlan have been among those whom I have encouraged.

It has long been my feeling that advances in the understanding of schizophrenia are most likely to be made by solid empirical research in which specific samples of patients are studied in systematic research programs. Empirical data collected in this way, using standardized instruments where possible, can advance the field. This model becomes much more powerful if it is combined with systematic follow-up of the same patients over time. A research program of this type can be designed to advance knowledge of state versus trait features in schizophrenia. In the settings that I have directed in the past, I have encouraged this type of research and attempted to supply the resources (including financial) to help. Harrow and Quinlan have conducted such an exploration, using systematic instruments, collected on large samples of patients over time. I believe this type of longitudinal approach to research on disordered thinking is unique to the field, can make major contributions, and can advance our state of knowledge.

Harrow and Quinlan have been among the nation's leading scholars in the area of thought disorder, as a result both of their consistent productivity in this area, and of the new ideas they have generated and new areas they have studied. Their research has explored a variety of areas concerning schizophrenic thought disorder. This includes their exploration of factors that underlie thought disorder, their longitudinal studies of schizophrenic thinking, and their study of how thought disorder has been erroneously identified only with schizophrenia. Thus, a major feature of importance to the field concerning Harrow and Quinlan's research, along with that of Andreasen and others, is that they have been able to identify thought disorder in both schizophrenia and in other psychiatric syndromes, such as bipolar affective disroders. Until now, however, their research findings have been spread among a variety of different psychiatric and psychological journals. This is one of the reasons why I have encouraged them to pull together current diverse aspects of their research into a single book.

Roy R. Grinker, Sr., M.D.
Chairman Emeritus,
Department of Psychiatry
Michael Reese Hospital and
Medical Center;
Professor Emeritus
Department of Psychiatry
University of Chicago.

Preface

T hought disorder, or disordered thinking, has long been viewed as one of the major features of schizophrenia. This has been true with patients regarded as schizophrenic according to the older DSM II system of classification and is still true for patients regarded as schizophrenic according to more current diagnostic systems.

Over the years extensive research has been conducted to answer major questions about thought disorder. Despite these efforts, thought disorder in schizophrenia is still not completely understood. There are large gaps in our knowledge of the types of disordered thinking that are most important, of the empirical relationships that exist, and there is considerable lack of certainty about the exact role of thought disorder in schizophrenia.

The present book contains a presentation of major aspects of a program of research studying schizophrenia conducted over a number of years by the two authors. This program began with our collaboration while we were both on the faculty at Yale University, and has continued since then when one of us (MH) left to assume a position in Chicago. Our continued collaboration has provided us with the advantages in our work of being able to study samples from two different geographical areas.

During this period of collaboration our goal has been to collect data systematically bearing on a number of different theoretical approaches concerning thought disorder in schizophrenia. We have also attempted to study schizophrenic patients at a number of different phases of their disorder in order to get a more rounded and complete picture of what schizophrenic patients are like. Our studies of thought disorder in schizophrenia have also lead us to explore, systematically, the presence of pathological cognition in other, nonschizophrenic patients, including manic patients. Major aspects of the data associated with our research program have been published previously in a number of psychological and psychiatric journals.

Our goal in this book has been to outline our research bearing on the classical theories of schizophrenic thinking, as well as some of the approaches we have adapted to explore our new formulations and hypotheses. We have tried to be clear as to which theories are supported by our data, and which theories our data question. We have also discussed our views on various types of thought disorder in schizophrenia, and how one should regard them in the light of our own and others' modern research.

Thus, our data have led us to adopt a theoretical position that bears on the potential importance of various types of thought disorders in relation to schizophrenic psychopathology, and to adopt a theoretical position on factors that we have proposed are involved in schizophrenic thought disorder. We have discussed this at various points in the book, with special emphasis on our position in the latter part of Chapter 5 and Chapter 16, although we also have included material on aspects of this position in Chapter 3 and in several other places.

We should note that our research on schizophrenic thinking has been facilitated by the active help of a number of key figures. Dr. Gary Tucker, Professor and Chairman of the Department of Psychiatry at Dartmouth Medical School has worked with us as a colleague during a number of years of our research, with the three of us actively directing the overall research program during that period. Our investigation of schizophrenic cognition, and of schizophrenia in general, our productivity, and our thinking in these areas have been enhanced considerably by his colleagueship.

We have also received strong continual administrative support and encouragement from our respective departmental chairmen, as well as from other professionals with administrative responsibility in our settings. While a number of key figures have been involved, this especially includes Drs. Malcolm Bowers, Jr., Robert Davies, Thomas Detre, Daniel X. Freedman, Roy R. Grinker, Sr., Daniel Offer, and Morton Reiser.

In addition to receiving strong administrative support, we have received considerable stimulation from regular discussion with a number of other senior investigators, among whom are Drs. Boris Astrachan, Sidney Blatt, Stephen Fleck, Philip Holzman, and Theodore Lidz. Possibly of most importance to us has been our work, at various points over the years, with a large number of other vigorous and talented investigators, some as colleagues, some as students, and many in combinations of these two. These investigators have taken major responsibility for implementing key aspects of the research program. They have included Drs. David Adler, Rima Brauer, Evelyn Bromet, Kathleen Carlson, John Colbert, Linda Grossman, Ilene Lanin-Kettering, Joanne Marengo, Joan Miller, Sally Ross Oldham, Larry Pickett Jr., Michael Pogue-Geile, Mel Prosen, Sue Wallington Quinlan, Francine Rattenbury, Arthur H. Schwartz, Martin Schwartzman, David Schultz, Paul Shield, Andrew Siegel, Marshall Silverstein, Jerry Westermeyer, and Arnold Wilson.

The research program has been aided by the very fine secretarial assistance provided by Ms. Yvonne Nelson, Ruth Strawder, Laura deCarvalho, Karen Heinold, and Louise Hall.

In addition to the excellent research atmosphere provided by our department chairmen and other key administrators at our settings, funding for major aspects of our data collection and analyses have been dependent on the support of research grant nos. MH-26341, MH-30929, and MH-30938, from the National Institute of Mental Health, research grant no. SIMH-8039-3 from the State of Illinois, DMH-DD, and grants from the John D. and Catherine T. MacArthur Foundation, and from the Carnegie Corporation.

Finally, we should note that during the very busy, at times almost hectic, period during which we have conducted this research, we have had the support, encouragement, and tranquil peace in our home lives that our industrious and supportive wives, Helen Harrow and Sue Quinlan, have provided, even while simultaneously pursuing their own productive careers.

We also would like to thank the editors of the following journals and books for their kind permission to reproduce tables of data and results which we had published in the articles and chapters listed below.

American Journal of Psychiatry, 128, 824–829, 1972; *130,* 702–706, 1973.
Archives of General Psychiatry, 20, 159–166, 1969; *27,* 40–45, 1972; *27,* 443–447, 1972; *28,* 179–182, 1973; *31,* 27–33, 1974; *34,* 15–21, 1977; *39,* 665–671, 1982.
British Journal of Psychiatry, 117, 509–515, 1970; *121,* 529–539, 1972; *127,* 240–246, 1975.
Comprehensive Psychiatry, 15, 57–67, 1974.

Journal of Abnormal Psychology, 83, 533–541, 1974.
Journal of Nervous and Mental Disease, 162, 105–112, 1976.
Journal of Personality Assessment, 40, 31–41, 1976; *42,* 401–408, 1978.
Psychiatric Quarterly, 48, 1–8, 1974.
Williams and Wilkins Company, *Human Functioning in Longitudinal Perspective,* Chapter 2, pp. 9–18, 1980.

## PART I

INTRODUCTION

1

The Nature And Status Of Disordered Thinking In Schizophrenia

A young schizophrenic woman was asked, shortly after being hospitalized, to talk about the events leading up to it:

I had a . . . I was . . . first, uh, I found myself constantly trying to find myself, and part of that got me into Alaska where I was fishing. And I enjoyed the work on the boat but some of the implications of that work . . . I made a lot of free associations about what I was doing, and how that pertained to myself or my image of myself, and when I lost the job on the boat . . . and later that fall my mother called several times and telegrammed—I flew down to her house and found that things that were going on between myself and her were very strange to me.

I felt very frightened about the idea of . . . of . . . of . . . uh . . . of what a supposition my taking the earth as being a universal woman image could mean as far as being much too heavy a burden for anybody and especially difficult, uh, for me and yet it seemed like a lot of people were on that kind of a merry-go-round—that was becoming increasingly destructive to life and to a sense of home which I liked to feel about being in. [slight pause] Also, I guess I probably felt some fear of being kind of left on my own, without any . . . uh . . . any patterns, really, it didn't make any sense to me . . . I seemed to be robbed of just the ability to go by my senses and what I thought was natural . . . that seemed to be something too . . . too demanding. Uh, what I was in was a relationship to someone else. And, uh . . . sometimes I'd feel like I wanted to hold on and stop, uh, that whole cycle, and other times I would feel kind of giddy about being involved in that whole cycle.

But it always seemed to kind of mean that I was a radius of something that was going on in my life . . . most of my friends and relations could talk to me even if they couldn't talk to each other . . . that was especially true between my mother and my father . . . they both felt close to me, concerned about me, but they couldn't bridge any gaps between themselves. And, uh. that made me feel to some extent that I'd like to be very strong, but I didn't like the idea of having to be that strong—it seemed very weighty . . . very heavy . . . a very heavy kind of load psychically to be carrying or whatever . . . emotionally . . . to try to be carrying.

Severe mental disorder, and psychotic thinking, have been aspects of human experience in almost all cultures known to man. Man's fear and awe of psychosis and his rudimentary attempts to make sense of the phenomenon have existed since antiquity. The approaches have been two-edged: marked by both fear of the unknown and a desire to extirpate or control it; on the other hand, people have held a sense of awe and fascination such that in some cultures, persons passing through a bout of psychotic behavior have become set apart as having magical or prophetic powers or being special. The modern counterpart of this fascination can be seen in the experimentation with hallucinogenic drugs.

Some early "hypotheses" to explain psychotic disorders emphasized the lack of apparent control the victim had—he or she was "taken over" by evil spirits, demons, or the like as if another person were in control of the body, often with malevolent intent. Treatment could range from banishment and avoidance, to invocation of religious figures to reintegrate the victim, to more violent means for "getting rid of" the disruptive presence. On the more benign side, poets and artists were at times regarded with awe for the "poetic frenzy" they were at times observed to display when "inspired by the muse." The nonrational behavior of poets, artists, and others placed them apart, perhaps in small part as objects of fear, but to an even greater extent as objects of fascination.

Two aspects of psychotic thinking that emerge in these accounts are noteworthy. First, there is the common assumption that a person "has" or "does not have" the phenomenon in question; possession, inspiration or witchcraft is usually regarded as an all-or-nothing state. Second, there is the belief that the victim or recipient has lost control to other forces; the behavior is not considered human. Other non-Western cultures evolved different conceptions of what we infer to be manifestations of mental illness, but the treatment of disordered or different behavior as due to an entity that is not human and not under control of the person is a common notion of psychotic disorders.

Psychology and psychiatry have shared the ambivalent attitude toward psychosis and disordered thinking. In the past, the view has been that a patient either "has" or does not have a *thought disorder*. A person afflicted with such a disorder is treated as if he or she has some entity, "schizophrenia" or "psychosis," that must be extirpated before recovery can be complete. Some writers have seen aspects in the nonlogical creative process and in dreams similar to the distortion of psychosis, such as Freud's *Interpretation of Dreams* (Freud, 1965), Kris's study of art (Kris, 1952), and Robert Holt's elucidation of primary and secondary process on such projective techniques as the Rorschach (Holt, 1977). The fascination with the nonlogical but at times insightful communication have induced some therapists to focus on this aspect of psychosis as a value that should be fostered, rather than "ameliorated" by such techniques as psychosis-reducing drugs.

There is tacit agreement on the presence of disordered thinking in psychosis. Disordered thinking is a prominent and nearly universally agreed upon feature of schizophrenia, and is frequently considered a part of psychosis in general. That illusory agreement breaks down as soon as we ask, "What is the disorder in disordered thinking?" Answers to such a question frequently illuminate more about how or where the responder was trained than about the nature of disordered thinking. Many hypotheses about the origin and nature of disordered thinking have been proposed. We have studied several of these hypotheses and will present them in detail. Kraepelin (1950) can be considered the originator of the modern classification of schizophrenia; he included dementia as an essential aspect of the disorder. Freud (1965) introduced the notion of continuity between normal neurotic and psychotic processes, and the psychoanalytic theories of Freud and others are rich in hypotheses such as the influence of drive, the breakdown of psychic boundaries, and general disintegration of ego. Other hypotheses have been more specific; for example, disordered thinking arises out of one or another particular aspect of thinking such as associations, logic, substitution of dominant meaning, overinclusion, interference by affect, concreteness, and attentional deficits.

GOAL OF THIS BOOK

Given the already enormous body of literature on schizophrenia and disordered thinking, how far advanced is our thinking on the topic? How much do we know? And are most of the key features already agreed upon? After all, most clinical and research efforts directed at schizophrenia have agreed that a disorder of thinking is a major and central aspect, either as a primary or causative factor, or as a key secondary exacerbating symptom. Further scrutiny, however, reveals a polyglot of interpretations as to what constitutes a "thought disorder." Bleuler (1950 emphasized the "loosening of associations" that he believed is a common factor. Cameron (1944) emphasized over-inclusion. Others, such as Goldstein (1944) and Benjamin (1944), have emphasized the schizophrenic's concreteness, and still others, such as Arieti (1974a) and von Domarus (1944), have noted the schizophrenic's problems in the formal use of logic. Thus, in many ways, there is a great deal of disagreement concerning which aspect of disturbed thinking is central to schizophrenia, and the label "a schizophrenic thought disorder" is being used by clinicians to describe different phenomena, some of which may even be unrelated.

While there is still no agreement on which aspect of thinking is disordered, a variety of possible "central disturbances" in the thinking disorder are associated with schizophrenia. This book is not a review of theories of thought disorders. Such reviews exist elsewhere (Buss and Lang, 1965; Lang and Buss, 1965; Chapman and Chapman, 1973, among others). Rather, this book describes a series of empirical studies of schizophrenics and other disturbed patient populations that have a direct bearing on the major theories of disordered thinking conducted in several successive populations of psychiatric patients. Many patients have been studied at early, acute phases of their illness, to assess the validity and utility of the various concepts of schizophrenia at the phase when initial clinical diagnoses occurs, although we also have studied other chronic schizophrenic samples. Our systematic investigations of these successive populations of patients have led to a series of formulatons about the nature of the cognitive disorder in schizophrenia, which we will present.

PLAN

In this chapter, we will briefly describe some of the major theories of disordered thinking. In the next chapter, we will discuss general methodological issues and the particular issues arising in the studies of schizophrenic thinking.

In Part II, Chapters 3 to 5, we will review our research on bizarre-idiosyncratic thinking, a concept we have employed to encompass various types of "positive" thought disorder. Chapter 3 covers our major findings in patients during the acute phase of their illness, the phase in which most diagnostic decisions are made. Chapter 4 addresses some of the issues raised by bizarre-idiosyncratic thinking— its prominence in schizophrenia, its occurrence in other disorders, and its discriminating power among diagnoses. Disordered thinking as a symptom shows distinct differences in various phases of psychiatric disorder. In Chapter 5, we examine the levels of bizarre-idiosyncratic thinking during different phases of the illness: the acute phase, the phase of partial remission, the posthospital phase, and the chronic phase. In Chapter 5 we also discuss some of our research studying factors that may influence bizarre-idiosyncratic thinking.

In Part III, we look at our research bearing on some of the major classical theories of schizophrenic thought patholgy. The presence of primitive-drive-dominated thinking and it relationship to schizophrenia and other disorders are detailed in Chapter 6. The hypothesis of concrete versus abstract thinking is presented in Chapter 7, while loose associations, so critical in early theories of schizophrenia, are explored in Chapter 8.

Part IV outlines our research bearing on a major area: hypotheses about the quality of boundaries in schizophrenic thinking. Evidence for the presence of disturbed boundaries is presented in Chapter 9. "Conceptual Overinclusion," one of a number of forms of the general hypothesis of overinclusion, is described and detailed in a series of studies presented in Chapter 10. Depersonalization, derealization, and *déjà vu*, forms of disturbance that have been described as boundary-related phenomena, are explored in relation to schizophrenia and dysphoric affect in Chapter 11. Attentional disorders, particular stimulus overinclusion, are described in Chapter 12.

In Part V, we explore facets of disordered thinking that are related not only to schizophrenia, but also to hallucinogenic drug use (Chapter 13), and disordered thinking in family members of both schizophrenic and nonschizophrenic patients (Chapter 14). In Chapter 15, the intercorrelations of various Rorschach responses indicating disordered thinking are compared with each other and with other measures of psychopathology. Finally, in Chapter 16 we present a review and summary of major facets of disordered thinking, including our own synthesis of major issues in the area. We have also presented, as an appendix, a detailed manual describing our assessment and measurement of the construct of bizarre-idiosyncratic thinking.

PSYCHIATRIC CLASSIFICATION
AND THOUGHT DISORDERS

Kraeplin

Kraeplin's early classification of psychiatric illnesses completed a century-long movement to take disordered "mental" behavior out of the spiritual realm into the medical. His key focus was on separating patients with *dementia praecox* (his term for the disorder we now label "schizophrenia") from other patients with manic-depressive psychosis. As he saw it, patients with *dementia praecox* had a disorder that began early (often as early as adolescence), and followed a progressive downhill course. In contrast to the downhill course of *dementia praecox*, manic-depressive patients had a circular disorder in which periods of free-functioning recovery were followed by relapses, by later recoveries, and by further relapses. Kraeplin's formulation of the disorder *dementia praecox* as an entity had several additional distinguishing features: its major identifying symptomatology was dementia, but in addition it was considered to be a separate identifiable medical condition, and was looked at as genetic in cause, and therefore not amenable to treatment. If the patient improved, it was assumed that the diagnosis had been wrong and that the patient "had" another illness. Kraeplin, with his careful emphasis on detailed description, also could be considered to have brought the focus for behavior disorders into a scientific-descriptive era.

CLASSICAL VIEWS OF THOUGHT DISORDER

Bleuler (1950) made one of the earliest contributions to understanding the nature of thought disorder in schizophrenia. In his view, the major symptoms of schizophrenia were the "four As" affect, association, autism, and ambivalence. While this included affective, interpersonal, and other dimensions of the schizophrenic's behavior, his central emphasis was on associations.

One of Bleuler's contributions to the study of schizophrenia was to introduce psychological principles to the study of schizophrenia, and of thinking disorders. He brought the then current attention to associations, which was popular in the psychology of his day, to the understanding of schizophrenic thinking. Bleuler believed that a loosening of associative links (the single major factor in his theory), combined with the presence of affective deterioration and a dominance of the person's inner life, could explain a whole range of phenomena in schizophrenia, including delusions and hallucinations. In particular, he felt that the weakening of associative links combined with a dominance of the patient's major problem areas, his wishes, conflicts, and complexes, are of crucial importance. He believed that these intrude into the patient's behavior, with this being the major factor in the forming of his psychosis. In this way he brought psychological principles into the picture, centered on the person's dynamic wishes and fears.

A second emphasis introduced by Bleuler was the deterioration of affect and blunting in schizophrenia. The very use of the term "schizophrenia," which has remained with us to this day, signified what Bleuler considered to be the central aspect of schizophrenia: the splitting and weakening of the various mental functions, and of the personality. Thus, theories of mental functions, most of which are subsumed under thinking, took a central position in theories of thought disorder.

One of the earliest attempts to operationalize "thinking" per se can be seen in work by von Domarus (1944), later developed more fully by Arieti (1974a, 1974b)—namely, that the disorder of schizophrenia is a failure of *logical* thinking, or "paleologic." In this view, schizophrenic symptoms proceed along the path of primitive but illogical thinking.

Another thrust in the early work on thinking disorder was to view schizophrenic thinking as the outcome of a different use of *language*. Symbolic meanings are taken as literal, and literal as symbolic; parts are taken for the whole and wholes for parts. This position and a number of other positions based on the study of the meaning of schizophrenics' speech and behavior can lead to the view that the disordered productions have meaning, albeit often private one, which, if understood, would make schizophrenic thinking intelligible.

PSYCHOANALYTIC THEORIES OF THOUGHT DISORDER

Many of the classical hypotheses about the nature of thought disorder are influenced by psychoanalytic models. As Freud, and later his followers, developed psychoanalysis, various models evolved for the conceptualization of thought disorder. Even Bleuler's emphasis on the later dominance of the patients's inner life and his conflicts reflects the influence of Freud and Jung.

Early theories of affect blocking suggested a difficulty with undischarged affect. Offshoots of these concepts persist in hypotheses involving interference theory, such as a disruption of thinking by affective stimuli (Lang and Buss, 1965; Buss and Lang, 1965). Beginning with his classical work on the interpretation of dreams, Freud's topographical model suggested that schizophrenic thinking along with normal states of altered conscoiusness were due to a dominance by primitive forms of drive-dominated thinking, or "primary process" thinking. Along with later drive theories, aspects of such a model are seen in notions of drive-dominated thinking and the use of primitive modes of thought (e.g., condensation, displacement). A somewhat later step placed heavy emphasis on developmentally early conflicts leading to the core symptomatology of schizophrenia.

With the emergence of emphasis on the ego and its role in defending against both drives and external stresses, the notion was advanced of defective barriers and boundaries, allowing too-free play to primitive impulses and failing to protect the psyche from too-intense stimulation. Later ego theories place more emphasis on the defective ego and its failure in one or more functions (e.g., Bellak & Loeb, 1968). Schizophrenia can be seen in this light as a generalized ego defect, resulting not only in the "negative" symptoms, but also the "positive" symptoms, the misdirected attempts to make sense of disordered inner representations and defective perception of reality. This latter view is the most comprehensive and general theory of schizophrenia. Unlike earlier forms that sought "core" or primary symptoms, theories of ego defects allow a multiplicity of symptoms of varying types to be subsumed under "ego defects." These more general theories are quite appealing, but have the disadvantage of not being specific as to which of many disordered features can be expected to be most frequent or specific in schizophrenia. Any manifestation can be interpreted as a sign of the disorder, without placing primacy on any specific aspect.

INTERPERSONAL THEORIES

While theories emphasizing thought disorder in schizophrenia have tended to focus on the internal mental "works" of schizophrenics, other theories have emphasized the distorted interpersonal relationships in the disorder. Sullivan, for example, in his theory focusing on personal insecurity (1953), emphasized the difficulty of the schizophrenic in forming nonpossessive relationships with others. Modern offshoots of "object-relations" theory have focused on the distortion of current relationships by attempts to re-create early infantile relationships. Diverse theorists such as Kaiser (Fierman, 1965), and Blatt and Wild (1976), have cited their belief in a simultaneous wish for and fear of fusion with others as a core element in the genesis of distorted interpersonal relationships. Views such as those of Blatt might be labeled as "boundary" theories.

"Transactional" theories emphasize distortions of communicaton in the schizophrenic's familial relationships (e.g., Lidz, Fleck, and Cornelison, 1965; Singer and Wynne, 1965a, 1965b; Bateson, Jackson, Haley, and Weakland, 1956). Theories such as that of Lidz emphasize that a thinking disorder is most clearly found in the distortions in communication patterned after inconsistent and deviant family patterns of communication, rather than in the schizophrenic's inability to reason about neutral objects. In a number of places in this book, we examine a view of disordered thinking as a breakdown in two aspects of interpersonal communication: the loss of perspective and the failure to monitor one's behavior. These two aspects of disordered thinking can be applied to a number of theoretical positions that emphasize the communicative element of thinking and speech.

SOME MAJOR HYPOTHESES ABOUT DISORDERED THINKING

Several attempts have been made to isolate the "central" defect in disordered thinking. Such attempts have agreed with Bleuler's distinction between "primary" and "secondary" symptoms in which a single or a few central symptoms start a chain of secondary effects that produce the final array of the clinical picture. To assert that one aspect of schizophrenic thinking constitutes a "primary" symptom implies a theory of thinking in which the central symptom is related to a core process of thought, or one that has very general relationships in the thought process.

Positive and Negative Symptoms

Symptoms of schizophrenia have been classified by some investigators as "positive" or "negative," using the following guidelines: (a) *positive symptoms*—floridly symptomatic behavior, or unusual or bizarre thoughts; and (b) *negative symptoms*—the absence of normal functioning, or a deficit state or defect state (Andreasen, 1979, 1982; Angrist, Rotrosen, and Gershon, 1980; Chapman and Chapman, 1973; Strauss, Carpenter, and Bartko, 1974). The terms "positive" and "negative symptoms" were first used by Hughlings-Jackson (1931). Among the more common positive symptoms are delusions, hallucinations, and "positive formal thought disorder" symptoms; these "positive" symptoms are characteristic of schizophrenia, but are present in some other disorders as well. In regard to disordered thinking, Fish (1962) originally defined positive formal thought disorder as "a wealth of unusual thoughts." Negative symptoms include reduced or impoverished speech; flattened affect; anhedonia; social isolation; cognitive and intellectual deficit; psychomotor retardation; and various other deficit symptoms. Kraeplin (1950) [originally published in 1919] initially identified dementia praecox as a disorder with a progressive downward course, implying an increase of negative symptoms.

Two "negative" symptoms, restricted (flat) affect and poor rapport were among the most discriminating symptoms in 1,202 patients in the International Pilot Study of Schizophrenia (Carpenter, Strauss, and Bartko, 1974), but several positive symptoms were almost as discriminating. Some investigators have suggested that negative symptoms are the outcome of the disorder and resulting relationships with individuals and the deleterious effects of living in institutions (Gruenberg, 1969; Wing, 1962; Wing and Brown, 1970).

Negative symptoms have also been associated with poor outcome (Astrup and Noreik, 1966), although this result could be due to confusion with chronicity (Strauss and Carpenter, 1974). In recent research we have conducted with M. Pogue-Geile on a sample of relatively young, early schizophrenics studied during the posthospital period, we found a subgroup of these schizophrenics with negative symptoms. Our data indicated that there was a significant relationship between the presence of negative symptoms and poor posthospital social and work functioning (Pogue-Geile and Harrow, 1984). Even here, however, the possible influence of early chronicity in this young sample cannot be completely ruled out. In addition we found a relationship between poor prehospital social functioning and subsequent negative symptoms at follow-up. Andreasen (1982) also found that schizophrenics with negative symptoms had poorer premorbid history, more and longer hospitalizaton, and had more frequently received ECT. Patients with negative symptoms also had more frequent signs of cortical atrophy on CAT scans.

Many of the positive symptoms are strongly associated with schizophrenia. Schneider (1959) identified eleven symptoms designated "first-rank" for the positive identification of schizophrenia. Most of these signs (e.g., audible thoughts and thought insertion) involve positive symptoms related to disorders of thought. The International Pilot Study, among others, has suggested that these positive signs are highly related to the diagnosis of schizophrenia (Carpenter, Strauss, and Bartko, 1974). The classification of schizophrenia in the new diagnostic system adopted in the country, DSM III, is based primarily on positive symptoms. The relationship of positive symptoms at the acute phase to later outcome is not clear (Harrow, Bromet, and Quinlan, 1974); in general, findings have tended to indicate little prognostic significance beyond the negative outcome of schizophrenia itself, when one restricts the sample being analyzed to only schizophrenics.

At times in this book we have placed aspects of our research on thought disorder within the framework of the concepts of positive and negative symptoms. Thus, a construct we have found most promising, bizarre-idiosyncratic thinking, is for all practical purposes a comprehensive measure of "unusual" thoughts or of positive thought disorder, and our detailed research using this construct will be discussed extensively.

Logic

From a historical standpoint, the logic involved in the schizophrenic patient's thinking has been the subject of considerable discussion. Von Domarus (1944) proposed a theory of schizophrenic logic, elaborated by Arieti, called *paleologic*, in which the identity of predicates is generalized erroneously to the identity of the subject. For example, "The devil influences some people, I feel influenced, I am therefore being influenced by the devil" would be a paleological origin of a delusion of influence. Logicians may be more familiar with this as a form of the fallacy of the undistributed middle term. According to this view, the schizophrenic is distinguished by the frequency of such illogical errors. A more general view would be that thought disorder originates by the frequent, pervasive, and unyielding quality of illogical thinking in the schizophrenic. These views have not yet been documented with large samples of patients, and our early research in this area has not tended to support them.

Associations

As noted earlier, since Bleuler's original formulations, the looseness of schizophrenics' associations has been noted as a major form of thought disorder, and has been the basis of one of the prominent theories of schizophrenia. An association shows overt signs of being "loose" when it involves shift of topic or content that is not predicted (presumably by an impartial observer) by the previous speech of the patient. Our research on loose associations is described in Chapter 8.

While concepts about loose associations in schizophrenia form one of the important theories of this disorder, they leave many questions unanswered. This formulation, if accurate, opens almost as many new questions as it purports to solve old ones. Thus, if hypotheses about loose associations are accurate, the important issue would be: What are the *major or most prominent characteristics* of such looseness?

If loose associations are important, is the material that sets off loose associations related to the patient's emotional concerns or is more neutral material just as likely to set off loose associations in the schizophrenic? Does the loose material come from the patient's personal life? If it comes from the patient's personal life, is it from material related to childhood events, or more recent events, or from some other source? If the loose material is related to the patient's personal life, does the loose material come from one central "complex" for each individual patient or from a variety of topics for each patient?

Chapman and Chapman (1973) have suggested a highly specific form of looseness. They believe that schizophrenics' associations are more frequently loose. When looseness occurs, the meaning of the word chosen by the schizophrenic is the more dominant meaning, usually defined as the more frequent use of a word. For example, "The problem weighed heavily on his shoulders," would sometimes be interpreted by a schizophrenic as, "He had something heavy around his shoulders," since this is the more common meaning of the term "heavy." While Chapman and Chapman's formulations are important, they only focus on one or two aspects of the hypothetical "looseness" of the schizophrenic. A number of other questions about the potential looseness of the schizophrenic would still need to be resolved, even after possible confirmation of their hypothesis.

Looseness of associations is usually defined in a more general fashion. Perhaps what appears "loose" for a patient is an intermingling into his verbalizations, and possibly into his thinking, of his personal concerns, at times idiosyncratically interpreted. We have presented aspects of our research studying this issue in Chapter 5. Disordered thinking may be overgeneralized or overpersonalized, such that the train of thought does not "make sense" to another person who is unfamiliar with the patient's concerns.

Overinclusion

On the basis of a series of detailed observations and experimental work, Cameron emphasized overinclusion as a key factor in the schizophrenic disorder (1939). At one point, Cameron defines over-inclusion as an "inability to maintain the boundaries of the problem and to restrict their operations within its limits (1944, p.56)." Examples of this given by Cameron include a patient's inability to limit himself to sorting colored blocks that were given to him in a sorting task; the patient instead inappropriately also sorted the experimenter's pencil, shirt, and watch, the telephone, and other objects outside of the experimental task, and commented that, "I've got to pick it out of the whole room. I can't confine it to this game" (Cameron, 1944, p.57). Cameron sometimes talked of overinclusion in terms of difficulty in thinking the boundaries should be "temporal as well as spatial, and apply as well to the structure of his thinking as to . . . " (Cameron, 1939, p. 1030). At another point Cameron defined overinclusion as a relative inability to exclude "contradictory, competing, and more or less irrelevant responses" (Cameron and Margaret, 1951, p.511).

Cameron and others have made careful, and possibly important, observations on the presence of overinclusion in schizophrenic pa-tients. Since this formulation about schizophrenic cognition was first posed in the late 1930s, it has been readily accepted by a wide number of clinicians and theorists, and a vast amount of research has been conducted on this concept.

While most would agree that overinclusion represents a potentially promising theoretical construct in looking at schizophrenic disorders, there has been considerable inconsistency in the definition of over-inclusion. At times overinclusion has been defined as a perceptual phenomenon (inability to exclude irrelevant stimuli), at times as a central phenomenon involving thought processes and a disorder of concept formation (difficulty in maintaining the usual conceptual boundaries and a tendency to include in one's concepts elements that are either not essential or are irrelevant), and at times as a *response* tendency (as in Cameron's second definition discussed above). Thus, interpretations about overinclusion have differed somewhat according to which theorist is involved, and sometimes even within the writings of the same theorist.

As can be seen by the above discussion one problem in the area is that of separating the different types of overinclusion, in terms of a clearer conceptual analysis, and then studying these potentially different types. A second, more essential question concerns the issue of whether overinclusion is a basic component in schizophrenia, or whether it is only a concomitant or byproduct or other, more essential schizophrenic features. Our research in this area, which is described in Chapters 10 and 12, was designed to explore this question of whether it has a fundamental and sustained role in schizophrenia, by using both conceptual and empirical analysis. The empirical analysis of conceptual overinclusion that we conducted, for instance, involved studying differences in overinclusion in samples of schizophrenics in a number of different phases of their disorder, to provide clues on overinclusion as a possible sustained and fundamental feature of schizophrenia.

Affect

Bleuler pointed to the disturbance of affect as one of the cardinal symptoms of schizophrenia. Many have observed that affective disturbance may take several forms: labile or unpredictable affect; blunted or "flat" affect; inappropriate affect; or consistent anxiety or depression. In each instance, the affect in schizophrenia is not a realistic response to appropriate stimuli.

While Bleuler's main emphasis was on blunted affect and deterioration in affective responsivity, a number of workers have emphasized emotionally loaded *stimuli*, and the schizophrenic's difficulty in dealing with this type of stimuli. Thus, some theorists have suggested that thought disorder and psychotic ideation emerges from disturbances by affective stimuli, and that the core of schizophrenia is in the breakdown of affect modulation and control. The thinking of the patient, this theory would hold, deals satisfactorily with affectively neutral ideas, but deviates when the topic approaches meaningful, affectively charged material.

Clearly, the affective patterns of schizophrenia are distorted, as are those of many other psychiatric patients. The thinking of patients with other psychiatric disorders is often distorted around affectively charged issues, and Beck (1967) has suggested that depression has a core distortion of cognition. Some believe, however, that unlike other syndromes, schizophrenic distortions of affect are not limited to specific topics and areas, but rather are widespread and often unpredictable. One question for investigation is whether affective distortions occur in conjunction with disordered thinking. We have examined in a number of places, the correlation of affect with aspects of disordered thinking, especially depersonalization (Chapter 11).

Drive-dominated Thinking

Related to the theory of affect intrusion is the formulation of the schizophrenic process as a loss of the usual barriers to primitive-drive-derived thoughts. Closely connected with the concept of "regression," this theory holds that schizophrenia represents a failure of the repression of direct drive expression, which has its origins in earlier childhood experiences or is similar in form to such experiences. With the fragmenting of the ego's fuctions, the failure of repression allows more primitive expressions to emerge. The result is that the ego must employ "emergency" defenses to defend against such impulses and ideas—including the distortions of hallucinations, delusions, and withdrawal. Robert Holt (1956; Holt and Havel, 1965) has elaborated a method of assessing the severity and frequency of such drive intrusion. A critical distinction is made in the level of socialization or defense against the drive. On the primitive level, the drive expression is direct and has the potential to "shock" the unsuspecting observer. On a more socialized level, the drive material is more neutralized and may in fact lend interest to the subject's verbalizations.

A question of considerable importance is whether or not drive-related thinking distortions are exclusive to schizophrenia. Sociopaths, for example, are frequently hostile and inappropriately aggressive in terms of their overt behavior. It is possible that in addition to their aggressive overt behavior there is an underlying core of drive-dominated thinking that might be influential as one determinant of their overt behavior. Our attempt to explore this area is described in Chapter 6. It is also possible that drive-dominated thinking is not unique to schizophrenia, but what is distinctive about schizophrenia is the degree to which drive-related material distorts the patient's thinking and relationship with reality.

The Abstract-Concrete Dimension

Concrete thinking and the loss of ability to abstract successfully occupy an important place in theoretical conceptualizations about schizophrenia. The schizophrenic's impairment in abstract ability was originally emphasized by Vygotsky (1962), by Benjamin (1944) and by Kurt Goldstein (1944). In Goldstein and Scheerer's (1941) research, concreteness or the inability to abstract from immediate perceptual stimuli was seen as characteristic not only of brain-damaged conditions but also of schizophrenia. What is seen as impaired in schizophrenics is the "abstract attitude." For example, when one patient was asked, "What brought you to the hospital?" her answer was, "the ambulance," reflecting an overly literal interpretation of "brought."

One issue related to the disturbance of abstract attitude is whether concreteness is characteristic of all schizophrenics, or only of some. Concreteness may, for example, be more characteristic of nonparanoid schizophrenics or of "process" schizophrenics. It may also be more characteristic of chronic schizophrenia than of the acute episode.

While hypotheses about the importance of concrete thinking in schizophrenia have been prominent for a number of years, most of the evidence to support these formulations is based on the study of chronic, institutionalized schizophrenics. If a concrete attitude is more prominent only in chronic deteriorated schizophrenics, and not in acute ones, this leaves open the possibility that concreteness is only a concomitant of the natural downhill course of those select chronic schizophrenics who are hospitalized on a long-term basis. We have attempted to resolve some of these problems, and our work in this area is described in Chapter 7.

ASSESSMENT OF DISORDERED THINKING

There have been many suggestions about how to assess the nature and extent of thought disorder. Chapman and Chapman (1973) have pointed out the utility and elegance of "objective" multiple-choice formats in assessing rival hypotheses of thinking disorder, although they have used both this and other techniques. Others have believed that the nature of schizophrenia is most clearly understood by interpretation of projective material, (e.g., the Rorschach). Thus, for instance, it is possible that one of the central features in the schizophrenic disorder might be these patients' difficulty in dealing with the boundaries between themselves and a) other people, and b) the world. If that were to be the case, then perhaps a major technique to clarify schizophrenic disorders would involve projective or other techniques to reveal the schizophrenic's underlying ways of representing people and the world, and by this means the basic disorder of faulty representations could be uncovered.

There are several intermediate grounds on which schizophrenic thinking can be observed. One of these involves the careful analysis of the patient's spontaneous productions to structured and unstructured situations. Some of the studies presented in this book examine the responses of patients in situations ranging from those as unstructured as a fifteen-minute period of free speech to the structure provided in response to an intelligence test. In some cases, we have used parallel data from the MMPI to allow comparison of ratings on a very structured task with those from other less structured situations.

Overall, we have evaluated a wide variety of types of cognitive functioning in schizophrenics, with a number of different assessment techniques, applied on a number of different types of schizophrenic variables, at various phases of these patients' disorders. Table 1.1 presents an outline of some of the various aspects of cognition, and the techniques and types of schizophrenic samples we have studied. A number of these studies are described in detail in the succeeding chapters. Others of these studies which we have reported elsewhere will be referred to in presenting our overall view of schizophrenic thought pathology.

While many plausible arguments can be advanced for any one form of data collection, the question we address is: Under what conditions and in what way do various types of thought disorder occur, and what does this tell us about the nature of the schizophrenic disorder? In reviewing the theories of thought disorder, one is frequently struck by the close tie between a theory and a single method of measurement used to support it. By assessing the multiple theories with multiple methods one can gain a broader and more comprehensive view of schizophrenic thought pathology.

PHASE OF DISORDER AND SCHIZOPHRENIC PSYCHOPATHOLOGY

In addition to our research on what type of schizophrenic thought pathology is important, and other related questions about the nature of disordered thinking, we found that another key factor, the particular phase of the disorder, must be dealt with. Thus, when conducting our research on schizophrenic cognition we have devoted much attention to the particular phase of the disorder the schizophrenic is currently in. Most of the older research on schizophrenia and even some of the more recent research seem to study "schizophrenia" as though it were a

TABLE 1.1
Overall Research Design

Factor Assessed	Technique Used	Type of Sample Assessed	Phase of Schizophrenia Studied
I. CLASSICAL DISORDERED THINKING			
1. Loose Associations	Free Verbalization Interview	Acute Schizophrenics Nonschizophren Pts. Chronic Hospit. Schiz Chron Ambulatory Schiz	Acute Phase Partial Recovery Chronic Phase
2. Conceptual Overinclusion (Disorganization)	Object Sorting	Acute Schizophrenics Nonschizophren Pts. Chronic Hospit Schiz.	Acute Phase Partial Recovery Posthospital Phase Chronic Phase
3. Autistic Logic	Rorschach Proverbs	Acute Schizophrenics Nonschizophren Pts.	Acute Phase Posthospital Phase

(continued)

TABLE 1.1 (continued)

Factor Assessed	Technique Used	Type of Sample Assessed	Phase of Schizophrenia Studied
II. *OTHER PSYCHOTIC ASPECTS OF THINKING*			
1. Boundary Problems	Rorschach	Acute Schizophrenics Nonschizophren Pts.	Acute Phase Partial Recovery Posthospital Phase
2. Idiosyncratic Thinking	Proverbs Test Comprehension Test Rorschach Object Sorting Free Verbalization Interview	Acute Schizophrenics Nonschizophren Pts. Outpatients Chronic Hospit Schiz Chron Ambulatory Schiz Normals	Acute Phase Partial Recovery Posthospital Phase Chronic Phase
3. Primitive-Drive-Dominated Thinking	Rorschach Figure Drawings Proverbs	Acute Schizophrenics Nonschizophren Pts.	Acute Phase Partial Recovery Posthospital Phase
4. Poor Reality Testing	Rorschach	Acute Schizophrenics Nonschizophren Pts.	Acute Phase Partial Recovery Posthospital Phase

TABLE 1.1 (continued)

Factor Assessed	Technique Used	Type of Sample Assessed	Phase of Schizophrenia Studied
III. LEVEL OF THINKING			
1. Abstract and Concrete Thinking	Proverbs Test Similarities Test	Acute Schizophrenics Nonschizophren Pts. Chronic Hospit Schiz	Acute Phase Partial Recovery Chronic Phase
2. Behavioral Overinclusion	Object Sorting	Acute Schizophrenics Nonschizophren Pts. Chronic Hospit Schiz	Acute Phase Partial Recovery Posthospital Phase Chronic Phase
3. Rich Associations	Object Sorting	Acute Schizophrenics Nonschizophren Pts. Chronic Hospit Schiz	Acute Phase Partial Recovery Posthospital Phase Chronic Phase
IV. PERCEPTION— ATTENTION—BOUNDARIES			
1. Stimulus Overinclusion	Interviews Perceptual Experience Inventory	Acute Schizophrenics Nonschizophren Pts. Normals	Acute Phase Partial Recovery Posthospital Phase
2. Depersonalization	Interviews Questionnaires	Acute Schizophrenics Nonschizophren Pts. Normals	Acute Phase Partial Recovery

single-phase illness in which the same picture is seen throughout the course of the disorder. This has been so despite some of the original conceptions (e.g., Kraepelin) of dementia praecox as a disorder in which there is a systematic change in the direction of deterioration.

Our own clinical observations have suggested that some of the confusion about what the schizophrenic patient is like arises precisely because various investigators have looked at patients at different phases of their disorders. In the past, generalizations have been made about a variety of different types of "schizophrenia" on the basis of such phase-limited research. Different investigators have then made statements and drawn conclusions from their data that are sharply at odds with each other. In effect, they have been studying what almost amounts to a different disorder (because patients are at different phases) and making observations at variance with each other from their research data.

During the course of our research, our initial observations (as well as observations made by others) about the importance of the particular phase have been confirmed by the more formal data we have collected in this area. Thus, our results have suggested considerable differences in the schizophrenic picture during various phases of the disorder. The data have also helped provide a more coherent picture of the various phases of the disorder, and provide clues as to the nature of schizophrenia.

THE USE OF SCHIZOPHRENIC SPEECH TO ESTIMATE SCHIZOPHRENIC THINKING

Over the years, studies of the verbal productions of patients, including studies of their verbal content, have made valuable contributions (Gottschalk and Gleser, 1969; Maher, 1972). However, in research on disordered thinking, a problem that has vexed many serious workers in the field is the lack of complete knowledge about the relationship between thought and language or speech (Chaika, 1982; Lanin-Kettering and Harrow, In Press). While some have tried to separate speech and thinking, others have proceeded as though they were identical. The two are obviously not the same or isomorphic with each other. In many aspects of practical research on thought disorders, however, the distinction between speech and thinking in schizophrenia is very difficult to maintain. Whether the emphasis is on intrapsychic mechanisms or on interpersonal relationships, the primary tool for assessing thinking is either the verbal productions and/or the nonverbal behavior of the patient. Certainly, in many situations speech cannot be wholly identified with thought. Abstract visual reasoning and visual artistic productions, among others, are activities that cannot be readily or even wholly reduced to verbal formulas. Yet, for many other situations, there is no presumptively better way to assess thinking than to use the patient's verbal productions as an index. Speech and thinking are sufficiently intertwined for much of everyday activity that this confusion is not entirely misleading. Nevertheless, in our own work we have attempted a slightly more balanced approach, involving a two-pronged attack on the problem as follows.

The first of these two steps involves our conducting some studies of schizophrenia in which the verbal behavior of the patient is the central focus, while we also recognize, at the same time, that inferences about thinking from the study and analysis of speech behavior alone are fallible. The assumption here, in this latter case, is that speech usually reflects thinking, but only provides a partial and incomplete estimate. The assumption is that because of this, in most cases the two are correlated, although imperfectly, and the study of speech behavior frequently does provide a valuable clue about thinking behavior.

The second step is based on the belief that one should also attempt other investigations of schizophrenics in which verbal behavior is not the only factor being investigated, such as employing tasks involving the manipulation of objects or of things used in real-life situations. Thus, attention to nonverbal aspects of thinking disorder is also relevant and of value if one wishes to attempt a balanced approach to the investigation of schizophrenic thinking. To maintain proper perspective on the situation, we should remember that this other method of studying schizophrenic thinking has been tried by many investigators, but so far it has not proven clearly superior to the study of speech behavior.

As noted above, in our own research we have used both approaches, frequently studying schizophrenic verbal behavior, but also at times employing instruments that allow the schizophrenic patient to display disordered behavior that is not as heavily dependent on language.

Later in this book, and in the manual on bizarre-idiosyncratic thinking included in the Appendix, we have discussed whether strange speech production typically reflects disordered thinking or is only a sign of a language disorder. As we have noted, our evidence suggests that while a phenomenon such as strange communication by schizophrenics is sometimes a consequence of faulty expression of reasonable ideas, more often it is a consequence of ideas that are strange or socially inappropriate (Lanin-Kettering and Harrow, In Press).

DISORDERED THINKING AND IMPAIRED PERSPECTIVE

In the course of our reseach on disordered thinking we have explored a conception of how to understand the various manifestations in the many spheres studied. We base our conceptualization of disordered thinking on the premise that such thinking often shows itself in the process of communication between the patient and another person. In "disordered" thinking, the patient fails to communicate in the fashion the audience anticipates and expects. Disordered thinking violates the implicit expectations of communication that govern what is appropriate, or conversely, what is "bizarre."

We have proposed that a major factor in the bizarre verbalizations of schizophrenics involves impaired perspective about the social appropriateness of their own speech and behavior. Cognitive psychologists have suggested higher organizing central processes to link together the multiple components of thinking. Important in these higher processes are "executive" processes selecting and governing behavior and modifying it in a continuous, ongoing process. We propose that an important aspect of disordered thinking is the failure to follow one's own productions successfully, from the viewpoint of, "Is this sensible in terms of what other people expect?" or more pointedly, "Will this sound odd to others?"

What we mean by "the generalized perspective of the other" is a set of tacit social expectations about what is appropriate in a particular situation. In the process of our research we have found that there is a high degree of consensus about "bizarre" behavior. Relatively untrained judges can rate samples of speech or behavior showing a high degree of agreement with trained clinical "expert" judges. Even schizophrenics can show reasonable agreement with clinicans' judgment, *except for their own responses*. The impaired perspective involved in bizarre speech and behavior is not usually a permanent skill deficit. Rather, it involves a temporary failure to use previously acquired, long-term, stored knowledge about what is socially appropriate in that particular situation effectively. Further, disordered thinking can fluctuate with the *phase* of the disorder, as well as being a persistent issue for some patients but not for others.

We will discuss this viewpoint more as we review our evidence from the multiple aspects of disordered thinking.

OTHER QUESTIONS OF THEORETICAL IMPORTANCE ABOUT THOUGHT PATHOLOGY IN SCHIZOPHRENIA

The research we are conducting on schizophrenic cognition, outlined in the succeeding pages, has been designed to answer the question of whether or not schizophrenics *have* disordered thinking, as well as the question of *what type* of thought pathology is most prominent in schizophrenia. We believe, however, that the questions of theoretical relevance and importance are not restricted to whether or not schizophrenics have disordered thinking. Thus, if schizophrenics have thought pathology, then a number of key issues that are of at least equal moment arise. Some of these issues are: What specific type of thought pathology is most prominent? Under what circumstances does the thought pathology appear? Why do schizophrenics have it? Which type of schizophrenic shows it most prominently? And how unique is the schizophrenic's disordered thinking as compared to the thinking of other disturbed patients?

Hence, in addition to our studies of what *is* the schizophrenic thought pathology, we have prepared a series of other important questions about schizophrenic thinking and its relation to psychopatholoy. Our research has been designed to provide clues on these questions. Some of the specific questions are:

1. How important and central a feature of schizophrenia is disordered thinking?
2. Are all types of thinking usually mentioned by various clinicians and theorists really disordered in schizophrenia?
3. Is schizophrenia the only source of disordered thinking (i.e., is disordered thinking unique to schizophrenia)?
4. Does the degree or level of severity of disordered thinking matter, and is the level of thought pathology important in distinguishing schizophrenic from nonschizophrenic patients?
5. Is disordered thinking a unique entity, or does it fit on a continuum with normal thinking?
6. Does disordered thinking in schizophrenia appear overtly under all circumstances?
7. Is disordered thinking a permanent characteristic of schizophrenia?

8. Is there one particular type of disordered thinking or disordered verbalizations that our research suggests is a key factor?
9. Is schizophrenic disordered thinking influenced by the specific concerns and preoccupations of the patients?
10. Is there a particular type of content or problem area specific to the schizophrenic patient's disturbed thinking?
11. Are the schizophrenic's idiosyncratic verbalizations "caused" or influenced by a general impairment in social knowledge and understanding of social conventions?
12. Do any specific types or subgroups of schizophrenics show more thought pathology?
13. What are some of the mechanisms that might influence disordered schizophrenic thinking?

Each of these questions is addressed, in the succeeding chapters, along with a number of other issues that have arisen in the course of exploring schizophrenic thought pathology.

2
Plan of Study

In this chapter we will cover those aspects of our data collection that will tend to affect interpretation of our outcomes. These methodological issues are important in understanding the limitations and the generalizability of our findings. We will summarize some of the major issues that affect our findings and trust that serious readers will further pursue these specific issues around populations, instrumentation, and outcome in the studies that we will cite in the references.

Most of the studies reported in this book were conducted in an inpatient setting in a general hospital. By and large, the patients were young, studied at an early phase of their disorder, frequently experiencing their first hospitalization, and in a setting that emphasized the reduction of overt pathology in the interest of recovery of social functioning. Other samples of patients were also studied for investigating specific questions; these included chronically ill inpatients, less severely disturbed outpatients, and nonpatient college students and families drawn from the New Haven and Chicago areas. In some instances, patients were assessed during hospitalization and followed up afterwards.

CLINICAL SETTING

The majority of the studies reported in this book were conducted over approximately eight years in the Psychiatric Inpatient Unit of the Yale-New Haven Hospital. Other facilities from which patients were selected for study included two state hospitals in Connecticut, one in the Chicago area, and two psychiatric inpatient settings in Chicago: Michael Reese Hospital and the Illinois State Psychiatric Institute. The Yale inpatient unit is typical of those units that are psychiatric facilities within a general hospital and for which the major sources of referral are from physicians, and other mental health practitioners, within the community as well as self-referrals. The general expectations of the Yale treatment program are that the immediate presenting problems and symptoms that prevent a person from functioning in the community are the primary goal for treatment in hospitalization. The unit consists of a single floor treating twenty-four to thirty inpatients at any one time within a general hospital that is part of the Yale University School of Medicine. The structure of the unit is organized along the lines of a therapeutic community and is discussed in detail by Almond (1971). The constitution of the unit, originally written by patients on the service, describes the ward as "a community whose goals are that each can learn how to be responsible for himself and is able to help himself through helping others." At times patients at the Yale setting enter the hospital in need of intensive supervision by the staff or the patients, and proceed through a "ladder" of privileges to the point where they spend extensive amounts of time outside the hospital on independent status looking for jobs, anticipating discharge and other therapeutic tasks required toward the end of the hospitalization. Passage from one step on the ladder to the next higher step is accomplished through a request reviewed by a patient advisory committee and then reviewed by a patient-staff community meeting which passes on or rejects the patients' requests. The statement of values and behavioral norms in the community are explicit and consistent in stating that patients are expected to behave normally; to socialize with each other; to discuss problems openly in the meetings and with each other as well as with the staff; and to take an active part in the ongoing process of running the community.

Multiple modalities of treatment are employed in the course of hospitalization in addition to individual psychotherapy with a primary clinician. The patient participates in several different types of group meetings and activities including small psychotherapy groups, leader-less group meetings, and large group patient-staff community meetings (Astrachan et al., 1967) There are also meetings of patients and families together in a group, various kinds of activity and planning meetings and meetings with the patient, his or her family, the patient's therapist, and the family's social worker. The philosophy of the hospital is oriented toward restoring the patient's adequate social functioning as directly as possible through alleviation of the major presenting symptoms, including use of psychotropic medications in most instances, and in restoring the patient's interpersonal social functioning to allow him or her to resume normal status outside the hospital as quickly as possible.

The mean length of hospitalization in the Yale inpatient setting during the periods of our studies was approximately nine weeks. Hospitalizations with symptom relief may range from as short as four weeks to as long as six months. Factors affecting the length of hospitalization are mainly based on the patient's clinical picture, but also include the capability of the patient's normal living group to receive him or her back and reintegrate him or her into everyday life, and whether or not sufficient financial resources, such as third-party insurance payments, provide for periods of hospitalization. Thus, length of hospitalization is a rough measure of degree of severity but can be affected by other aspects in the patient's life.

Research measures on the patients' clinical and social functioning at the Yale setting were collected during the course of hospitalization, with the data collection integrated into the patients' ongoing schedule of meetings. Two 1½-hour periods per week are set aside for group psychological testing (e.g., MMPI). In addition, when individual testing is scheduled, it is generally conducted by a person who is part of the ongoing treatment group, such as a psychologist who is familiar to the patient in the treatment setting. On entering the hospital, patients are informed that they are in a teaching hospital, that research occurs within the context of the teaching hospital, and are asked for informed consent for participation in the research procedures. Thus, most of the patients, to a greater or lesser degree, are involved in one or another aspect of research so that the inclusion in one study or another does not single out a patient by virtue of his or her unusual symptom status.

CLINICAL RATINGS

Extensive ratings of patients were made on a variety of symptoms and behaviors. Each patient's primary therapist completed a checklist of symptoms and behavior on a weekly basis as part of the standard routine of recording the patient's progress. In addition, a brief checklist of observable behaviors was completed by a nurse on each of the three shifts on a daily basis for each patient. These ratings were used at a number of points in the research.

CHARACTERISTICS OF THE PATIENT POPULATION

Two important aspects of selecting of patients for study are the *time* of hospitalization and the nature of the comparison groups. As we will discuss in Chapter 5, the phase of hospitalization has an important effect on the degree of pathology observed in patients' responses. The early phases reflect not only the effects of acute pathology, but also the turmoil and upset that often accompany the process of hospitalization. It is important that all patients used for comparisons be at a similar period in their hospitalization so that these factors are approximately equivalent for all patients.

Secondly, in studying the varieties of disordered thinking in schizophrenia, it is important that comparisons be made with other inpatients in comparable (preferably the same) settings. Without nonschizophrenic inpatient comparison groups (e.g., if only "normal" controls are used) disordered thinking and other disturbances might be attributed to the disruptive effects of being removed from one's usual environment, being confined in a hospital, and being a "psychiatric patient."

Since the patients in the Yale setting were drawn from the general referrals in the psychiatric community to an adult inpatient unit, the patients present a broad spectrum of age, social class, and presenting clinical picture. While the median age of all patients is twenty-one years, groups of patients tend to cluster in early adolescence, young adulthood, and a smaller but significant group of patients in middle age or somewhat older. The predominant classes from which patients come are lower-middle and upper-middle class with a number of working- and upper-class patients. Since the unit operates at a private hospital, it is available to those who have either self-sufficient means of payment or third-party insurance that covers inpatient hospitalization. In various samples, the mean estimated IQ of the patient population has ranged between 108 and 115; the usual mean is approximately 110.

The diagnoses given to the patients include a broad variety of psychiatric diagnoses from among the major psychiatric disorders that require inpatient care. In a sample of 171 patients, which is typical of the hospital patient population, 28% were diagnosed as schizophrenic, 22% as borderline schizophrenic patients (a number of these patients who show schizophreniclike features but are not overtly psychotic have been labeled as "latent" schizophrenics), 22% as having depressive disorders, 21% as having various personality or character disorders, drug abuse and substance abuse (most with secondary depression), and 7% as having miscellaneous other diagnoses. Most patients (60–70%) were experiencing their first psychiatric admission. Only rarely would a patient who had been chronically ill and hospitalized for extensive periods be admitted in the Yale setting. Most patients are discharged to their homes, with a small number, less than 10%, being transferred to other institutions for longer terms of care. Thus, the patients we are describing are primarily in the acute phase of their illness, have not had chronic symptomatology, and by and large, present with symptoms that are amenable to milieu therapy along with individual psychotherapy and psychotropic medications.

CHARACTERISTICS OF THE SETTING

Of particular relevance to the study of disordered thinking are the steps taken by the therapeutic setting with regard to manifestations of psychopathology and disordered thinking. When patients display pathological behavior, it is labeled as a symptom, whether it be in terms of language, overt behavior, or withdrawal. Responses to patients are oriented toward redirecting their behavior toward more appropriate expressions within the therapeutic community. Hospitals vary widely on the way in which such behavior, particularly disordered thinking, is responded to. Within this setting, disordered thinking is perceived as a symptom that is within the patient's control and the patient is asked to communicate more directly, rather than in symbolic form. Thus, when disordered thinking appears in such patients, it appears in the context where disordered thinking, bizarre speech, and the like are perceived as deviations from the norm, as symptoms, rather than communication, and as behaviors that are contrary to the explicit goals of the community. We are not suggesting here that disordered thinking does not, at times, have a communicative aspect, or that it does not contain some symbolic clues concerning aspects of conflicts; rather, our research has suggested to us (see Chapter 5, describing our investigation of "intermingling") that in a large number of cases of disordered language, the *content* of the deviant verbalizaton is partly based on the patients' individual needs, concerns, preoccupations, and conflicts.

What we are suggesting here is that within the goals and method of the main setting (the Yale inpatient setting) in which this research was conducted, there is a lack of encouragement for the overt expression of disordered thinking in social situations. This point is important in evaluating the implications of the appearance of disordered thinking in the various forms of psychopathology. A minority of other settings that we have worked in and studied in greater detail do not actively discourage overt expression of psychopathology. In these settings we have usually observed a slightly greater degree of expression of disordered and deviant thinking in the routine ward situation and in social situations. In the test situation in these settings, however, we have only found about an equal level of disordered thinking. In this minority of settings where freer expression of disordered verbalization and language is allowed, other factors in the test situation seem to be more important influences on the level of disordered verbalization than the encouragement of the expression of psychopathology in the more social ward situation. Thus, within limits, in test situations where patients are closely observed and are being assessed as to how "sick" they are, the ward atmosphere may exert some influence but it does not seem to be the major factor. In these "test" situations, patients usually try to behave "at their best," or not to show as much overt psychopathology or much deviant language, even when they do exhibit psychopathology in the "freer" ward situation.

DIAGNOSIS

One of the major issues in the study of disordered thinking is arriving at consistent empirically valid criteria by which classifications can be made. Of equal importance to the question of criteria is the method by which information was gathered for arriving at a diagnosis. In the studies reported here, the clinical diagnosis was arrived at by the consensus of two senior clinicians working on a daily basis in a supervisory capacity on the ward, at least one of whom was a board-certified psychiatrist; other diagnostic teams included a clinical psychologist. In arriving at the diagnosis, material was reviewed after the patient was discharged, and relevant information from the presenting picture, course of hospitalization, and discharge picture were also included. Information from research procedures and testing was *not* included in the material used in arriving at the diagnosis; in no instance did the two diagnosing clinicians participate in the direct collection of the data in such a way that they could be influenced by material arising out of the research procedures.

An issue that has been of concern in the study of schizophrenia has been the reliability and verifiability of the diagnosis across clinical settings. We have dealt with this issue by using, in addition to standard clinical diagnosis, the New Haven Schizophrenia Index (NHSI; Astrachan et al., 1972). Thus, for the diagnosis of schizophrenia, this additional procedure was employed to verify the existence of symptomatology sufficient to warrant the diagnosis of schizophrenia. The NHSI was developed by a panel of psychiatrists and psychologists, including members of the present research team, to study diagnostic criteria from a variety of inpatient and outpatient settings. None of the patients in the research studies reported in this book was included in the criteria panel on the basis of which the index was validated. The NHSI involves a number of specific symptoms that investigators and clinicians consistently identify as being associated with schizophrenia, and that could be easily retrieved from charts or clinical interview schedules and reliably rated. In addition, the symptoms had to have a high degree of construct validity, that is to say, to be related to prominent, widely accepted theoretical work in the field of schizophrenia. The panel agreed on minimal and sufficient criteria for the diagnosis of schizophrenia; the symptoms used for the NHSI are shown in the box on p. 34.

Thus, for almost all studies, patients diagnosed as schizophrenic met a minimum criterion score of at least four on the NHSI, as well as being clinically diagnosed as schizophrenic by two senior clinicians.

Most of the patient samples were collected before the advent of the third edition of the *Diagnostic and Statistical Manual* (American Psychiatric Association, 1980). Some variations may have occurred had we used the DSM III criteria. All of our schizophrenic patients met the NHSI criteria, and were clearly psychotic. Some would possibly fall into such related diagnoses as schizo-affective. Any studies of schizophrenia and disordered thinking face the problem that most of the literature is based on earlier nosological practices using DSM II or similar criteria. While DSM III presents many improvements in consistency of diagnosis, it by no means brings us to nosological nirvana (Harrow and Silverstein, 1981; Pawelski, Harrow, Grinker, and Grossman, in press). Our use of "schizophrenia" is consistent with DSM II practice and includes the added safegard of the NHSI criteria. It is too early to judge, with any finality, the impact of the new criteria on the study of disordered thinking.

New Haven Schizophrenia Index Checklist and Scoring System

Checklist of Symptoms
1.
    (a) Delusions (not specified or other than depressive)
    (b) Hallucinations (auditory)
    (c) Hallucinations (visual)
    (d) Hallucinations (other)
2. Crazy thinking and/or thought disorder
    Any of the following:
    (a) Bizarre thinking
    (b) Autism or grossly unrealistic private thoughts
    (c) Looseness of association, illogical thinking, overinclusion
    (d) Blocking
    (e) Concreteness
    (f) Derealization
    (g) Depersonalization
3. Inappropriate affect
4. Confusion
5. Paranoid ideation (self-referential thinking, suspiciousness)
6. Catatonic behavior
    (a) Excitement
    (b) Stupor
    (c) Waxy flexibility
    (d) Negativism
    (e) Mutism
    (f) Echolalia
    (g) Stereotyped motor activity

Scoring System

To be considered part of the schizophrenic group, the patient must score on either Item 1 or Items 2a, 2b, or 2c, and must attain a total score of at least 4 points.

He can achieve a maximum of 4 points on Item 1: 2 for the presence of delusions, 2 for hallucinations.

On Item 2, he can score 2 points for any or all symptoms a through c, 1 point for either or both symptoms d through e, and 1 point each for f and g. He can thus score a maximum of 5 points on Item 2.

Items 3, 4, 5 and 6 each receive 1 point.

Note: Where the 4th point necessary for inclusion in the sample is provided by 2d or 2e, these symptoms are not scored.

From Astrachan, Harrow, Adler, et al. *British Journal of Psychiatry, 121,* 529-539, 1972. Reproduced by permission of the publisher.

In our more recent research, however, we have studied positive thought disorder in samples of schizophrenics using the newer, "narrow" criteria of schizophrenia, such as those found in DSM III and in the Research Diagnostic Criteria (RDC) (Harrow, Grossman, Silverstein, and Meltzer, 1982; Harrow, Grossman, Silverstein, Meltzer, and Kettering, in press; Harrow, Silverstein, and Marengo, 1983). In this research we have found similar levels of thought disorder in schizophrenics diagnosed according to DSM III and the RDC criteria, as in the samples we have reported in this book using samples of DSM II schizophrenics. Even our follow-up research, in which we specifically compared DSM III samples of schizophrenics with DSM II samples of schizophrenics, have found a great deal of similarities in the post-hospital adjustment of DSM III versus DSM II samples of schizophrenics (Pawelski, et al., in press).

In general, a number of factors, such as diagnosis and other variables, may influence the degree of expression one may find, and the degree of deviance represented by any given instance of disordered thinking. For example, Wild (1962) found that a group of artists gave responses that were rated on objective measures of pathology as equally disturbed as those given by schizophrenics. The context for these two groups, however, was quite different. The expectations in testing for an artist might be to discover creativity in the looser aspects of thinking or possibly even a straining to be "different" as evidence of creativity. For schizophrenics being detained in an institutional setting and being evaluated by an authority figure, it may be reasonably interpreted that manifestation of pathology would be a way of contributing to a negative evaluation of one's treatment status and prognosis, and they would be regarded as "sicker."

MEDICATIONS

Psychotropic medications, particularly the phenothiazines and similar compounds in the treatment of thought disorder, were used on virtually all of the patients in our studies who were diagnosed as schizophrenic. The use of such medication could pose a problem in the study of disordered thinking. Behavior observed in such patients is a product not only of the underlying clinical state but also of changes and modifications brought about by the psychotropic medications (Detre and Jarecki, 1971; Klein and Davis, 1969; Spohn, 1973). Complicating matters further is the fact that many of the patients in the other diagnostic groups (for example, patients with neurotic or psychotic depression) are often receiving another family of psychotropic medications, the antidepressants. In such a situation, sorting out the effects of underlying disorder from those effects that might be produced by the psychotropic medications is difficult. This is a problem that almost all modern studies face. Other factors that we note suggest, however, that phenothiazine use does not eliminate schizophrenic thought pathology, or prevent its study. Ideally, one would want to study disordered thinking not only in schizophrenics but also in other patients before they are put on a treatment regimen for psychotropic medications.

Fortunately, we have been able to collect such a sample of unmedicated patients. On the whole, the schizophrenics from this sample, studied at an early acute phase of hospitalization, showed considerable thought disorder (see Table 4.3). However, a larger sample of patients including both the unmedicated patients and an additional smaller group of medicated patients in the same setting at the same time showed similar levels of thought disorder (Harrow, Grossman, Silverstein, and Meltzer, 1982). Apparently, medicated schizophrenics show as much or almost as much positive thought disorder as parallel unmedicated schizophrenics. Much of the improvement in thought disorder during the early acute phase of schizophrenia with the use of phenothiazines seems to take a week and a half or longer before becoming prominent. Most of the acute schizophrenic samples reported in this book were assessed early enough in the course of their hospitalization so that severe thought disorder still appeared, despite the use of phenothiazines.

Most of our comparisons, however, are subject to the limitation that some of the effects we observed might have been due to unknown underlying effects of the medication the patients are receiving, although the severe thought disorder found in our medicated schizophrenics suggests that this problem was a limited one.

In addition, there are other indications that these problems are not undermining the validity of our diagnostic comparisons. First of all, the generally observed clinical effect of such medications, particularly the phenothiazines and related compounds (e.g., Haldol), is to suppress and reduce the level of disordered thinking. This may reduce the variance between schizophrenics, who generally receive more medication, and the nonschizophrenic group. Consequently, the effect of medication may be to decrease the likelihood of finding schizophrenic-nonschizophrenic differences in thought disorder, making estimates of differences between these groups conservative.

Second, the observations made in the studies reported here constitute what can be the expected appearance of patients in an active treatment program that incorporated psychotropic medications. Thus, even though the differences obtained may be differences of the combination of schizophrenia plus medication versus depression and other symptoms, plus medication this nonetheless corresponds to the picture that would more typically be seen in modern clinical practices.

Last and certainly not least, there is a group of patients in whom there is some variation in the practice of prescribing medication, namely the personality and character disorders. In several of our studies in which it was possible to make comparisons of nonschizophrenic patients on medications with those who are not on medication, no significant differences were obtained between those patients who were medicated and those who were not. This does not totally dismiss the possibility that some differences may arise out of medication, but it does suggest that the degree of differences that we observe among our clinical groups during early acute phases of disorder cannot be accounted for solely by the differences that would arise out of the administration of psychotropic medications.

Some Considerations on Measurements Used for Assessment of Disordered Thinking

The literature on the study of disordered thinking is by no means so consistent as to recommend what the ideal instrument would be for the assessment of these aspects of thinking. Different techniques present advantages for some areas of study and disadvantages for others. Chapman and Chapman (1973), for example, have used a variety of techniques, including both objective and projective methods. Some of their research has suggested some advantages for the use of objective tests with clear response alternatives, where some responses support one hypothesis about disordered thinking while other choices support alternative hypotheses or check for sources of error. Multiple-choice procedures offer distinct advantages; the stimuli are clearly defined, the response choices are unequivocal, and clinical judgment and ambiguity are greatly reduced. However, they also present, several difficulties: (1) they set up artificial, non-real situations for the responder; (2) they may require different cognitive processes from those used by patients in their everyday life; (3) they change the situation in which much of what is noticeable about schizophrenia (psychotic verbalization, bizarre language, etc.) may be eliminated since the patient is not given the opportunity to manifest these phenomena, or in some cases they may not appear on the record even when there is underlying thought pathology.

Other theories of thinking disorders, such as Blatt and Wild (1976), have emphasized the need for open-ended projective testing in order to elicit those aspects of disordered thinking that underlie schizophrenia. Wachtel (1973) observed that many of the occasions from which we assume disordered thinking arises are occasions when there is no clear structure provided by the environment. Thus, within the field of study of disordered thinking, there are quite diverse opinions about what constitutes the appropriate research instrumentation for study.

Our approach has been to sample a spectrum of instruments varying from structured multiple-choice tests through open-ended projective tests and free open-ended interviews, in order to determine not only the nature of disordered thinking but also to assess where such disordered thinking will and will not arise. The instruments used in studying disordered thinking are described in detail in the specific chapters covering them, but the following is a brief introduction to some of the measures we have employed: (1) *personality instruments:* a number of studies have been used that employ instruments requiring the subjects to make a reply to a structured format provided by the researcher, such as the Rotter Locus of Control Scale (Internal versus External control) (Harrow & Ferrante, 1969), and questionnaires devised within this research project to study such phenomena as depersonalization and derealization also are employed as instruments of this type; (2) *semistructured instruments;* and (3) *projective tests and open-ended interviews.*

One example of a semistructured interview would be our use of the Perceptual Experiences Interview to assess disordered attention (Chapter 12). Another example would be the Wechsler Adult Intelligence Scale Subtests for Information and Comprehension. These subtests have an accepted "right" answer, but allow a great deal of variety for the form of the response. On such instruments, one can look to see whether or not the objective criterion of the correct response has been met; one can also take a look at the form in which the response is given. Thus, for example, we have developed a manual for the scoring of bizarre and idiosyncratic thinking based on the answers given to items on the WAIS Comprehension subtest that allow the patient considerable latitude and require him or her to give relatively unpracticed answers. A similar kind of issue arises out of the degree to which the test taps relatively unpracticed, unlearned responses. In general, our findings have pointed to the fact that somewhat well-practiced and/or shorter responses (of only one or two words), such as those required on the WAIS Similarities subtest, tend to show fewer obvious manifestations of disordered thinking. Other tests measure a similar underlying cognitive dimension such as the Proverbs Test, which requires the patient to formulate a longer answer (typically two or three sentences) based much more on his or her own personal experience, knowledge, and ability to reason abstractly in the here and now. Such tests tend to elicit more of the idiosyncratic, unusual, and bizarre concrete thinking that has so frequently been observed within schizophrenia (see Appendix and Part VI below).

We have employed much more open-ended procedures, including such instruments as the Rorschach and the open-ended interview. In such instruments there is a minimal degree of structure provided by the testing setting. One of the critical factors on instruments such as these is the strategy used by the investigator on evaluating the responses given to these instruments. In our study of loose associations, for example, we looked at the degree to which spontaneously loose association occurred in an open-ended, free-format clinical interview setting in which the patients talked without interruption or clarification by the interviewer. Ratings were made according to a detailed scoring manual with definitions of multiple types of looseness and other speech disturbances. On the Rorschach, the material was presented in the standard format by the examiner and responses were recorded in a standard inquiry procedure. We applied objective rating scales for different facets of psychopathology (Quinlan, Harrow, Tucker and Carlson., 1972). Open-ended interviews and projective interviews are not "tests" as such. The psychometric properties of reliability and validity apply to the *rating scales* used by the investigator and the degree of accuracy and precision with which aspects of disordered thinking can be scored.

RELIABILITY

Much emphasis has been placed, especially in recent work in classification, on the reliability of instruments in clinical research. For many of the measures employed, our strategy has been to compile a manual in which we define our terms and giving examples, and then to train raters to the point where acceptable interscorer reliability is obtained. These manuals will be cited at relevant places in the subsequent chapters. Reliability in and of itself does not assure that the ratings are either valid or useful. Interscorer reliability does, however, assure that, in principle, trained raters can assess the phenomenon studied in a consistent and reproducible fashion.

Test-retest reliability on measures of disordered thinking poses an unusual problem. Psychotic thinking generally shows a reduced level of severity during the acute phases of the disorder. There is some patient-to-patient variability in the *rate* of improvement. Thus, test-retest reliabilities would not be expected to be high in measures that reflect clinical improvement over time. By and large, we are forced to rely on intertest correlations to assess for both reliability and construct validity: measures of similar phenomena show a high degree of intercorrelation at similar time periods.

SOME GENERAL CONSIDERATIONS OF ADMINISTRATION

Those investigative procedures that required individual administration included the open-ended interview, the Object Sorting Test, the Information and Comprehension subtests, the Proverbs Test, and the Rorschach. In each instance the procedure is given near the beginning of hospitalization, usually within the first week and a half or two weeks (when specified by the research protocol), or after a given period of hospitalization in the case of pre and post studies. The subjects' responses were recorded either by audiotape recording with subsequent transcription or by verbatim written recording by the examiner at the time of the testing, or both. The identity and diagnosis of the patient were disguised and all test responses were scored by persons other than those who had administered the instruments. When reliabilities were obtained, they were obtained by two raters who did not have specific clinical responsibilities for the patients involved, and who were not aware of the identity of the patients whose records they were scoring. Some specific instructions for each of the instruments are described below:

1. *The Object Sorting Test.* The Object Sorting Test (described in detail in the next chapter) is administered with the materials provided in the standard kit for the Goldstein Sheerer Object Sorting Test. The format of administration (Part 1) is: standard stimulus objects, or "starting objects," are presented to the subject, one object per trial, and he or she is required to sort the remainder of the objects into a class conceptually related to the first one (Himmelhoch et al., 1973). After the objects are noted in terms of order of sort and total number of objects included in the sort, the experimenter makes a routine inquiry into the rationale for the sort and the response to this inquiry is recorded verbatim for subsequent scoring.

2. *Wechsler Adult Intelligence Scale subtests (WAIS).* Complete or abbreviated versions of the Information, Comprehension, and Similarities Subtest are used frequently within the research. These are

administered according to the standard format suggested within Wechsler's manual, with inquiries used to elaborate on points that are unclear. The answers used are those that would be obtained in ordinary clinical administration of these tests without any modifications of inquiry, but answers are recorded verbatim for further rating (e.g., for bizarre-idiosyncratic responses).

3. *Open-ended Interview.* In the open-ended, free-response interview, patients were told that they would be asked to speak on each of two topics for a period of about seven and a half minutes for each topic. Once the tape recorder was turned on, the test administrator began the period by introducing the general topic (e.g., about events leading to hospitalization) and intervened only to encourage the person to continue talking about each topic. The free verbalizations of the subject were transcribed from the tape, with any identifying information deleted before judges rated the protocols.

4. *Rorschach.* The Rorschach was administered by a person trained in the scoring and interpretation of the Rorschach who was not informed of the clinical diagnosis of the patients being tested. The Rorschach was administered within the first two weeks of hospitalization (except for follow-up studies) and was presented with the instructions recommended by Rappaport, Gill, and Schafer (1968), namely, "What does this look like?," "What do you see?," without further elaboration of the nature or purpose of the test. Responses to the first card were recorded according to the method of Rappaport and others, with the exception that the subject was encouraged to give at least two and no more than three responses on a card. After the free response to the first card, inquiry immediately followed, along with a separate period for the location of the responses. After the first Rorschach card had been given, the free-response period, inquiry, and location of the second card were then presented. All ten Rorschach cards were presented in the same session and the patient was asked to speak at a pace that made it possible for verbatim recording to be made. Scorers for the Rorschach were trained prior to scoring of actual protocols (Quinlan, Harrow, Tucker and Carlson, 1972). For this training phase, protocols from patients not included in the main body of the study were utilized. Scoring did not begin until an acceptable level of reliability had been reached.

SUMMARY

Information obtained during the course of procedures was not utilized as part of the patient's treatment. When psychological testing was requested on each of the patients, a separate battery of psychological tests was administered by someone who had not administered the procedures as part of the research.

In summary, we conducted much of our study of disordered speaking on acute psychiatric patients admitted (many for the first time) to inpatient facilities. We also used outpatients, chronic patients, and normals. Although most of our patient samples were medicated, we also observed a sample of medication-free inpatients to allow a separate, controlled assessment of such patients. Extensive clinical ratings and other information were used for the purpose of comparison with test-derived scores. This other information was gathered after testing and without knowledge of test results, and thus separate sources of information were gathered "blind" to reduce possible effects of prior information in the rating of any of the variables. Diagnoses of schizophrenia were further verified by the use of the NHSI. Testing for most of the patients occurred in the context of a milieu therapy unit in which disordered thinking was labeled as a symptom and was not encouraged. The personnel administering the instrument to the patients were very often personnel familiar to them from other aspects of hospitalization but were not the primary therapist who had been involved in formulating their diagnosis. A broad spectrum of instruments ranging from objective to projective techniques was employed to assess the different types of disordered thinking that are potentially elicited by different types of research instruments. Thus, the research attempted to assess disordered thinking in a context that allowed for the generalization to both acute schizophrenic and nonschizophrenic patients, and to chronic patients, with careful attention to the specificity of the diagnosis, utilizing a broad spectrum of instruments, assessing several facets of disordered thinking.

## PART II

BIZARRE-IDIOSYNCRATIC
THINKING

3

Bizarre-Idiosyncratic Speech and Thinking During Acute Stages of Schizophrenia

A disordered schizophrenic patient responded to the proverb, *Speech is the picture of the mind* with the following answer: "You see the world through speech. Like my grandfather used to speak to me of Alaskans and Alsatians and blood getting thicker and thinner in the Eskimo. He was against the Kents in England. I can't smoke a Kent cigarette to this day." A second disordered schizophrenic responded to the proverb, *Barking dogs seldom bite*, with "A bear in a tree is worth two in a zoo." A third patient responded to the proverb, *Don't count your chickens until they're hatched*, with "One chicken might go bad, and if it had twelve, but only eleven, don't count on it," A fourth patient responded to the following social comprehension question, "Why should we keep away from bad company?" with: "Is that a question? Why is Jesus to me. It sounds like you are asking Jesus to me. Like asking Jesus the question—so it's none of my business. You know how he hung on the cross like a Y. So he's 'why' to me. You'll have trouble with every 'why' question you ask me until I have this straightened out." In this case, the patient is interpreting the word "why" as referring to the shape of the letter "Y," and hence as a symbol of the crucifixion. All of these schizophrenic patients had one or more forms of disordered thinking.

In at least one of these instances the verbalizations could be classified as showing loose associations, in another two as showing confused and disorganized communication or thinking, and in the last instance as showing an example of a disorder in logic, or predicate logic. Are these the best ways of classifying these particular verbalizations? Perhaps. One problem is that a number of very disordered schizophrenic verbalizations can be classified in three or four different ways. Thus, simultaneously they may be loose *and* illogical *and* confused *and* perhaps disordered in other ways as well. The question that appears most prominent is: On which dimension of the disordered verbalization should one focus? The answer should center on what is the most fruitful or productive way to classify these verbalizations, in order to get the most complete and general picture of schizophrenia, and perhaps most important, to begin to approach the underlying processes responsible for generating these disordered verbalizations. Many diverse types of disordered schizophrenic verbalizations would fit fruitfully under the label of being "bizarre" or "idiosyncratic," and we have focused a major part of our research efforts on this particular aspect of thinking.

In terms of our definition of *bizarre-idiosyncratic* speech, the one we have proposed, as a temporary working definition, is: *(a) verbalizations or speech which are unique to the particular subject, (b) deviant in respect to conventional social norms, and (c) frequently hard for an unfamiliar audience to empathize with, or understand where the utterance came from. other general (but less common) characteristics which may sometimes occur are: (d) the verbalizations may appear as confused, contradictory or illogical, (e) the verbalizations or responses may involve sudden or unexpected contrasts, and (f) they are usually inappropriate or unresourceful in relation to the task at hand.*

During our early research on thought pathology we had analyzed a number of other, more traditional aspects of potential disordered thinking in acute schizophrenics, including overinclusive thinking, primitive-drive-dominated thinking, autistic thinking, disordered logic, concreteness, and loose associations. While we have tended to emphasize the construct of bizarre-idiosyncratic thinking, these other dimensions of disordered thinking cannot be dismissed out of hand, and some of them represent potentially important components of the overall thought pathology found in many psychotic patients. We have studied them also and our research focusing on them is described in Chapters 6 though 12. They represent traditional dimensions on which disordered thinking can by scrutinized and evidence can be found to support some of these traditional dimensions. From our standpoint, however, looking at disordered thinking in terms of more general concepts such as bizarre-idiosyncratic thinking is an alternate way of viewing it that can be quite productive.

Thus, it gradually became clear to us during our early research in this area that a factor of potential importance involves bizarre and/or idiosyncratic verbalizations, which presumably reflect bizarre and idiosyncratic thinking. This is not a unique discovery peculiar to our research group; others have at times written about it, frequently in an offhand way. As we have observed in Chapter 1, Fish (1962) has used a similarly broad construct of "positive formal thought disorder" to classify "unusual" thinking, although he has not conducted formal research using this construct.

Often, bizarre-idiosyncratic speech has been an implicit factor influencing decisions about what types of verbalizations reflect disordered thinking, but it has not usually been the central focus in large investigative studies, partly because it is difficult to handle conceptually. We cannot explain away its presence as being merely a product of loose associations, as some might hypothesize. In certain cases, loose associations seem to be involved in bizarre verbalizations, and there is often a statistically significant difference between schizophrenics and nonschizophrenics in the overt appearance of loose associations. But in many other cases bizarre verbalizations occur without any noticeable looseness. This can be seen most clearly in some verbalizations that involve poor communication, as well as in some verbalizations that are extremely stilted or verbalizations that are inappropriate to the level of discourse; for example, Q: *"Don't judge a book by its cover."* A: "A facade of regal compliance bides an etiology of ire."; Q: *"Discretion is the better part of valor."* A: "Pliant recititude is a trait more appropriate for successful living than hot-headedness which is either stubborn or crusady."

"BIZARRE-IDIOSYNCRATIC SPEECH AND THINKING," AND WHAT IS BIZARRE?

In our original review of this area, we had tried to assess what is the most frequent referent of the terms "thought disorder," "thought pathology," and "disordered thinking," Our observations were that the language and behavior that we have labeled as "bizarre" or "idiosyncratic" were the type of phenomenon that would fit most frequently, although at times other nonbizarre behaviors (such as concreteness) also have been viewed as aspects of a "thought disorder." While theorists frequently have attended (at some level of awareness) to bizarre behavior in classifications of what is thought disordered, some have not seemed to recognize overtly that the dimension of bizarreness was a major criterion.

In our research we have come to the position of using the terms "bizarre-idiosyncratic speech and thinking" to describe a variety of diverse types of speech and behavior that are sometimes labeled by others as bizarre, peculiar, and odd, and sometimes are given other labels to indicate how strange they are (e.g., Johnston and Holzman, 1979; Lang and Buss, 1965; Rapaport, Gill, and Schafer, 1968; Shimkunas, Gynther, and Smith, 1967). Thus, also fitting into this category of "bizarre" would be most types of languages that are classified as autistic, loose, and illogical. We would *not* consider other categories, such as concrete and incorrect responses to a question (e.g., responses to a proverb), bizarre, except in those special cases where, in addition to being concrete or incorrect, they *also* are odd, strange, or out of place.

Bizarre-idiosyncratic verbalizations and thinking can be viewed as a slightly different way of "cutting the pie" concerning disturbed verbalizations, or as focusing on a slightly different aspect of disordered verbalizations and thinking. By focusing on bizarre-idiosyncratic verbalizations, one cuts across some of the usual lines discussed in this area concerning disordered cognition. At the same time, the concept of bizarre-idiosyncratic verbalizations excludes some types of verbalizations and thinking that are often included as disordered, such as concrete thinking, and drive-dominated thinking (except insofar as such thinking violates certain boundaries of social appropriateness).

Looked at more specifically, the concept of bizarre-idiosyncratic speech also includes other types of cognitive behavior that have not been formally focused on as much in the past, such as verbalizations involving odd meanings or outlooks (e.g., *Q: "One swallow doesn't make a summer?"; A:* "Just because a bird says it's summer and acts like it's summer, maybe it really isn't. Sometimes a bird could say it's summer, and it would really be winter."), and many types of verbalizations that are socially inappropriate or taboo.

As we have noted above, some clinicians have commented on schizophrenics' "bizarre language," and it undoubtedly has influenced many of their judgments about psychosis and about what is "schizophrenic." However, whether or not language is "bizarre" is not a dimension along which most workers have, in an overt manner, tended to cut the pie of "thought disorders," even though it does fit much data that have been collected in the field. A focus on bizarre-idiosyncratic speech as a central dimension offers a way of viewing in a uniform manner a range of different types of disordered verbalizations and strange and inappropriate communication and thinking that are usually studied separately. These include, among others, disordered logic;

neologisms; loose associations; some overinclusive behavior; autistic thinking; and certain types of communicative disorders (Arieti, 1974; Bleuler, 1950; Goldstein et al., 1978; Lewis, Rodnick, and Goldstein, 1981; Lidz, Fleck, and Cornelison, 1965; Payne, 1970; Rapaport, Gill, and Schafer, 1968; Singer, Wynne, and Toohey, 1978; Von Domarus, 1944; Wynne, Singer, Bartko, and Toohey, 1977). By unifying these different aspects of disordered thinking under the label "bizarre-idiosyncratic," it is possible to begin to analyze this type of disordered speech, and to search for one cognitive mechanism, or a small group of cognitive mechanisms, common to the above varied aspects of thought pathology.

DOES BIZARRE THINKING REPRESENT A FORMAL THOUGHT DISORDER?

In terms of how, or along which dimension, one should classify various aspects of disordered language and thinking, a major difficulty has been the common conception of a "formal" thought disorder, which many feel is a basis of the schizophrenic disorder. Discussions of "formal" disorders of thinking have at times led to confusion, since various investigators have used different definitions of terms such as "formal." Some have used the term "formal" in relation to thinking to describe the *style* of thinking (e.g., a fragmented versus an amorphous style; Wynne and Singer, 1963a, 1963b), others have used it to refer to the structure of thinking, and some have used it to refer to other aspects of thinking. Probably the most commonly used definition of the term "formal" in relation to disordered thinking is in terms of the rules or structure of thinking. It is possible that the structure of thinking is disordered for schizophrenics. As of now, however, there is not substantial evidence as to whether or not the form or structure of thinking is involved.

Actually, there are large gaps in our knowledge about what the rules or structure of thinking are for everybody, normals or patients. Research on normal cognition has resulted in considerable progress in our understanding of thinking. Despite major advances in our knowledge on human cognition made by a variety of investigators, there are still large gaps in our understanding of the mechanisms involved in many aspects of higher-level executive functioning involving problem solving, judgment, and short- and long-term decision making.

When we turn to the attempt to understand the rules or structure of normal thinking, in order to get a better grasp on schizophrenic thinking, we find that there have been a number of recent advances in our knowledge of normal thinking and cognition. Despite these advances, nobody seems to be quite sure of what the formal rules and structure of thinking are for normals or patients, particularly when they involve verbal productions, which do not follow the rules of grammar and logic as closely as written language. In terms of the formal structure of thinking, some theorists seem to feel that a disorder in logic, or possibly even concrete thinking, would fit under the term "formal." It is unclear, however, why a disorder in one of these particular areas must be a "formal" one, or whether there is any strong empirical evidence about the importance of a formal thought disorder. In addition, our early data did not show a striking disorder in logic, providing us with negative evidence in this area, and, as outlined in Chapter 7, the data showed a mixed picture concerning concrete thinking in schizophrenia.

We could sum up our position in this area by saying that although many theorists talk about the importance and centrality of a "formal" thought disorder in schizophrenia, there is much inconsistency and little empirical evidence on this issue. Even the conceptual and theoretical basis of this belief has not been spelled out fully. We have some doubts about this frequently unquestioned belief in the centrality of a "formal" thought disorder, at least until there are more compelling theoretical and empirical arguments.

While issues about a "formal" thought disorder are still unresolved, our research (and our informal observations) has continually provided us with examples of what we would call bizarre or idiosyncratic thinking. Unlike some other aspects of disordered cognition, idiosyncratic thinking does not fit neatly under some uses of the term "formal thought disorder," nor does it even lend itself to a neat definition or an easy set of specifying operations.

DEFINITION OF BIZARRE SPEECH

The observation that bizarre speech does not lend itself to a neat set of specifying operations presents an interesting problem. When people talk of overinclusive thinking, they usually refer to a difficulty in maintaining conceptual boundaries, and with concepts such as over-inclusive thinking the definition can be neat and precise. It is much more difficult to set up specifying operations or criteria concerning bizarre-idiosyncratic verbalizations and thinking, or about related concepts such as positive thought disorder. When we did set up the definition of idiosyncratic verbalizations and idiosyncratic thinking that we have outlined earlier, we observed that it depends heavily on two components: (1) What types of verbalizations, and presumably what types of thinking that underlie it, does one have difficulty *empathizing* with, understanding, or quickly seeing where it originated? And (2) it also depends to a large extent on a difficulty or failure in grasping and utilizing social *norms* at that particular instant of saying something bizarre. Thus, it is closely tied in to one's perspective and judgment in recognizing the social consensus about what is idiosyncratic or deviant in our society, or within our society's subcultures. On this latter feature, the utilization of social norms, our informal observations, and more formal research by our own group and by others (Brown, 1973; Hunt, Jones, and Hunt, 1957) have shown a surprising degree of consensus within both our society and its subcultures as to what is typical or normal and what types of verbalizations or behavior are expected. This general agreement seems to cut across various intellectual levels, and is not limited to well educated or intelligent people. Even when one cuts across different social classes, one finds much more agreement than disagreement as to what types of verbalizations are very bizarre or very idiosyncratic.

A question frequently asked by students and colleagues is if, because of their unique and sometimes unusual features, creative, novel solutions to a problem would be included under "bizarre-idiosyncratic" thinking. The answer is no, they would not. There are a number of differences between unique, creative responses and bizarre-idiosyncratic responses. "Creative" verbalizations communicate to the observer. Perhaps of key importance, creative verbalizations may contain unusual or unique features, but they are very much "in tune," and it is usually not hard to empathize with or understand both the basis of the creative verbalization and where it came from.

There are rare instances in which aspects of the unusual features of creative, novel responses appear similar to, or even overlap with the unusual features of bizarre-idiosyncratic responses. Creative verbalizations, however, are not confused or illogical. In addition, creative verbalizations and/or behavior usually are goal directed and oriented toward task achievement. To be "creative," responses must be resourceful and appropriate to the task.

While the definition we cited above may be somewhat controversial, the underlying processes involved in judging what is bizarre or idiosyncratic seem to elicit remarkable agreement among most people in our society; most examples of idiosyncratic speech or behavior are easily agreed upon by observers. Some examples of idiosyncratic behavior that we encountered in responses to the Object Sorting Test show this consensus quite clearly: in one instance, a schizophrenic patient was given *a pipe* and was told to sort objects that belong with it. He sorted a bicycle bell as belonging with the pipe because "I'm afraid father is going to die of lung cancer and the bicycle bell could warn him." Or, when a patient sorted an unusually wide variety of objects as belonging with the pipe because "they're for therapy, for maintenance therapy," or when a patient was handed *a red paper circle* and put a red ball with it because " the red symbolizes the passion of Christ. The ball is Christ's heart."

Similarly, when one looks at proverb interpretations, and responses to Social Comprehension questions, one can find numerous examples of responses that would be generally considered bizarre or idiosyncratic. Some have already been presented above; others include such verbal responses as the following:

Q: *The grass is always greener in the other fellow's yard.* A: Don't trouble trouble til trouble troubles you. [The question was repeated.] People are always—it's like you're always getting a raw shake and you're always trying to keep up with the Joneses. My response is don't touch that question of comparison and competiton. It's killing the world.

Q? *It never rains but it pours.* A: God's rule comes in huge storms.

Q: *A drowning man will clutch at a straw.* A: 1 could say I'm a drowning man right now. Anyone who asks for help. Ask and you shall receive. Seek and you shall find. It all has to do with Christ.

Q: *The proof of the pudding is in the eating.* A: Say you have two bottles. One contains hemlock and one contains 7-Up which equals pudding. There's only one way to know which is which, and that is to drink one or the other or both. No matter what the food looks like it's the taste that counts.

Q: *A rolling stone gathers no moss.* A: Could be a grave or anything. You could sit on a stone, see a gang and everything.

Q: *Rome was not built in a day.* A: It's love, I think of it as love. I have to work towards love and love has to work towards me. And this has to gradually come.

Q: *A rolling stone gathers no moss.* A: You can't sit still on life. You must go on to one and ask another or you'll be indecent.

THE RELATIONSHIP BETWEEN BIZARRE-IDIOSYNCRATIC THINKING AND THE VARIOUS TYPES OF THOUGHT PATHOLOGY VIEWED AS IMPORTANT IN DSM III

Almost all of the various types of thought pathology listed in DSM III as potential features that may be found in schizophrenia are included in the construct of bizarre-idiosyncratic thinking that we employ. In particular, DSM III discusses looseness of association, incoherence, neologisms, blocking, clanging and illogical thinking as features that involve disturbances in thinking. All of these types of cognitive disturbances would fit under our definition and criteria for bizarre-idiosyncratic thinking. Finally, DSM III also includes poverty of content of speech as a type of disordered thinking. On the surface it might seem as though this latter feature does not fit under the construct of bizarre-idiosyncratic thinking. However, the specific examples of poverty of content of speech provided in DSM III and other diagnostic manuals have usually included speech that is both bizarre and idiosyncratic. In that respect, many cases of poverty of content of speech also involve bizarre and idiosyncratic thinking and would be classified as such.

CONSENSUS IN OUR SOCIETY ON WHAT IS BIZARRE AND IMPLICATIONS OF THIS CONSENSUS

In the above examples of bizarre-idiosyncratic thinking, and in countless other examples that we have come across in schizophrenic patients, the "bizarre" or "idiosyncratic" nature of the verbalization (and presumably of the thinking) was quite clear. In every one of these cases the statement or response differs from the more typical or the consensual responses in our society. In addition to deviating from what is socially typical, it is also often hard to empathize with the response, in that it is not easy to discern how it was derived or the ideas to which it was connected.

As we have observed, instances of idiosyncratic verbalizations are agreed upon surprisingly easily when raters sit down to assess specific examples (Hunt, Jones, and Hunt, 1957). (Further data and discussion of reliability and validity are provided in the manual to assess this construct in the appendix in Part VI). With very little training, people can usually reach a high level of consensus as to whether something is idiosyncratic or bizarre. Apparently, in our society a wide range of professionals (and nonprofessionals) do share a number of common experiences and there is surprisingly good agreement as to what is common to our culture and what is out of place, bizarre, or idio-syncratic, and even what is idiosyncratic to a subculture. This would suggest that a relatively common set of standards concerning what is socially appropriate (and even socially tolerable) have been developed, and is shared by almost everyone in our society.

It would appear to us that this relatively high agreement as to which comments are bizarre and which are not may offer a valuable clue to some of the underlying processes involved in decisions about what things can be said in our society, and what should not be said or should be screened out. A relevant question that is of considerable theoretical importance here is whether the acute schizophrenic patient recognizes that what he is saying is bizarre in terms of the social consensus, at the time that he says it. If he does not recognize it, then one important component in the process of the acute schizophrenic's saying bizarre things may be a breakdown in his judgment or *perspective* about what is socially appropriate as opposed to what is strange or bizarre. A second and less important breakdown might be a difficulty in being able to *monitor* or regulate his speech on a moment-to-moment basis by adjusting it as it emerges to conform to correct standards of speech behavior (e.g., correct selection and use of words, correct pronuncia-tion, correct syntax, etc.). Problems in these areas, including difficulty in recognizing which of his own verbalizations are strange (because of impaired perspective), are especially prominent when the patient (and even the "normal" person) is acutely upset or overinvolved in his conflicts.

We have labeled this potential problem as difficulty in *perspective* and *monitoring* (Harrow and Miller, 1980; Harrow and Prosen, 1979). A factor implicated in the underlying processes involved in disordered language and thinking concerns the maintaining and effective use of an internal sense or perspective about what is "normal," and what is "deviant" or "strange" in our society. Most of the acquisition of this function occurs during growth and development in childhood, but it continues throughout the course of adult life. This ability, involving the moment-by-moment integration of previously acquired knowledge about society with current information about the immediate situation, allows one to interpret what the immediate situation or context is, and to make judgments about how to behave in it. The continual integration of past knowledge and experience with current stimuli allows one, under normal circumstances, to recognize strange comments or responses by others, and to monitor oneself by screening out and preventing these inappropriate comments from occurring in one's own behavior. We believe that this is a basic, higher-level, executive type of cognitive process in adults, and that it involves metacognitive behavior. It has not, however, been given sufficient focus in research on normal human cognition or in the study of disordered cognition.

Beginning evidence of our research group suggests that this ability to recognize (and to screen out) strange or inappropriate comments, and impairment in this ability during certain periods, may be one of several central factors involved in schizophrenic psychosis. Even during an acute or active schizophrenic episode, this ability to maintain perspective and to recognize what is appropriate (and to engage in adequate monitoring to make it conform to the usual social standards) may be diminished primarily in respect to one's own behavior and verbalizations, and not be as impaired in judgments of others' behavior and verbalizations. We would propose that the schizophrenic does have the potential for this ability, although its effective utilization may be more sporadic. It is our belief that this ability has been developed, either to some extent or completely, in the schizophrenic, and is lost, diminished, or not utilized effectively in relation to monitoring one's own speech in certain instances, as during an acute or an active psychotic episode. For most schizophrenics, the impairment in perspective during an active episode appears to have selective elements, in that the difficulty does not appear in relation to all topics, or in all situations. Other components of our research tentatively suggest that during periods of partial recovery or remission there is a restoration, for many schizophrenics, of this ability to maintain perspective and to recognize which aspects of their own verbalizations are appropriate or "normal." Aspects of our research in this area are discussed in greater detail in Chapter 5, which reports our attempts to explore factors that may influence bizarre-idiosyncratic thinking.

PLAN OF STUDIES ON BIZARRE-IDIOSYNCRATIC THINKING

Our empirical work in this area was focused on three goals. The first step involved studying the frequency of bizarre-idiosyncratic speech and thinking during acute phases of schizophrenia. This research is outlined in the current chapter. The second step involved analyzing their potential importance in schizophrenic disorders, and as diagnostic indices. Much of this research is outlined in Chapter 4. We have also included in Chaper 4 a summary of our research and thinking on a series of related issues, such as the process-reactive dimension and its relation to thought disorders in schizophrenia, whether bizarre language and thinking are unique to schizophrenia, and whether bizarre speech and thinking are discrete phenomena or lie on a continuum with normal thinking. The third goal in our research on bizarre language has been to assess its course over time, particularly during periods of partial recovery and remission, to determine whether bizarre speech and thinking are permanent, nonremitting features of schizophrenia, or whether they are only associated with active episodes of the disorder. In addition, our work on bizarre speech has been designed to begin to explore possible factors that might influence or determine bizarre speech and thinking. The research and our conclusions from these latter two stages of our studies in this area are outlined in Chapter 5.

During the course of our investigations in this area we have attempted to determine which techniques are the most efficient for studying bizarre-idiosyncratic speech and thinking; toward this end, we have used a variety of methods. After initial efforts with some less fruitful methods, our research has involved the use of five related techniques to evaluate idiosyncratic speech. These are based on assessing responses to proverbs tests, to the Rorschach Test, to the Object Sorting Test, to a test of social comprehension, and a series of free-verbalization interviews. Our patient populations have consisted of four samples of acute schizophrenic and nonschizophrenic psychiatric patients, with these patients usually being assessed during the acute phase of their disorder and then during the phase of partial recovery. Three samples have also been assessed during the posthospital period, to evaluate their thinking during what, for many schizophrenics, was a postpsychotic phase, and also to relate their level of thought pathology to their level of functioning and symptom status, and to their frequency of rehospitalization. In addition, we have studied three samples of chronic, multiyear, hospitalized schizophrenics, and two samples of "normals."

BIZARRE-IDIOSYNCRATIC VERBALIZATIONS AND THINKING AT THE ACUTE PHASE

Overview

The first stage of our studies in this area involved research on samples of acute patients, to explore the presence and frequency of bizarre-idiosyncratic verbalizations and thinking in these types of patients. Along these lines we conducted a series of investigations of different samples, using a variety of instruments, and studying bizarre-idiosyncratic thinking at several early phases of the patients' disorders. Aspects of our earlier research in this area on acute patients, some of which is outlined in this chapter, are described in greater detail in a series of reports (Harrow, Himmelhoch, Tucker, Hersh, and Quinlan, 1972; Harrow and Quinlan, 1977; Harrow, Tucker, and Adler, 1972; Quinlan and Harrow, 1974; Quinlan, Harrow, & Tucker, 1972; Reilly, Harrow, Tucker, Quinlan, and Siegel, 1975; Tucker, Quinlan, and Harrow, 1972).

The results with each of the five major instruments we used produced a similar picture. Each instrument produced data indicating that schizophrenics are more bizarre or show more positive thought disorder than nonschizophrenic patients when assessed at the more acute phase of their disorders. When evaluated with a combination of several of our major instruments, and a composite index of bizarre-idiosyncratic thinking has been used, a large majority of the schizo-phrenics at this phase showed signs of bizarre verbalizations or of disordered thinking. When assessed at the most acute phase with our composite index, from 65 to almost 85 percent of the schizophrenics showed abnormal thought at either moderate or severe levels of bizarre-idiosyncratic thinking. Whether the rate of bizarre thinking is at the lower end of this estimate or reaches the 75 to 85 percent level seems to depend in part on whether we were able to assess the schizophrenics during the first week of hospitalization, at the height of the acute phase, or instead waited until they had been in the hospital for two to four weeks. As with other aspects of the clinical picture, after two to four weeks in the hospital some of the more severe thought pathology had diminished and the patients no longer showed as much flagrant psychopathology. The rate of disordered thinking is also influenced by whether we assess medication-free samples. While medicated samples (e.g., patients receiving phenothiazines or pheno-thiazinelike medications) frequently showed less thought pathology, even among medicated samples as many as 80 percent of the schizophrenics still showed abnormal thinking, when they were assessed at the height of the acute phase.

It can not yet be clearly ascertained whether the few remaining schizophrenic patients who show no signs of bizarre-idiosyncratic thinking are or are not actually disordered in their thinking. It is possible that these patients also have tendencies toward bizarre-idiosyncratic verbalizations and thinking, but that the particular test instrument used was not the optimal instrument for eliciting such responses from them. The particular tests used are, obviously, not the last or only word in providing material to elicit bizarre verbalizations, and it is possible that a more sensitive instrument might have elicited bizarre verbalizations from these patients. However, since this minority of schizophrenics (15 to 20 percent at the most acute phase) did not show evidence of abnormal thinking in terms of moderate or severe levels of bizarre verbalizations, it is our belief that this minority of schizophrenics would be less bizarre, or perhaps not bizarre at all, under any circumstances. Thus, we believe that not all schizophrenics will show such bizarre-idiosyncratic thinking, and that a small percentage of schizophrenics do not have major thought pathology.

It should be noted that while the schizophrenics showed a high level of bizarre verbalizations on our five major types of instruments, a percentage of nonschizophrenics also showed some signs of bizarre verbalizations, although this was true of a smaller percentage of these patients. This type of data bears on the question of whether or not nonschizophrenics also have idiosyncratic or bizarre thinking; this is discussed more fully in Chapter 4.

The type of verbalizations and thinking that appeared in the patients' responses included a wide variety of different kinds of bizarre verbalizations. However, no single type of bizarre-idiosyncratic thinking or positive thought disorder that others have hypothesized to be important has tended to predominate in the strange verbalizations that have appeared. Some of these verbalizations could be classified as reflecting one aspect of disordered thinking hypothesized by others to be important (e.g., conceptual overinclusion, or communicative difficulty, or disordered logic), and some have reflected other hypothesized types of disordered thinking. Many of the more disordered verbalizations seem to reflect, simultaneously, several of the diverse types of thought pathology that have been observed as important in schizophrenia. While no single type of bizarre verbalizations proposed by others has predominated in all the responses, or even in the great majority of disordered comments, two different features, which at times overlap, have been frequent: (1) at least a moderate percentage of the bizarre verbalizations might be viewed as involving loose associations or loss of goal-directed thinking; and (2) at least a moderate percentage seem to be connected in some way with the patients' personal material, personal concerns, or conflicts that were intermingled with their speech and thinking at a time when such intermingling was inappropriate, and thus made the patients appear strange or bizarre. When viewed from a different dimension, and looked at from the standpoint of higher-level cognitive processes, almost all of the disordered verbalizations of these *young acute patients* involved some loss of perspective by the patients concerning which aspects of their verbalizations were socially appropriate and which were strange and inappropriate. These features are discussed in the latter part of Chapter 5.

Results from Comprehension and Proverbs Tests

The results, bearing on issues concerning bizarre thinking and positive thought disorder in acute schizophrenia, included data from our use of two types of short verbal tests, the (social) Comprehension Scale of the Wechsler Adult Intelligence Scale (WAIS), and several proverbs tests. The comprehension scale of the WAIS contains fourteen questions, eleven of which are related to aspects of social comprehension (e.g., "What would you do if while in the movies you were the first person to see smoke and fire?"; "Why does the state require people to get a license in order to be married?") (Wechsler, 1955). The proverbs tests we used in our research involved both the Benjamin Proverbs Test, containing fourteen common proverbs (Benjamin, 1944), and the Gorham Proverbs Test, which includes three parallel sets of proverbs, or three proverbs tests (Gorham, 1956).

Two closely related scoring systems were constructed to rate the proverbs and comprehension tests. The second and more modern of these two systems, which we employ in our current research, is described in considerable detail later in the Appendix in Part VI. Both of these two scoring systems are based on assigning scores for bizarre-idiosyncratic speech for each proverb (or comprehension item) in which the response contains one or more of the following features: (a) lack of shared communication; (b) an inappropriate verbalization, often involving cognitive slippage; (c) an inappropriate, overly elaborate response; (d) peculiar logic; (e) inappropriate intermingling into the response of personal (or other irrelevant) material; (f) a grossly incorrect interpretation, unrelated to the original question; (g) a response that is deviant in respect to social convention; (h) a response involving an odd meaning or outlook; (i) a confused or disorganized response, and (j) other strange or bizarre behavior.

The original scoring system used in our initial research at Yale-New Haven Hospital involved scoring responses to each proverb and comprehension item along a five-point scale for a bizarre-idiosyncratic response. Scores for each response ranged from zero for a response that is not bizarre to 4 for a very severe bizarre response. (Further details on our initial scoring system and extensive examples are available in Adler and Harrow, 1973.) We have already noted a number of examples of bizarre-idiosyncratic responses in this chapter. Two additional examples follow. First is an example of a lack of shared communication: *Q: He who laughs last laughs best; A:* "The one who knows what the issues are and doesn't presume to know, but makes a study, is the one." The second involves a grossly incorrect interpretation that is unrelated to the original question: *Q; He who laughs last laughs best; A:* "I think if you have a principle and don't believe in it, never back out."

The results from one of our very early studies, using the proverbs and comprehension tests, are presented in Table 3.1. In this research, assessing ninety-five acute inpatients from our inpatient setting at Yale-New Haven Hospital, we found that the schizophrenics showed significantly more bizarre-idiosyncratic verbalizations and more positive thought disorder. These relatively young patients, who were evaluated during their first ten days in the hospital, at the most acute phase, showed evidence of severe levels of thought pathology. Thus, when assessment was made early in the course of hospitalization, there were very large, significant differences between the schizophrenic and nonschizophrenic patients on both the comprehension and the proverbs tests. This trend toward significantly more bizarre-idiosyncratic verbalizations in schizophrenics on these short verbal tests has been repeated in several other studies we have done of early-phase schizophrenic samples.

TABLE 3.1
Mean Scores on Bizarre-Idiosyncratic Thinking from the Comprehension and Proverbs Tests at the Acute Phase (Yale-New Haven Sample)

| | *Bizarre-Idiosyncratic Thinking* | | | |
| | *Comprehension Test* | | *Proverbs Test* | |
Sample	*N*	*Mean*	*N*	*Mean*
Classical schizophrenics	25	6.24	25	5.56
Latent schizophrenics	23	3.09	23	2.22
Nonschizophrenic patients	47	1.77	47	2.09
Classical schizophrenics versus nonschizophrenics (*t* test)	*t* = 4.70*		*t* = 3.59*	

*P < .001

From Adler, & Harrow. "Idiosyncratic Thinking and Personally Over-involved Thinking in Schizophrenic Patients During Partial Recovery," *Comprehensive Psychiatry*, 15, 57–67, 1974. Reproduced by permission of the publisher.

In one of our recent samples of young schizophrenics and non-schizophrenic patients from our Chicago settings, we found similar, but less powerful, trends. In that sample, we assessed the patients at the second to fourth weeks of hospitalization, using a modified and improved version of our scoring system (see Appendix in Part VI for a detailed description). Scores for each response in this revised system range from 0 (not bizarre at all) to 3 (very severe bizarre responses). The results showed significant differences between the schizophrenic and nonschizophrenic patients on the proverbs test. On the comprehension test the results were not significant, although the mean differences were in the expected direction. It is our belief that the smaller differences between the schizophrenic and the nonschizophrenic patients (although still significant on one of the two tests) were attributable to the fact that the patients were assessed during the second to fourth weeks of acute treatment and hospitalization, after some of their more marked, acute psychopathology had diminished.

This view has been supported by our most recent results from the same Chicago settings. We again found large, significant, schizophrenic-nonschizophrenic differences when we controlled more carefully for phase of disorder by assessing patients early in their hospitalization during the most acute phase of disorder.

In addition to analyzing schizophrenic-nonschizophrenic differences, we looked at the relationship between scores on the comprehension test for bizarre-idiosyncratic verbalizations and the parallel scores on the proverbs test. The result was a correlation of $r=0.62$, indicating that patients whose scores are high on one of these indices of bizarre-idiosyncratic verbalizations will usually show high scores on the other index. This suggests that bizarre-idiosyncratic responses and positive thought disorder at the acute phase of psychopathology, as assessed on short verbal tests, are not specific to one test instrument alone. There is a high level of agreement between scores on the two types of tests, and this reflects on the generality of the construct involved. There is also agreement between test scores and other observations of the patient's behavior, with these two sets of results suggesting that there is consistency of behavior across situations when bizarre-idiosyncratic verbalizations are assessed at the acute phase.

We analyzed the relationship between bizarre-idiosyncratic thinking and delusional activity at the acute phase in our Yale New Haven Hospital sample. We found a tendency for those patients highest on bizarre-idiosyncratic verbalizations, using the proverbs and comprehension tests, to show the greatest degree of delusional activity. The correlations between delusions, as rated by independent clinicians (psychiatrists) and bizarre-idiosyncratic verbalizations and thinking varied from $r=0.40$ to $r=0.57$, depending on the test involved in assessing bizarre-idiosyncratic verbalizations.

The data on the strong relationship between the two verbal tests of bizarre-idiosyncratic thinking suggest that different measures of the same construct show agreement at the acute phase. The relatively high correlations between bizarre-idiosyncratic thinking and delusions relate to the validity of the construct at the acute phases. The data also may suggest, however, that *at the acute phase* there is a general psychosis factor for schizophrenics that heavily influences the clinical picture, and that may provide clues to some of the underlying processes at that phase of disorder.

Results from the Object Sorting Test

The third major instrument we used to assess bizarre-idiosyncratic behavior and to gain clues about disordered thinking is the Golstein-Scheerer Object Sorting Test (Goldstein and Scheerer, 1941). This test consists of a set of common objects that can be looked at in terms of a number of different concepts (e.g., a spoon, a toy knife, a red poker chip, a bicycle bell, a screwdriver, a cigar, a white candle, a sugar cube, and others). The classical system of administration of Part I of the Object Sorting Test was used as the basis for obtaining the measure of bizarre-idiosyncratic thinking that we devised. Part I involves presenting the subject with an object (called the "starting object," or SO) and asking him to sort with the starting object all the other objects that belong with it. After he has completed this, the subject is asked his reasons for his selections. This procedure was carried our separately with each of the following seven starting objects: (1) a sink stopper; (2) a fork; (3) a pipe; (4) a bicycle bell; (5) a red paper circle; (6) pliers; and (7) a red rubber ball.

High ratings for bizarre-idiosyncratic thinking were assigned when a patient engaged in the following behavior: (a) using the starting object in reference to oneself or one's own experience (for example, the subject is given the *bicycle bell* as SO; he responds by sorting the toy dog, and explaining, "Whenever I ride my bike Spotty comes along"); (b) linking the starting object to other objects for strange, illogical, or socially unshared reasons (for example, given the SO, *fork,* the subject sort the *red paper circle,* and explains, "It's part of my personal cosmogeny"; or for the SO, *pipe,* the patient sorts the dog and explains, "The dog signifies death and the pipe signifies comfort") (c) using the starting object as a cue that is understandable only to the patient (e.g., given a *red ball* as SO; a patient sorts tools, "To build a place to play");

and (d) inappropriate or strange behavior toward the test or tester (such as strange asides or comments, or inappropriate behavior).(Further details on this scoring system are provided in Himmelhoch, et al., 1973.)

The results on bizarre-idiosyncratic thinking and positive thought disorder from our first sample of sixty-seven acute patients from the Yale-New Haven inpatient setting showed significant differences between our schizophrenic and nonschizophrenic patients, with more bizarre scores for the schizophrenics. These results are presented in Table 3.2 which reports the mean scores for the schizophrenics and the major types of nonschizophrenic patients (depressives and severe personality disorders). Our subsequent results from several other samples of acute patients have similarly shown schizophrenics as higher on bizarre-idiosyncratic thinking than nonschizophrenic patients.

Again, the schizophrenic-nonschizophrenic differences were most striking when we assessed patients at our Yale-New Haven Hospital setting in the first week to ten days, at the most acute phase. Some of our later samples of patients from Chicago were evaluated during the second to fourth weeks in the hospital. While these first four weeks may still be an acute phase, such evaluation is often after the height of the acute phase of psychosis. As was the case for the results from some of

TABLE 3.2
Mean Scores of Schizophrenic and Nonschizophrenic Patients on Object Sorting Measure of Bizarre-Idiosyncratic Thinking at the Acute Phase (Yale-New Haven Sample)

| | | Bizarre-Idiosyncratic Thinking | |
Sample	N	Mean	t (Schiz. versus Nonschiz.)
Classical schizophrenics	28	3.00	3.75*
Nonschizophrenic patients	39	1.74	
Depressives	20	1.75	
Personality disorder and neurosis	14	1.36	
Other nonschizophrenic patients	5	2.80	

*P < .01

From Harrow, Tucker, Himmelhoch, & Putnam. *American Journal of Psychiatry, 128,* 824–829, 1972. Reproduced by permission of the publisher.

our other instruments, score differences between schizophrenic and nonschizophrenic patient samples at this time of testing were smaller, although the differences were still statistically significant.

Utilizing an important independent index of psychotic activity again, namely an index of delusional activity, we found a correlation of $r=0.51$, ($P< .001$) between psychiatrists' ratings of delusions and the scores for idiosyncratic thinking on the Object Sorting Test, using our Yale-New Haven sample of patients. Again, these results bear on the validity of the construct, and also might suggest that there is a general acute psychosis factor at the acute phase of schizophrenia.

Results from the Rorschach Test and from the Free Verbalization Technique

The Rorschach Test provided us with an additional opportunity to assess the construct of bizarre-idiosyncratic language and thinking in patients. The Rorschach is usually viewed as an unstructured or projective test because the stimuli (ink blots) do not provide the subject with clear or socially familiar guidelines concerning the stimuli and the expected responses. In this test the subject is asked to tell "what things you see in the inkblots." Responding to unfamiliar and vague stimuli, subjects must draw on their own internal associations, or supply more of their own structure to the stimuli in order to make sense of them. In all situations, including everyday familar ones, subjects must decide how to understand and integrate current stimuli with previous experience. However, with vague stimuli, such as the Rorschach, subjects must make a more difficult and ambiguous decision about which aspects of their previous public and private experience are linked with the current (inkblot) stimuli. Subjects must also choose their responses without clear guidelines from their own experience as to what answer is the most socially appropriate one in the unfamiliar Rorschach situation.

Our discussion of the Rorschach in this and subsequent chapters is based on an index we have developed of *deviant thought quality* (*TQ*), which is similar in many respects to our measure of bizarre-idio-syncratic thinking. Further information on our use of the Rorschach scales to assess various aspects of cognition are presented in Chapters 5, 6, 9, and 15, and more complete details of our use of this test to assess disordered cognition, with extensive examples, are reported in a manual available to the interested reader (Quinlan, Harrow, and Carlson, 1973). A brief summary of our measure of deviant thought quality from the Rorschach is outlined below.

The measure of deviant thought quality is scored according to the coherence of the responses and whether the responses have strange, peculiar, or illogical components. During the course of our research we found that this Rorchach measure of deviant thought quality was a good index of the concept of bizarre-idiosyncratic language and thinking and of positive thought disorder. In addition, the measure of deviant thought quality also permits us to assess separately the *degree* or *severity* of the particular bizarre verbalization, since all responses are scored on a five-point scale, based on the severity of the bizarre features. Hence, scores on our Rorschach index of deviant thought quality may vary from *TQ0* for nonbizarre responses to *TQ1* for mildly strange or mildly "peculiar" responses, all the way up to *TQ4*, which usually involves the most severely bizarre responses, and at times extremely disordered logic as well.

An example of a Rorschach response that is scored *TQ1* (a mildly strange response) is the following response to card VI: "These could be two . . . what do you call them technically, balls" (the mildly strange part of this response is the use of "technically" to describe "balls"). An example of a Rorschach response scored *TQ3* (a severely bizarre response) is the following response to card IX: "A paranoid cow. (?) Because it had two big eyes and it was staring out from behind a bush so it couldn't be seen." An example of a Rorschach response scored *TQ4* (a very severe bizarre response) is the following response to card III: "Two predatory carnivorous insects doing a ballet around a carcass of an animal or insect that they've killed and will consume in one way or another . . . (What made it look like they will *consume* it?) I think what it was, way my eye went to center and saw open mouths and I related identity of central figure to outer. I relate myself to being eaten alive, by my parents I guess." This response contains autistic logic in relating the center to the outer details of the blot, and extreme fluidity, compounded by overspecific tendencies emerging in an illogical and bizarre sequence.

When we used the Rorschach Test to compare schizophrenic and nonschizophrenic patients at the acute phase, the results were similar in principle to those obtained with our other tests of bizarre-idiosyncratic language and thinking. Our initial analysis using our Rorschach overall index of deviant thought quality at the Yale-New Haven inpatient setting with twenty-eight patients showed significantly more bizarre responses for the schizophrenic than for the nonschizophrenic patients. When this patient sample was enlarged, subsequent analysis with an enlarged group of 159 acute inpatients again showed significant diagnostic differences. These significant results, using a two-way ANOVA on this sample (diagnosis $\times$ sex) involved a comparison of forty-eight classical schizophrenics, thirty-five latent schizophrenics, thirty-eight severe personality disorders, and thirty-eight depressives. After obtaining a significant F for diagnosis ($P< .001$), subsequent Newman-Keuls tests indicated that the "classical" schizophrenic group was significantly higher on deviant thought quality than each of the other three diagnostic groups. These results are presented in Table 3.3.

More recently we used the Rorschach Test to assess another sample of patients from our inpatient settings in Chicago. These patients were not evaluated as early in the acute phase as we had done at Yale-New Haven Hospital; they were instead typically given the Rorschach during the third to fifth weeks of hospitalization. Here again, there was a trend towards differences between schizophrenic and disturbed nonschizophrenic patients ($P< .10$), but the differences were smaller than those from our Yale-New Haven Hospital samples. Our assumption again is that the narrower differences between the schizophrenic and nonschizophrenic patients were a consequence of a diminishing of acute psychopathology by the third to fifth weeks in the hospital.

In the Yale-New Haven setting we also used our data-collection system to assess the relationship between the Rorschach scores for deviant thought quality and independent ratings by the patients' psychiatrists on bizarre behavior for a small subsample of forty-eight patients. The correlation of $r= .79$ between the Rorschach Test scores on deviant thought quality and independent clinicians' ratings of

TABLE 3.3
Mean Scores of Schizophrenic and Nonschizophrenic Patients on Rorschach Measure of Bizarre-Idiosyncratic Thinking at the Acute Phase (Yale-New Haven Sample)

| | | Deviant Thought Quality | |
Sample	N	Mean*	S.D.
Classical schizophrenics	48	21.90	17.11
Latent schizophrenics	35	12.23	12.72
Personality disorders	38	9.55	10.43
Depressives	38	5.76	9.54

*Results from two-way ANOVA (Diagnosis × Sex): F for diagnosis = 11.29, df = 3,151, $P< .001$. (The F values for sex, and sex by diagnosis, were not significant.)

From Harrow, Quinlan, Wallington, & Pickett. *Journal of Personality Assessment, 40,* 31–41, 1976. Reproduced by permission of the publisher.

bizarre behavior during the week of Rorschach testing for this small subsample indicate a strong relationship between the test scores and observers' ratings of behavior. Again, these results provide positive evidence on the validity of the construct involved.

We have reported above in some detail our results from four of our measures of the concept of bizarre-idiosyncratic thinking or positive thought disorder. We will now briefly outline the results from our fifth measure, based on a free-verbalization interview. These interviews were conducted with several of our samples of acute patients from the Yale-New Haven inpatient setting, and with several other samples of chronic schizophrenic patients. In this fifteen-minute, tape-recorded, free-verbalization interview, patients were encouraged to speak for seven and a half minutes in response to a question about their emotional problems, and also to talk for seven and a half minutes about any topic other than mental health problems. Half of the patients were instructed to talk on the mental health problem first, and half on the other topic first. The taped interviews were then rated for various types of speech and thought pathology.

The results obtained with the free-verbalization technique, which apply at this point, are based on a measure of overall deviant language and communication, rated from the tapes of the interviews. Adequate reliability was obtained on the overall ratings of the patients' deviant language and communication. The concept rated was a global one, which was primarily based on a series of factors that fit under the heading of bizarre-idiosyncratic speech or positive thought disorder.

Using this summary index of bizarre-idiosyncratic speech from the free-verbalization technique, we obtained results similar in principle to those obtained with our other major instruments. Thus, we again obtained large significant schizophrenic-nonschizophrenic differences at the acute phase. A more detailed account of this aspect of our research with acute patients can be found in a separate report (Reilly, Harrow, Tucker, Quinlan, and Siegel, 1975); our research using this technique with chronic patients can also be found in a recent report (Siegel, Harrow, Reilly, and Tucker, 1978), and is reviewed in Chapter 5.

We should note in this case that the significant results were obtained using a different type of technique to assess bizarre-idiosyncratic thinking—and one that has some similarity to free conversation (verbalizations by subjects about themselves and their thoughts about other things). However, this technique also *differs* in some ways from routine conversation. In this technique, patients are encouraged to talk with less feedback from the listener, so that the interviewer does not influence the patients by nonstandardized interview material, and to minimize the possibility of potential examiner bias as a factor influencing the patient's comments. This deviation of the free-verbalization technique from routine conversation (i.e., the lack of feedback) seems extremely sensitive for eliciting bizarre speech, but also has some disadvantages in terms of being a novel, artificial, situation for most subjects.

OVERVIEW

Overall, our scores for bizarre-idiosycratic thinking and for positive thought disorder at the acute phase, using a variety of different types of measures, and sampling various aspects of behavior, show consistent patterns. These results show severe thought pathology for the schizophrenic-nonschizophrenic patients, and they also suggest significant schizophrenic-nonschizophrenic differences. As we moved away from the most acute phases of the patients' disorders, however, the differences tended to narrow.

As can be seen by the material presented in this chapter, one can derive a conceptual basis for looking at bizarre-idiosyncratic thinking. Further, when examining the presence of this type of thinking in schizophrenia, one finds that it is present at the acute phase in most schizophrenic patients, if the patients are examined early enough in the course of their hospitalization. This type of result was prominent with five different techniques to assess bizarre-idiosyncratic thinking, and it occurred in both our Yale-New Haven inpatient sample and our Chicago setting at Michael Reese Hospital. The next step in our research in this area is to look at a number of issues that are important for an understanding of the role of bizarre-idiosyncratic thinking in schizophrenia; these are described in Chapter 4. Chapter 5 carries our analysis of bizarre-idiosyncratic thinking one step further as it describes the results of our research studying bizarre-idiosyncratic thinking over time, at other phases of the schizophrenic disorder, as well as our attempt to study factors that may influence or determine bizarre-idiosyncratic thinking.

4

Major Issues in Understanding the Role of Bizarre-Idiosyncratic Thinking in Schizophrenia

W e have discussed the concept of bizarre-idiosyncratic thinking in Chapter 3, and have also presented consistent results indicating the presence and relatively high frequency of bizarre-idiosyncratic thinking in schizophrenia during the acute phase. Our next step is to analyze some of the prominent issues related to the appearance of this type of thinking. This includes analysis of differences in implications between mild and severe levels of bizarre-idiosyncratic thinking and analyzing whether positive types of thought disorder such as bizarre thinking are unique to schizophrenia. It also involves a series of studies on bizarre-idiosyncratic thinking in process versus reactive schizophrenia. In addition, it includes an analysis of bizarre speech and thinking as possible diagnostic indicators, as well as consideration of several other major issues.

DOES THE SCHIZOPHRENIC'S BIZARRE SPEECH
APPEAR UNDER ALL CIRCUMSTANCES?

The results reported in the preceding chapter, and other data we have collected, can be used to further our understanding of positive thought pathology such as bizarre verbalizations along several major dimensions. This includes issues concerning whether or not bizarre verbalizations are an invariant feature of the schizophrenic, or whether they only appear under certain circumstances.

In addition to the tests and techniques presented in Chapter 3, we have used other tests, including the Information subtest of the Wechsler Adult Intelligence Scales (WAIS). These other instruments also elicit bizarre-idiosyncratic language, but the occurrence of such language is rarer with this type of test. Thus, in contrast to our results with instruments such as the Rorschach, the probability that deviant schizophrenic verbalizations will appear is diminished when a carefully structured stimulus is presented to the patient. The opportunity for bizarre response is also diminished when the patient is allowed to select a response in a multiple-choice situation, or when a stereotyped response, which has been well rehearsed, is demanded. The schizophrenic does not behave bizarrely in all situations. Bizarre behavior is much more likely to appear in situations where unstructured stimuli are used, or nonstereotyped responses are called for. Our results indicate that the particular type of situation presented to the patient is a very important factor; some situations or stimuli arouse bizarre-idiosyncratic language much more readily than others. The overt appearance of bizarre verbalizations depends heavily on the type of stimuli present, and on the opportunity for a schizophrenic patient's tendency toward disturbed thinking to show itself in his or her verbalizations.

The type of *response* demanded of the patient is also of central importance. In the major instruments that we have used successfully to detect possible bizarre or idiosyncratic language and behavior the patient must respond in the absence of a socially stereotyped answer or well-rehearsed response to that particular stimuli. Much emphasis has been placed on the vague and unstructured nature of the stimulus as the key factor is producing disordered verbalizations and thinking with instruments such as the Rorschach. It is our belief that a factor of equal importance in eliciting disordered language and thinking on the Rorschach and on other tests such as a proverbs test, is the subject's lack of experience in choosing and knowing which type of reply or which specific response is called for in that particular test situation, and the absence of familiar guidelines concerning potential responses to give.

To assess bizarre verbalizations and thinking (and differences between diagnostic groups) at the most fruitful level, the means of assessment (e.g., a proverbs or comprehension test) should be sensitive enough to elicit bizarre language in many patients. It also should not be too sensitive, or too difficult, or too vague such that too many people (including many normal and nonpsychotic patients) will show bizarre language.

This carries certain implications about the nature of bizarre speech. It suggests that some material may be too sensitive, so that it elicits verbalizations that are slightly "off," or mildly bizarre, or strange, from too many people, including nonpathological people. For this reason, such a task may be less capable of distinguishing disturbed groups of people. Here we suggest that under conditions that elicit bizarre speech to a high degree, a large number of people may show signs of such strange verbalizations. Our evidence indicates that the appearance of bizarre speech is heavily influenced by the situation in which the patient or normal person is placed. It also suggests that most people are capable of emitting some language that is slightly "off," strange, or even bizarre, depending on the circumstances. In the typical, routine, social situation, most people have well-rehearsed responses in their repertoires and are not likely to emit much bizarre speech. In more stressful situations, more complex situations, and more unfamiliar situations, bizarre speech is somewhat more likely to be emitted by some normals, although even here, the degree or level of idiosyncracy of the bizarre speech may only be mild.

Many schizophrenics (in active phases) will produce some bizarre speech even in routine social situations. The issue is a matter of degree, depending on the extent of psychopathology or disturbance, the particular kind of psychopathology (e.g., schizophrenia), and the context of how difficult and how unfamiliar the situation is. In the context of a strange, unfamiliar, and possibly threatening situation, we would expect some deviant speech occasionally, even from normals. Obviously, the social context and degree of departure from a routine social situation is a major consideration here. However, also to be recognized and dealt with is the fact that many schizophrenics and nonpsychotics may be capable of producing bizarre verbalizations, and in this respect the appearance of bizarre speech might be viewed as a potential that could appear in their behavior under certain circumstances. This potential for bizarre verbalizations in nonschizophrenics, especially milder levels of bizarre speech, touches upon two central issues. These two issues—(1) mild versus severe levels of bizarre speech and thinking, and (2) bizarre speech in nonschizophrenics—are important ones, and are discussed more completely in several later sections of this chapter.

Context and Social Expectations

In regard to the importance of the social context, a question that is frequently posed by colleagues and students is whether the idiosyncratic and bizarre verbalizations may not be due to playfulness or "creativity"? Indeed, as we have noted in Chapter 2, Wild (1965) studied the Rorschach responses of schizophrenics, artists, and for comparison, schoolteachers. In comparison to schizophrenics, the artists produced a surprising number of responses that were scored for "primary process" thinking. The differences between the artists and the schizophrenics emerged on the affect the subjects reported for their responses: artists reported more positive affect than schizophrenics; they enjoyed their bizarre and idiosyncratic responses more; and when asked to respond in a normal fashion, they were able to give an ordinary, nonbizarre response. The artists showed both enjoyment and control.

The Wild study points to the critical nature of the *social context* when studying bizarre and idiosyncratic thinking. In some contexts, "artistic" students may see themselves as being evaluated to assess how creative they are, and in such instances they may extend themselves further to come up with original, and even unusual, responses. In addition, "control" subjects—be they artists, college volunteers, or staff members—may not anticipate the same consequences for manifesting bizarre and idiosyncratic responses as patients, given test stimuli in a clinical setting, may anticipate. In clinical settings when patients are assessed they usually see themselves as being interviewed or tested by an authority figure who is evaluating them for potential deviance and psychopathology. With a few exceptions, patients do not respond to test stimuli given by hospital or clinical staff, to study their potential psychopathology and "sickness," as an opportunity to be playful and "creative." And relatively few people, patient or nonpatient, can be as creative as the highly select group of people who are capable of producing truly aesthetically pleasing products. Again, we must emphasize that appropriate comparison subjects are those who are in some type of situation that they perceive as an evaluative one. Ideally, such an evaluative situation will make patient controls, or even normal controls, feel that their responses will have some consequences for them, in terms of making them appear nondeviant or "sane" to other observers.

BIZARRE-IDIOSYNCRATIC THINKING IN PROCESS AND REACTIVE SCHIZOPHRENIA

The Concept of Process and Reactive Schizophrenia

A major issue concerning disordered cognition in schizophrenia involves the process-reactive dimension. For a number of years formulations about the importance of the distinction between process and reactive schizophrenia have been prominent, and an extensive literature has developed on this way of categorizing schizophrenic patients (Garmezy, 1970; Higgins, 1971; Putterman and Pollack, 1976; Strauss, Klorman, Kokes, and Sacksteder, 1977). In order to assess these formulations, we have looked at our data in several different areas of cognition in terms of variables such as premorbid social-sexual competence, and other related variables usually viewed as assessing good and poor prognostic factors in schizophrenia. While formulations about process versus reactive schizophrenia and good versus poor premorbid schizophrenics are related, they are not identical, and the present discussion will deal with our investigations into bizarre-idiosyncratic thinking in process versus reactive schizophrenia.

Process schizophrenia is usually seen as being characterized by poor premorbid or prepsychotic adjustment, especially in the area of social-sexual competence. The process schizophrenic is viewed as one whose functioning either began to decline at a relatively early period in adolescence, or else did not show adequate development in the first place. The psychosis develops gradually or insidiously, after a prolonged downhill course, with no overt precipitants necessary for the psychotic phase. Subsequent prognosis for possible full recovery and later functioning is seen as poor. This type of schizophrenic would presumably come closest to the picture of a deteriorating course originally drawn by Kraepelin.

In contrast, the *reactive schizophrenic* is viewed as an individual with relatively adequate or "normal" prepsychotic functioning and satisfactory social adjustment. The prototype reactive schizophrenic would thus be one with adequate premorbid functioning who had a clear external precipitant or difficult stress that led to an acute onset, psychotic, "break." Prognosis for the reactive schizophrenic is usually seen as favorable.

While etiological theories of process and reactive schizophrenia vary, there are at least three (not necessarily disparate) views concerning the process-reactive dimension. They are:

1. A developmental view, in terms of reactive schizophrenics having achieved a satisfactory developmental level, and process schizophrenics being immature and never having achieved a satisfactory level. The developmentally immature process schizophrenic, having achieved fewer social skills or personal resources at earlier stages of development is likely to "break down" earlier and to have a poorer prognosis (Zigler and Phillips, 1961, 1962; Phillips, 1966; Harrow, Tucker, and Bromet, 1971; Bromet, Harrow, and Tucker, 1971).
2. A more "organic" view in terms of process schizophrenics having an organic etiology, and reactive schizophrenics having a psychodynamic origin and/or an origin arising from family psychopathology.
3. A view that process schizophrenia is a consequence of having had early developmental difficulty due to lack of adequate parenting, or lack of adequate figures for satisfactory parental identification, whereas reactive schizophrenics have had more adequate parenting, and/or parental figures allowing for more satisfactory identification (Rodnick and Garmezy, 1957).

A number of different measures have been used in the past to assess the process-reactive construct, with the most commonly used one being Part I of the Phillips Scale, which assesses premorbid social-sexual adjustment (Phillips, 1953).

A key question is whether process and reactive schizophrenia should be viewed as a dichotomy of two separate types of schizophrenia, or whether they should be seen as a continuum representing two ends of a common dimension, with many schizophrenics falling somewhere along this continuum. If process and reactive schizophrenia represent two basically different types of schizophrenia (or even two different disorders), the field would be simplified in that data showing apparent differences between process and reactive schizophrenia on premorbid functioning, on current functioning, and on prognosis and outcome could be explained.

This issue has not been resolved with any finality, and arguments have been advanced to support both positions. Currently, most people in the field believe that the process-reactive dimension and the adequacy of premorbid adjustment should be regarded as a *continuum* rather than as a dichotomy, although this issue is still open to question (Keith and Buchsbaum, 1978).

Our evidence has begun to suggest that the process-reactive dimension is more likely to represent a continuum than a dichotomy. We believe, however, that it is still possible that a select *subsample* of "reactive" schizophrenics, with good premorbid histories, may represent a separate group of reactive psychosis patients who are not necessarily schizophrenics. If this is the case, then the "true" schizophrenic disorder would consist of (1) the remainder of the "reactive" schizophrenics with good premorbid histories, and (2) all of the process schizophrenics with poor premorbid histories, with schizophrenic patients from these two combined groups falling on a process-reactive continuum of premorbid social-sexual adjustment. In this latter case (and it is still only one of several possibilities), the process-reactive dimension would represent a continuum for the majority of patients who are presently labeled "schizophrenic" by workers in the field.

A central belief tied in with the concept of the process-reactive dimension involves hypotheses about its utility in predicting schizophrenic outcome (e.g., reactive schizophrenics' having favorable outcomes). However, there are almost no *prospective, long-term* follow-up studies in this area to support these assumptions.

Some of our research that is unrelated to our work on cognition was designed to investigate potential links between the process-reactive dimension and outcome. In this research we have studied short-term outcome (length of hospitalization) and slightly longer-term outcome (adjustment eight to nine months after hospitalization). The results on the relationship between the process-reactive dimension and short-term outcome were quite positive (Bromet, Harrow, and Tucker, 1971; Harrow, Tucker, and Bromet, 1969). However, we found only mildly positive evidence to support the utility of the process-reactive dimension as a predictor of posthospital adjustment (Bromet, Harrow, and Kasl, 1974). Our recent research with a larger sample, studied over a longer time period, and controlling for chronicity by using young, nonchronic schizophrenics has not produced uniformly positive evidence in this area when we control for marriage. Thus, the early results from this recent research would seem to question these assumptions about a strong relationship between the process-reactive dimension and outcome in schizophrenia.

Process and Reactive Schizophrenia—Results on Bizarre-Idiosyncratic Thinking

In looking at our measure of positive thought disorder—namely, bizarre-idiosyncratic thinking—we have also analyzed whether this type of thinking is more common in schizophrenics who fit on the process side of the process-reactive dimension or of those who are more on the reactive side.

In the past, disparate types of findings have emerged in relation to the results on the process-reactive dimension and bizarre thinking in schizophrenia. A large sample of VA Hospital schizophrenics was studied by Kantor, who concluded from the sample that process schizophrenics are more bizarre and idiosyncratic (Kantor and Herron, 1966) The data from Kantor's sample have been loaned to other investigators for further analysis in other areas of cognition. The investigators reanalyzing these data for other aspects of cognition have also felt that their results support a position of process schizophrenics as being more bizarre. It should be remembered of course that these several different studies are all based on the same original sample of patients, rather than representing several independent samples replicating each other and showing similar trends. Tutko and Spence (1962) have also reported results on the process-reactive dimension, but in contrast to the work of Kantor, their results suggest that reactive schizophrenics are more bizarre.

In a review of a series of his own and other research reports, DeWolfe (1974) has interpreted his studies as indicating that reactive schizophrenics, prior to their schizophrenic break, have relatively normal thinking. He proposes that during the psychotic break, the thinking of these reactive schizophrenics shows temporary fragmentation. He believes that their disordered thinking, in this case fragmented and disorganized thinking, is a reaction to a period of stress or acute upset (i.e., associated with acute schizophrenic breaks). In contrast, he believes that process schizophrenics should be viewed as never having achieved a satisactory level of cognitive development, with unusual, idiosyncratic, and underdeveloped thinking being more prominent, and persisting in this type of schizophrenic patient.

Our own research in this area is based on the relationship between levels of premorbid adjustment on the Phillips Scale and scores from our measures of bizarre-idiosyncratic thinking, for both the Rorschach and the Object Sorting Tests. These two tests were administered at the acute phase and at follow-up, to our samples of patients from the Yale and the Chicago hospital settings.

When we analyzed our own data on bizarre-idiosyncratic thinking in young schizophrenics, our results were mixed. Tentative results on our first sample of schizophrenics, studied in our Yale inpatient settings, showed overall a slight (nonsignificant) tendency for more bizarre-idiosyncratic thinking in the process schizophrenics at the acute phase of their disorder. We reassessed a sample of the same schizophrenic patients as they began to enter into partial recovery (seven weeks later), and then again eleven months later after they had left the hospital (postacute and posthospital phase). The results at the phase of partial recovery showed a trend ($P<$ .05) for more bizarre-idiosyncratic thinking among the process schizophrenics. The data at follow-up again showed a significant trend for more disordered thinking among the process schizophrenics ($P<$ .05). Although the results for the schizophrenics at follow-up did not show extremely powerful process-reactive differences (partly as a result of the small sample size), they were significant, with process schizophrenics being more thought disordered. Overall, the results on our sample of schizophrenics from our Yale settings could be interpreted as showing mild support of the DeWolfe hypothesis, although several aspects of the data did not fit in neatly with his hypothesis. While confusion and disorganized thinking may be a part of the acute psychotic break in some "reactive" schizophrenics, beginning evidence of ours suggests that for select reactive schizophrenics, disorganized thinking may be a permanent, or at least long-term, characteristic of their thinking.

In contrast to our results from the Yale inpatient setting the data from our second larger sample of patients, those from Michael Reese Hospital in Chicago, have not shown strong differences in bizarre-idiosyncratic thinking between the process and reactive schizophrenics, at either the acute phase or the follow-up phase. Thus, in our Chicago setting, using our Index of Bizarre-Idiosyncratic Thinking from the Object Sorting Test, we assessed a sample of fifty-six schizophrenic patients at the acute phase, and also assessed a second sample of forty-five schizophrenic patients an average of three years after their "index" hospitalization. The schizophrenic patients' scores on bizarre-idiosyncratic thinking did not show a significant relationship to their ratings on the process-reactive dimension at either phase of their disorder. Similarily, we used the Rorschach with a subsample of schizophrenics assessed at the acute phase from our Michael Reese Hospital setting in Chicago. There was not a significant relationship between their scores on the process-reactive dimension and their scores on the Holzman-Johnston Revised Delta Index derived from the Rorschach Test, with this index being a measure that taps areas of cognition closely related to our construct of bizarre-idiosyncratic thinking (Johnston and Holzman, 1979).

Is There a Relationship between Process-Reactive Schizophrenia and Positive Thought Disorder, Such as Bizarre-Idiosyncratic Thinking?

We would interpret the data presented above as indicating that several different, and at times opposing, factors or influences associated with the process-reactive dimension may be operating to determine the results. Thus, at the acute stage, possible greater disorganization and some confusion in the more reactive schizophrenics might lead to a tendency toward more bizarre-idiosyncratic thinking in the reactive schizophrenics. Our contention is that acute fragmentation and disorganization can at times lead a patient to appear bizarre and idiosyncratic. This could, however, be counterbalanced by a tendency in the process schizophrenics toward more bizarre-idiosyncratic thinking as a consequence of the greater longevity of their disorder. The greater longevity and the more chronic nature of their disorder could be accompanied by greater loss of contact with reality, and for select process schizophrenics, trends toward the beginning of withdrawing into a more private world. If there is any beginning impoverishment of thinking in the more chronic, or process, schizophrenics, this could lead to less *overt* signs of disordered thinking (even in patients with considerable amounts of bizarre-idiosyncratic thinking), as a result of a paucity of *verbal responses* to test material.

These several sets of factors could counterbalance each other during the acute phase, leading to no significant differences between process and reactive schizophrenics at that stage. Our research in other areas has suggested that most schizophrenics' disorganization and confusion begin to diminish as they emerge from the acute phase and enter into stages of partial recovery, and then later enter the posthospital phase. The diminishing of confusion and disorganization could occur to a greater extent among the reactive schizophrenics. This could tend to reduce the level of bizarre-idiosyncratic thinking in these reactive schizophrenics, as they emerge from the more acute phase of their disorder, leading us to expect a tendency for less bizarre-idiosyncratic thinking in the reactive schizophrenics after the acute phase. As we have noted, the results from our Yale sample of patients have suggested such a tendency for more bizarre-idiosyncratic thinking in process than in reactive schizophrenics after the acute phase, although this was not confirmed in our Chicago sample.

We believe that since a number of different factors may be operating to determine these results on the relative differences between the amount of bizarre-idiosyncratic thinking in process and reactive schizophrenics, a slight shift in one or several of these factors could influence the results in either direction, and process-reactive differences could at times be small and nonsignificant. Our view here is that the picture of process and reactive schizophrenia is influenced by factors such as greater chronicity (and earlier onset of the disorder) in "process" schizophrenia, and by a host of other factors that may at times counterbalance each other. According to this view, we would propose that some of the results obtained for the process-reactive continuum are a second-order consequence of other, more basic factors, and in the cognitive area one should not always expect significant differences in bizarre-idiosyncratic thinking between these two types of schizophrenics.

The lack of a significant difference between the process and reactive schizophrenics in our Chicago sample would fit in with the hypothesis that the differences in bizarre-idiosyncratic thinking between these types of schizophrenics are not basic. They will sometimes be nonsignificant, with the significance level, or lack of it, shifting in different studies, owing to seemingly minor changes in other areas of the patients' functioning (e.g., more impoverishment, or less confusion, or more withdrawal, etc.). Thus, we do not view the process-reactive dimension as a prime influence on bizarre-idiosyncratic thinking; rather, we consider the results in this area a consequence of several different factors that operate on the process-reactive dimension, and that influence bizarre-idiosyncratic thinking in opposite directions.

A problem that arises in relation to the process–reactive dimension is that, unlike some of the neat schemes proposed for this dimension, most schizophrenics or even psychotic patients, do not fit on extreme ends of the process-reactive dimension. Many of our "reactive" schizophrenics, even those with reasonable levels of socialization, had not been completely free of previous psychological or social difficulties prior to their current disorder. Similarly, many of our "process" schizophrenics have not been completely isolated, detached, schizoid patients who had started downhill in early adolescence and deteriorated at a steady pace since then. Thus, a number of our process schizophrenics seem to have had some select areas of premorbid competence. This lack of clearly process and clearly reactive patients may be a general characteristic of currently hospitalized schizophrenic patients, or it may be more specific to upper-middle-class patients of the present decade. However, we also have seen this trend in a sample of lower-middle- and lower-class patients whom we are currently studying.

Overall, we can observe that we have found a few scattered positive findings concerning the process-reactive dimension and disordered thinking in schizophrenia, such as the current trends on bizarre-idiosyncratic thinking. Our results on cognition, and also our follow-up data on posthospital adjustment (Bromet, Harrow, and Kasl, 1974; Westermeyer and Harrow, in press), suggest that the process-reactive dimension may be less important than had been hypothesized some years ago. Thus, data from our research on posthospital adjustment, both at Yale and also in Chicago, have suggested that the power of the process-reactive dimension, and other classical prognostic indicators used by Vaillant (1964), Stephens and Astrup (1963), and Stephens

(1973), to predict subsequent outcome for young, relatively early schizophrenics, is not as strong as theories in the area have predicted. Recent data reported by Vaillant (1978) and by Strauss and Carpenter (1974) would lead to similar conclusions. We would propose that some of the potential strength of the process-reactive dimension as a predictor in schizophrenia may be a consequence of other factors often associated with it, such as chronicity or longevity of the disorder, that can influence scores on process-reactive scales (Strauss and Carpenter, 1974; Westermeyer and Harrow, in press).

Mild versus Severe Levels of Bizarre Thinking

In addition to providing data on the possible relationship between the process-reactive dimension and bizarre schizophrenic thinking, our research design also permitted us to examine a number of other questions, including the issue of mild versus severe levels of positive thought disorder, or of bizarre-idiosyncratic thinking. As we noted in Chapter 3, our Rorschach measure of bizarre verbalizations (deviant thought quality) was constructed to permit us to score individual responses that reflect mild versus severe levels of bizarre language and thinking, allowing us to assess this factor in relation to the diagnostic groups. The five-point scale used to score Rorschach responses ranges along a continuum from no strange or bizarre speech, to very mild strange or bizarre speech, and continues up to very severe levels of bizarre speech.

Our detailed separation of different levels of bizarre thinking on the Rorschach was partly based on analysis of ours suggesting that at times overall scores in this area can hide, disguise, or obscure the presence of individual responses reflecting mild as opposed to severe levels of bizarre verbalizations and thinking. Thus, for instance, even among patients who receive high overall scores in this area, this can arise via two or three severely bizarre verbalizations, or by means of a much larger number of mildly bizarre verbalizations that add up to a high overall score. Our initial impression that this distinction of mild versus severe levels of bizarre verbalizations is important was later confirmed. In previous observation we had noted that milder levels of thought pathology (e.g., what some would call mild cognitive slippage) could often be found in nonschizophrenic patients and normals, especially during periods of general upset and disturbance. This has included the observation that experienced and intelligent normal speakers, such as leading political figures, and even presidential candidates, show evidence of mild cognitive slippage during times of stress and upset, such as in major television debates.

Table 4.1 presents the results for various diagnostic groups using our Rorschach measure of positive thought pathology, namely deviant thought quality, to assess mild and moderate levels of bizarre-idiosyncratic thinking (Quinlan, Harrow, Tucker, and Carlson, 1972, 1973). The data were collected from an inpatient sample of 171 acute patients at our Yale Hospital inpatient setting. The great majority of nonschizophrenics in this sample were nonpsychotic patients. Table 4.2 presents these 171 patients' parallel results using our Rorschach measure of deviant thought quality for severe and very severe levels of bizarre-idiosyncratic thinking.

As can be seen in Tables 4.1 and 4.2, when the results for diagnosis were broken down into mild versus severe levels of strange verbalizations on the Rorschach, we found considerable differences in results, depending on the level of thought pathology assessed. At the very mildest levels of responses indicating deviant thought quality, there was little difference between schizophrenic and nonschizophrenic patients during the acute phase. Both diagnostic groups showed considerable signs of mild cognitive slippage. In contrast, at the moderate and at the more severe levels of deviant thought quality there were considerable (significant) differences between schizophrenic and nonschizophrenic patients.

The distinction between milder, subtle signs of thought pathology and more severe degrees is an important one. Both schizophrenics and nonschizophrenics show evidence of disordered thinking during the acute stages, and it is only at the more severe levels that schizophrenics differ significantly from nonschizophrenics.

In terms of the absolute frequency of positive thought disorder, or of idiosyncratic language, our results show that mild levels of disordered thinking are very frequent in many types of psychopathology. This includes both the schizophrenic and the nonschizophrenic groups. In contrast, at the more severe levels, positive thought pathology is less frequent among the nonschizophrenics, and the differences between schizophrenic and nonschizophrenic patients are significant.

It is difficult to determine from our data whether the distinction between mild and severe levels of thought pathology involves two different types of phenomena (mild versus severe) and thus reflects qualitative differences. The alternate possibility is that it represents a continuum from *no* thought pathology, to *mild* levels of thought pathology, and extends on the same continuum to severe levels of thought pathology. This issue is discussed further in a later section.

TABLE 4.1
Frequency of Occurrence of Responses Indicating Milder
Levels of Deviant Thinking (Rorschach)

No. of Occurrences of Deviant Responses	Classical Schizophrenia (N = 48)	Latent Schizophrenia & Borderline (N = 35)	Nonschizophrenic Patients (N = 88)	Depressives (N = 38)	Personality Disorder & Neurotics (N = 40)	Others (N = 10)
TQ1 (very mild deviant thinking)*						
0	0	0	8	5	2	1
1	5	6	11	6	4	1
2–3	17	7	17	8	6	3
4–6	15	14	27	9	15	3
≥7	11	8	25	10	13	2
Mean	4.79	4.80	4.59	4.00	5.20	4.40
t (each diagnosis vs classic schizophrenia)	...	0.01	0.35	1.13	0.59	0.33
TQ2 (moderate level of deviant thinking)†						
0	2	7	32	18	13	1
1	3	7	12	6	4	2
2–3	15	9	17	8	6	3
4–6	17	9	22	5	15	2
≥7	11	3	5	1	2	2
Mean	4.48	2.74	2.36	1.58	2.70	4.00
t (each diagnosis vs classic schizophrenia)	...	3.03‡	4.58‡	5.55‡	3.22‡	0.49

*One-way ANOVA for TQ1: $F = 0.85$; $df = 2,168$; NS.
†One-way ANOVA for TQ2: $F = 10.76$; $df = 2,168$; $P < .001$.
‡$P < .01$.

From Harrow, and Quinlan. *Archives of General Psychiatry, 34*, 15–21, 1977. Copyright 1977, by the American Medical Association, and reproduced by permission of the publisher.

TABLE 4.2
Frequency of Occurrence of Responses Indicating Severe Levels of Deviant Thinking (Rorschach)

No. of Occurrences of Deviant Responses	Classical Schizophrenia (N = 48)	Latent Schizophrenia & Borderline (N = 35)	Nonschizophrenic Patients (N = 88)	Depressives (N = 38)	Personality Disorder & Neurotics (N = 40)	Others (N = 10)
TQ3 (severe deviant thinking)*						
0	11	18	55	29	20	6
1	9	5	13	4	9	0
2-3	13	6	10	2	7	1
4-6	9	5	7	2	3	2
≥7	6	1	3	1	1	1
Mean	2.73	1.49	1.03	0.66	1.15	2.00
t (each diagnosis vs classic schizophrenia)	...	2.65‡	4.47‡	4.38‡	3.35‡	0.80
TQ4 (very severe deviant thinking)†						
0	30	25	79	34	36	9
1	5	4	4	3	1	0
2-3	6	5	5	1	3	1
4-6	6	1	0	0	0	0
≥7	1	0	0	0	0	0
Mean	1.21	0.57	0.19	0.16	0.20	0.30
t (each diagnosis vs classic schizophrenia)	...	2.15§	4.25‡	2.89‡	2.81‡	1.28

*One-way ANOVA for TQ3: $F = 10.05$; $df = 2,168$; $P < .001$.
†One-way ANOVA for TQ4: $F = 9.02$; $df = 2,168$; $P < .001$.
‡$P < .01$.
§$P < .05$.

From Harrow, and Quinlan. Archives of General Psychiatry, 34, 15–21, 1977. Copyright 1977, by the American Medical Association, and reproduced by permission of the publisher.

Is Bizarre Language and Thinking Unique to Schizophrenia?

A critical issue concerning the role of positive thought pathology in schizophrenia involves the question of whether bizarre-idiosyncratic speech is also found in nonschizophrenics, and this issue has been touched upon in previous sections, using one of our indices of disordered thinking. In the present section we have attempted to focus on this question, employing the results from several of our measures.

If positive thought pathology such as bizarre-idiosyncratic speech is only present in schizophrenic patients, then its centrality in schizophrenic disorders would be affirmed, and this would provide strong evidence for this type of thinking as a possible primary symptom of schizophrenia. Questions in this area become all the more important in standard formulations about psychopathology, since if disordered thinking is present in nonschizophrenics, this would cast doubt on the validity of some common assumptions in the field and raise issues concerning several areas of psychopathology. The presence of bizarre-idiosyncratic thinking in nonschizophrenic patients also raises questions concerning whether thought pathology should be included among the criteria for separating schizophrenic from nonschizophrenic patients.

Despite the beliefs of some theorists and many astute clinicians about the uniqueness of thought disorders to schizophrenia, our observations and the observations of others in this area have led us to the contrary belief, namely that bizarre-idiosyncratic verbalizations and thinking are not exclusive to schizophrenia. We believe and have obtained evidence that they are common in acute manic patients, and occur sometimes in other acute psychotic patients who are not schizophrenic. This is discussed further later in this chapter.

Perhaps of equal importance to theory is the issue of whether bizarre-idiosyncratic thinking can be found in nonpsychotic patients. A series of formal investigations by our own research team and by others have also begun to provide formal evidence on the presence of thought pathology in nonpsychotic patients (Braff and Beck, 1974; Harrow and Quinlan, 1977).

In order to focus in a more exhaustive way on the issue of bizarre-idiosyncratic thinking in nonpsychotic patients, we studied our data in this area using four of our major types of instruments: the Rorschach Test, the Proverbs and Comprehension Tests, and the Object Sorting Test. Of particular value here was the data from the Rorschach Test, which was used to assess mild versus severe levels of bizarre-idiosyncratic language. These data are presented in Tables 4.1 and 4.2, and their results have been analyzed in the previous section. The large sample of nonschizophrenic patients that we employed to focus on the issue of mild versus severe levels of bizarre-idiosyncratic thinking was primarily a nonpsychotic patient group.

As we have noted earlier, instances of mild levels of speech pathology were relatively frequent in the response of both our nonschizophrenic and our schizophrenic patients (see Table 4.1). The difference between these two diagnostic groups was not significant. While the lack of a significant difference between these patients is of interest, even more important for thinking about the current issue is the relatively common occurrence of mild idiosyncratic language in a variety of different types of nonschizophrenic patients. As we have found in other areas, acutely disturbed nonpsychotic patients can show various types of disturbed thinking, including considerable cognitive slippage.

Looking at the data for the moderate and more severe levels of bizarre-idiosyncratic verbalizations (in Tables 4.1 and 4.2), we find significant differences between the schizophrenic and nonschizophrenic (mostly nonpsychotic) patients when they are assessed at the most acute phase. Again, however, the important point for the present topic is whether or not nonschizophrenic patients show any thought pathology at this phase of their disorder. Here we found significantly fewer instances of moderate and severe bizarre-idiosyncratic language among the nonschizophrenic patients, but again we did find some of the nonschizophrenic patients with evidence of severe bizarre verbalizations. While severe levels of bizarre verbalizations and positive thought pathology are less frequent in most types of disturbed nonschizophrenic (and especially nonpsychotic) patients, they are not unique to schizophrenics.

Our earlier scoring of the Object Sorting, Proverb, and Comprehension Tests from the inpatient sample at our Yale Hospital setting did not allow as fine-grained an analysis of each patient's individual levels of bizarre-idiosyncratic responses. Recently, we have employed a revised scoring system with our newer samples of inpatients from the Chicago-area hospital settings. This revised system does permit such an analysis of mild and severe levels of bizarre-idiosyncratic language on the Proverbs and Comprehension Tests. When we have looked at our results from the nonpsychotic patients for their scores on these two tests, we found results similar in principle to those reported from the Rorschach. Again, we found less bizarre speech among these patients than among schizophrenics, but we did find a certain percentage of these patients with bizarre verbalizations. Our overall results in this area on a variety of different tests are clear. Bizarre language, and presumably bizarre thinking, are not unique to schizophrenia.

In addition to our research on the presence of mild and severe levels of thought pathology in nonschizophrenic and in nonpsychotic *patients*, studies of nonpsychotic *family members* of schizophrenic patients by other research teams also have shown evidence of communication disorders in some of these family members. This line of research was initiated by Wynne and Singer, and Lidz, in the 1950s and 1960s (Lidz, Fleck and Cornelison, 1965; Wynne and Singer, 1963), and continues into the present by Wynne and Singer, M. Goldstein, and others (Goldstein, Rodnick, Jones, McPherson, and West, 1978; Hirsch and Leff, 1975; Lewis, Rodnick, and Goldstein, 1981; Singer, Wynne, and Toohey, 1978). Our research, and that of others, has indicated that measures of communication deviance used in family studies show high correlations and have much overlap (in an item-by-item analysis of the specific behaviors rated) with major measures of thought disorder, such as our index of bizarre-idiosyncratic thinking (Quinlan, Schultz, Davies, and Harrow, 1978). Aspects of our own research in this area are discussed in Chapter 14.

Potential Thought Disorder in Manic and Other Psychotic Patients

As we have noted earlier, the most striking negative evidence on views that positive types of thought disorder are unique to schizophrenia can be found in investigations of acute manic patients. During the last few years, formal research by Andreasen (1979), Andreasen and Powers (1974, 1975), and our own investigations (Harrow, Grossman, Silverstein, and Meltzer, 1980, 1982; Rattenbury, Silverstein, De Wolfe, Kaufman, and Harrow, 1983) have provided evidence of severe thought pathology in acute manic patients. The clearest example of this can be found in a recent study we conducted employing patients from our own research center at Michael Reese Hospital, and from a Mental Health Clinic Research Center based at the University of Chicago and at the Illinois State Psychiatric Hospital. In the clinical research center, strong efforts are made to keep the patients unmedicated during the first week and a half in the study. This allows us to conduct research with a medication-free sample during the acute phase.

One of our recent studies of fifty-five acute patients who were medication-free included fifteen manic patients, twenty-five schizophrenics, and fifteen nonpsychotic patients. The measure of bizarre-idiosyncratic thinking we utilized involved a composite index of positive thought pathology, based on three of our tests, the Proverbs Test, the Comprehension Test, and the Object Sorting Test. Our results with this acute-phase, medication-free sample are presented in Table 4.3. The three most important aspects of our results were: (1) extremely high levels of positive thought pathology in both the manic and the schizophrenic patients; (2) no significant differences in extent of thought disorder between the manic and the schizophrenic patients; and (3) significantly higher levels of thought disorder for both the manic and the schizophrenic patients than for the nonpsychotic group. In our continuation of these studies we have found evidence suggesting that some manic patients show persistent thought pathology after the acute in-hospital phase (Grossman, Harrow, Lazar, et al., 1981; Harrow, Grossman, Silverstein, et al., in press). Thus, we have found considerable evidence indicating that positive thought pathology is an important factor in schizophrenia, but also that it is common in acute manic patients.

While we have found positive thought disorder to be extremely frequent in acute phases of schizophrenic and manic disorders (and, our early results suggest, possibly in some types of schizoaffective disorders), our initial explorations do not suggest that severe thought pathology is just a function of psychosis, regardless of the type of disorder. We found that severe positive thought disorder is less frequent in other types of psychotic disorders than in schizophrenic and manic patients in our recent exploration of this area. Our ongoing investigations are beginning to provide tentative evidence that "other

TABLE 4.3
Level of Thought Pathology in Unmedicated Patients during the Acute Phase*†

	% of Patients with Thought Pathology				
Patient Group	None	Minimal/ Mild	Moderate	Severe	Very Severe
Manic (N = 15)	0	6	20	27	47
Schizophrenic (N = 25)	4	20	28	20	28
Nonpsychotic (N = 15)	13	40	27	13	7

*Overall index based on all three tests.
†One-way analysis of variance: $F = 6.85$; $df = 2.52$; $P < .001$.

From Harrow, Grossman, Silverstein and Meltzer. *Archives of General Psychiatry, 39*, 665–671, 1982. Copyright 1982, by the American Medical Association, and reproduced by permission of the publisher.

psychotic" patients are more thought disordered than nonpsychotic patients, but less thought disordered than schizophrenic and manic patients.

Bizarre Thinking and Continuity Between the Thinking of Schizophrenic and Nonschizophrenic Patients

Our findings on bizarre speech in both schizophrenic and non-schizophrenic patients raise the question of whether bizarre speech and thinking can be placed on a continuum with normal speech and thinking. The alternate view would be that bizarre and normal thinking are discrete and separate types of behavior. The results we have cited to indicate the presence of bizarre speech and thinking in nonschizophrenics and in select nonpsychotics, and our results on mild versus severe levels of bizarre thinking, have led us to emphasize that bizarre speech and thinking lie on a continuum with that of normals (Harrow and Quinlan, 1977). Holzman's (1978) analysis of his research results also led him to emphasize that thought disorder lies on a continuum with normal thinking.

The data we have collected could support a picture in which: (a) mild levels of bizarre thinking are common and occur in many disturbed nonschizophrenic and nonpsychotic patients, as well as being present, perhaps even more frequently, in schizophrenics; (b) as one moves further out on the hypothetical continuum from normal to bizarre-idiosyncratic thinking, more severe levels of positive thought pathology are relatively infrequent among nonpsychotics, but still can be found in select nonpsychotics; (c) more severe levels of thought pathology occur to some extent in most overt schizophrenics during their most acute phases; however (d) severe levels are not exclusive to schizophrenics, and occur in some other psychotic patients as well.

While we have data that fit in and support theses views, the overall evidence on the issue of whether bizarre-idiosyncratic thinking and normal thinking actually lie on a continuum is indirect and involves some degree of inference. Formulations about whether or not features such as bizarre-idiosyncratic thinking fit along a continuum or are discrete are often difficult to resolve. Without clear knowledge of the underlying factors involved, it is difficult to obtain evidence that answers, with any certainty, questions about whether or not a "true" continuum exists in this area.

In the next chapter we will discuss our research and our positive evidence on two factors that we believe influence bizarre-idiosyncratic thinking: namely, (1) impaired perspective, and (2) severe emotional turmoil-upset that can lead to disorganization. Our tentative evidence concerning both of these factors would support a continuum hypothesis more readily than a dichotomy hypothesis of thought disorder. However, our evidence in these areas is tentative and incomplete. Thus, at present the issue of bizarre and disordered thinking as a continuum or as a discrete and separate phenomenon cannot be resolved with any finality. In the future, other techniques may have to be explored to help analyze this question. Currently, either alternative is possible, although the bulk of the evidence would support the view of bizarre and disordered thinking as fitting along a continuum with normal thinking.

Bizarre Speech and Thinking as Diagnostic Indicators

Early cognitive slippage and mild evidence of bizarre speech, as well as severe levels of bizarre speech, have frequently been used as early signs of schizophrenia. In one form or another, disordered speech and thinking have appeared as criteria of schizophrenia in numerous diagnostic systems, such as in the older *Diagnostic and Statistical Manual* of the American Psychiatric Association (DSM II), as well as in the Research Diagnostic Criteria (RDC) adopted for use in a number of large research programs and in the new revised *Diagnostic and Statistical Manual,* (DSM III), which has recently been adopted in the United States.

Our data in this area provide both positive and negative evidence. They suggest that any formulations based on distinguishing or diagnosing early schizophrenia on the basis of whether or not the patient or person is showing *beginning* signs of cognitive slippage is impractical and will not be effective. It will be ineffective because many other diagnostic groups, and some normals, show *mild* signs of strange-idiosyncratic speech and/or cognitive slippage. Many of the older formulations about cognitive slippage in schizophrenia are a consequence of astute observations by sensitive clinicians of cognitive slippage in schizophrenia. These formulations, however, are not based on systematic detailed examination and comparison of large samples of disturbed nonschizophrenic patients, or even on upset "normals," many of whom also show signs of mild cognitive slippage.

In contrast, the use of severe positive thought disorder or flagrant signs of bizarre-idiosyncratic speech and thinking as possible diagnostic indicators or signs to separate schizophrenics from nonpsychotic patients holds more promise.

Severe manifestations of bizarre-idiosyncratic thinking also occur in nonschizophrenics, but they are found less frequently in most types of nonschizophrenic patients. The most important exception to this may be acutely disturbed manic patients (those whose disorders are severe enough to warrant their hospitalization) who very frequently show evidence of bizarre speech.

Despite these indications of bizarre speech and thinking in some nonschizophrenic patients, signs of bizarre-idiosyncratic speech still have some utility as diagnostic indicators with the exceptions noted above.

It can be seen from the data we have presented in this and the last chapter that, despite the observations of some astute clinicians, disordered thinking is not a certain way to distinguish schizophrenics from nonschizophrenics. At our currrent stage of knowledge the concept of schizophrenia is a disjunctive one, depending on a combination of features. Bizarre speech and disordered thinking is one of the most prominent of these features, along with nondepressive delusions (Astrachan et al., 1972). Until our knowledge and understanding of psychosis are advanced further, and more precise criteria for schizophrenia are developed, severe levels of bizarre speech and positive types of thought pathology can be used as ranking among the *better*, high-probability signs of schizophrenia, although they are not infallible ones. Thus, overall, severe levels of bizarre speech are still reasonable tools that can be used profitably as possible diagnostic signs of schizophrenia, in practical clinical situations.

5

Bizarre-Idiosyncratic Thinking: Its Longitudinal Course and Factors That Influence Bizarre Thinking

The first few stages of our research on bizarre-idiosyncratic thinking, which are described in Chapters 3 and 4, involved studies of its prominence in schizophrenia at the acute phase, and analysis of a number of important features related to positive types of thought disorder and their appearance in schizophrenia. The next two objectives of our reseach program in this area involved the following:

1. A study of bizarre-idiosyncratic thinking over time to determine its longitudinal course, whether it persists past the acute phase and during periods of seeming recovery, and whether it is a permanent characteristic of schizophrenia;
2. A study of variables that may lead to or influence bizarre-idiosyncratic thinking, to gain further clues about factors involved in this type of psychopathology that may underlie the schizophrenic disorder.

In this chapter we have outlined our investigations centered around these two objectives, and the conclusions derived from them.

BIZARRE-IDIOSYNCRATIC SPEECH DURING
THE PHASE OF PARTIAL RECOVERY

The initial step in our program of longitudinal research was to study several samples of patients for bizarre-idiosyncratic thinking during the phase of partial recovery. Our research into this phase of partial recovery, which is presented in this chapter, has been described more completely in a series of reports (Adler and Harrow, 1974; Harrow, Grossman, Silverstein, and Meltzer, 1982; Harrow and Quinlan, 1977; Harrow, Tucker, Himmelhoch, and Putnam, 1972; Reilly, Harrow, and Tucker, 1973). The study of several samples of patients at two different phases during their hospitalization has allowed us to evaluate our informal observations about reductions in thought pathology with diminishing psychopathology in other areas, and about the importance of factors associated with the acute phase of disturbance. Thus, the study design we chose to meet this objective involved assessing patients at the acute phase during the first two weeks of hospitalization (described in Chapter 3), and then reassessing these patients six to seven weeks later at a stage that our evidence suggests is a period of partial recovery for many patients.

First, evidence was obtained that the period six to seven weeks later, which we have labeled the phase of partial recovery, really does involve a reduction in psychosis and in psychopathology in general for most patients. Thus, a sample of patients from our Yale inpatient setting who were studied for bizarre-idiosyncratic thinking were also assessed on several key components of psychosis, at the acute phase and six to seven weeks later, using psychiatrists' rating. Table 5.1 presents these data on reduction in psychosis for schizophrenia at the phase of partial recovery. The results showed significant or near significant declines in psychotic symptomatology over time for the schizophrenics, while the borderline patients and the nonschizophrenic patients showed small, nonsignificant changes in these symptoms. The very low initial levels of psychotic symptoms for these latter two groups would make it difficult for them to show much further decline in psychotic symptoms as they emerge from the acute phase.

However, in our research with other samples of nonpsychotic patients, assessing different symptoms such as depression, anxiety, and various other aspects of behavior, we found considerable improvement by the phase of partial recovery for nonschizophrenic patients, as well as for schizophrenic patients. Thus, in addition to the data in Table 5.1 on major psychotic symptoms, other data we collected on a sample of eighty schizophrenic and depressive patients whom we studied also indicate significant or near significant reductions in various other aspects of psychopathology. These data, assessing a variety of aspects of psychopathology, are based on psychiatrists' ratings of the patients, on nurses' ratings of the patients, on subjective ratings of the patients concerning various aspects of their mood level, and on performance tests. These data are presented in our research on postpsychotic depression, reported elsewhere (Shanfield, Tucker, Harrow, and Detre, 1970).

The analysis of a sample of patients at both the acute phase and then at partial recovery allowed us to focus on potential reductions in bizarre verbalizations as patients emerged from the most acute phase into a

TABLE 5.1
Means and Tests of Significance on Psychiatrists' Symptom Ratings at Each Phase of Disorder

	Bizarre Speech or Behavior	Delusions	Hallucinations
Classical schizophrenics (No.=25)			
Acute phase (mean)	12.44	9.44	6.75
Partial recovery (mean)	7.71	6.63	4.17
Change over time (*t*-Test)	(3.32)†	(1.86)	(2.34)*
Latent schizophrenics (No.=23)			
Acute phase (mean)	5.91	5.33	5.33
Partial recovery (mean)	4.73	4.73	4.73
Change over time (*t*-Test)	(0.97)	(0.55)	(0.55)
Nonschizophrenics (No.=47)			
Acute phase (mean)	4.83	4.65	4.26
Partial recovery (mean)	4.09	4.09	4.09
Change over time (*t*-Test)	(1.46)	(1.07)	(0.80)
Total sample (No.=95)			
Acute phase (mean)	7.14	6.11	5.17
Partial recovery (mean)	5.21	4.92	4.27
Change over time (*t*-Test)	(3.38)†	(2.15)*	(2.25)*

*$P < .05$
†$P < .01$.

phase of diminished stress and turmoil, and during a period of decreasing psychopathology. Using this study design with our samples of inpatients from the Yale inpatient setting, we were able to assess several samples of patients, employing the Object Sorting Test with one sample of ninety-patients, and the Comprehension and Proverbs Test with another, partially overlapping sample of ninety-five patients. The assessment of patients at two time periods with three different instruments allowed us to look at positive thought disorder in terms of bizarre-idiosyncratic speech and behavior in response to three different types of stimulus situations.

The results from the Comprehension and Proverbs Tests on our samples when we compared schizophrenics with nonschizophrenics at the phase of partial recovery are presented in Table 5.2. Not all of the diagnostic comparisons were statistically significant at the phase of partial recovery. As we reported in Chapter 3, when these patients were assessed at the acute phase with both of the short verbal tests (the comprehension subtest and the proverbs test), there were significant differences between the schizophrenic and nonschizophrenic patients. In contrast, during the phase of partial recovery for these young, relatively early patients (median age = 21 years), the differences between the diagnostic groups became smaller. Thus, as patients emerged from the more acute period of severe disturbance and psychopathology, the schizophrenics still scored significantly higher on idiosyncratic verbalizations on the WAIS Comprehension Scale than did the nonschizophrenic group ($P < .01$), but the differences for the Yale sample on the Proverbs Test at this phase were nonsignificant.

Perhaps most important, as schizophrenic patients emerged from the more acute phase and entered into a phase of partial recovery, their scores on bizarre-idiosyncratic thinking improved significantly on both the Proverbs Test and the Social Comprehension Subtest ($P < .001$). Table 5.2 also reports the significance tests associated with the change scores for each of the major types of patient groups. These data on bizarre-idiosyncratic thinking provide strong evidence against theories that this type of positive thought disorder is an invariant feature of schizophrenia that remains constant over time.

Table 5.3 reports the results on the Object Sorting Test during the phase of partial recovery, for the sample reported in Chapter 3, who had been assessed early in the acute phase. As we noted in Chapter 3, the results of the Object Sorting Test for this sample had shown very large, significant, diagnostic differences at the acute phase. Table 5.3 shows that at the phase of partial recovery, these differences between schizo-phrenic and nonschizophrenic patients also had diminished, although they were still significant.

TABLE 5.2

Mean Scores on Bizarre-Idiosyncratic Thinking from the
Comprehension and Proverbs Tests at the Acute Phase and
the Phase of Partial Recovery

Sample	Comprehension Test			Proverbs Test		
	Acute Phase Mean	Partial Recovery Mean	Change Scores t Tests	Acute Phase Mean	Partial Recovery Mean	Change Scores t Tests
Classical Schizophren. (N = 25)	6.24	2.96	3.44**	5.56	2.12	3.58**
Latent Schizophren. (N = 23)	3.09	1.35	2.67*	2.22	1.44	2.55*
Nonschizophrenics. (N = 47)	1.77	1.28	1.62	2.09	1.83	0.67

*P < .05
**P < .01

From Adler, & Harrow. "Idiosyncratic Thinking and Personally Over-involved Thinking in Schizophrenic Patients During Partial Recovery," *Comprehensive Psychiatry, 15*, 57-67, 1974. Reproduced by permission of the publisher.

TABLE 5.3

Distribution of Scores on Bizarre-Idiosyncratic Thinking from the Object Sorting Test at the Acute Phase and the Phase of Partial Recovery

	Acute Phase			Phase of Partial Recovery		
	No Biz.-Idios. Thinking	Mild-Moder. Biz.-Idios. Thinking	Severe Biz.-Idios. Thinking	No Biz.-Idios. Thinking	Mild-Moder. Biz.-Idios. Thinking	Severe Biz.-Idios. Thinking
Classical Schizophren.	6	7	15	12	8	8
Latent Schizophren.	16	3	5	17	4	3
Nonschiz. Patients	24	8	7	26	10	3

From Harrow, Tucker, Himmelhoch, & Putnam. *American Journal of Psychiatry, 128,* 824–829, 1972. Reproduced by permission of the publisher.

To answer questions about potential changes in the level of bizarre-idiosyncratic thinking on the Object Sorting Test as patients emerged from the more acute phase, the differences over time of the patients' scores on this variable were analyzed. The results again indicated that the classical schizophrenics declined significantly in bizarre-idiosyncratic thinking as they emerged from the acute phase. Thus, we have a general picture of patients in each diagnostic group, and especially the schizophrenics, as showing less idiosyncratic thinking on each of the major indices of thought pathology as they emerge from the more acute phase of their disorder.

Overall, at the phase of partial recovery, the differences between schizophrenics and nonschizophrenics were significant on two of the indices (the Object Sorting Test and the Comprehension Test of the Wechsler Scales) and nonsignificant on the third index used (the Proverbs Test). These positive and mixed results at the phase of partial recovery reflect a situation in which the type of disorder or underlying psychopathology (e.g., schizophrenia) exerts an influence on bizarre and idiosyncratic behavior in the direction of more pathological scores for schizophrenics on most of the indices. However, the phase of the disorder also proves to be an important influence on the level of bizarre behavior, with smaller diagnostic differences at the phase of partial recovery. The trend toward a reduction in bizarre-idiosyncratic thinking was much more prominent for the schizophrenic samples. Since the initial level of idiosyncratic speech was more severe for the schizophrenics, there was more room for these patients to show decreases in idiosyncratic thinking as they emerged from the more acute phase.

IMPLICATIONS: RESULTS ON BIZARRE-IDIOSYNCRATIC THINKING AT PHASE OF PARTIAL RECOVERY

These results on schizophrenics at the phase of partial recovery contain data that bear on several key questions about bizarre-idiosyncratic speech and thinking. Two of these questions are:

1. Are bizarre speech and thought pathology permanent, invariant features of schizophrenia?
2. Are bizarre verbalizations and thinking a function of factors other than just diagnosis, or is this the main determinant?

In response to these questions, the less severe scores on bizarre verbalizations and thinking during the phase of partial recovery indicate that bizarre-idiosyncratic verbalizations are not invariant features of schizophrenia, but rather that the level of bizarre verbalizations is partly a function of the phase of the disorder. Similarly, in response to the other question, if the same results are looked at from another angle, the data also suggest that bizarre thinking is influenced by other factors in addition to schizophrenia. The data begin to suggest that for a large number of schizophrenics, during early phases of their psychopathology, many aspects of their disorder diminish after the acute phase and may be intermittent or phasic. Both of these questions are important ones to help put the role of bizarre-idiosyncratic speech, and disordered thinking in general, in proper perspective concerning their importance to schizophrenia.

The preliminary answers we obtained with our samples from Yale at the phase of partial recovery needed further replication with patients at a later posthospital phase, and also needed to be supplemented with other samples for further verification. Later in this chapter, we will present our data from samples followed up at subsequent phases of their disorder.

Correlations Over Time

Before turning to our data on bizarre-idiosyncratic thinking at a later follow-up period, it would be appropriate to look at our data on the relationship (or correlations) between bizarre-idiosyncratic verbalizations at the acute phase as compared to the same type of bizarre thinking at the period of partial recovery. These correlational data offer an opportunity to begin to assess questions about the relative stability of bizarre verbalizations over short periods of time.

The results indicate relative consistency during this period, in that patients with bizarre language/thinking at the early stages of their hospitalization are more likely to show at least some signs of bizarre-idiosyncratic thinking seven weeks later. Thus, the correlation over this time period were $r = 0.59$ for our measures of bizarre-idiosyncratic thinking from the comprehension subtest, $r = 0.54$ over time for our measure of bizarre verbalizations from the proverbs test, and $r = 0.61$ for our measure of bizarre speech and thinking from the Object Sorting Test. These results can be contrasted with the stability of scores over this time period on our brief measure of intelligence. Our brief IQ measure, the Information Subtest of the Wechsler Intelligence Scales, showed an even higher correlation of $r = 0.73$ for the same time period, using the same sample of ninety-five patients to whom we administered the comprehension and proverbs tests.

Overall, while the absolute pathology scores on our major measurements of bizarre speech and thinking shift downward or decrease as patients begin to emerge from the most acute phase of their disorder, the *relative* position of the patients remains surprisingly constant, considering the turmoil and instability usually associated with this early phase of the patients' disorders. Our data suggest that there is at least moderate stability over this seven-week period. Stability and replicability do not guarantee that these measures of bizarre verbalizations are valuable as primary or fundamental features of schizophrenia. Other types of data on the relationship between these indices of thinking and other aspects of schizophrenia would be needed to place bizarre-idiosyncratic verbalizations and thinking in their proper context as features of schizophrenia that may or may not be important. The data do suggest, however, that these indices of bizarre thinking capture one aspect of acute or active schizophrenia that has some short-term consistency, although it is not clear how high the correlations would be over a longer period of time.

The consistency is not as high as that found in standard measures of intelligence. However, people high in bizarre verbalizations and thinking at one phase of their disorder do tend to be high on this characteristic at other phases of their disorder several months later, even though the absolute scores have tended to decline somewhat.

Does Bizarre-Idiosyncratic Speech Persist During the Posthospital Period?

As we have noted, one of the goals of our overall research program is to study thought pathology over an extended period of time in a series of schizophrenics, to determine potential shifts in disordered thinking over the course of schizophrenia. The plan is to obtain clues about basic processes in schizophrenia by answering such questions as the following, based on longitudinal research:

1. What is the longitudinal course of positive types of thought disorder in schizophrenia?
2. Is there an underlying thought disorder or process, significant traces of which persist when the schizophrenic patient is no longer overtly psychotic, or is in the "recovery" stage?
3. Do specific types of thought disorders that persist over time differentiate psychotic patients into "true" schizophrenics and reactive psychoses?

4. What is the prognostic significance of different types of thought pathology and what does this tell us about the nature of primary symptoms in schizophrenia? Do different types of thought pathology relate to patients' future clinical courses, such as the rate of rehospitalization, neurotic and psychotic symptomatology, or other areas of functioning?

Toward this end, we have begun to answer some of these questions by following up and studying schizophrenic and nonschizophrenic patients for potential thought pathology during the posthospital period. More detailed accounts of our research in this area, studying schizophrenic patients over more extensive periods of time, have been presented in a series of reports (Bromet and Harrow, 1973; Harrow, Bromet, and Quinlan, 1974; Harrow, Harkavy, Bromet, and Tucker, 1973; Harrow and Silverstein, 1980; Harrow, Silverstein, and Marengo, 1983). This line of research has involved following up two samples of schizophrenic and nonschizophrenic patients who had previously been studied as inpatients, using the Object Sorting Test. We also used the Rorschach test for the first of these two populations, a sample of former patients from the Yale setting.

The results on our index of bizarre-idiosyncratic thinking, or positive thought disorder, from the Object Sorting Test from our first follow-up are reported in Table 5.4. These data on the Object Sorting Test scores of former inpatients from our Yale Hospital setting did not show significant differences between schizophrenic and nonschizophrenic patients at an eleven month follow-up. There was, however, a trend for schizophrenics to show more bizarre-idiosyncratic verbalizations than nonschizophrenic patients on the Object Sorting Test at follow-up ($P < .15$). When we analyzed the Rorschach test results with the first of these two samples from our Yale setting, we also found there was a nonsignificant trend for schizophrenics to show more thought pathology than nonschizophrenic patients at the eleven month follow-up on our Rorschach measure of bizarre-idiosyncratic responses.

Table 5.5 presents the results on bizarre-idiosyncratic behavior from the Object Sorting Test from our second follow-up sample, a group of seventy-five young, relatively early schizophrenic and nonschizophrenic patients from our Michael Reese Hospital setting in Chicago. The mean age of this young sample at the time of their index hospitalizaton was 21.9 years. The scoring system using the Object Sorting Test with this second follow-up sample represents a slight modification and improvement of the scoring system we had used earlier. Despite the modification of our scoring system, the overall trend of the results and the *general* categories of level of bizarre behavior are comparable across the different samples, although the *individual* object

TABLE 5.4

Mean Scores on Bizarre-Idiosyncratic Thinking from the Object Sorting Test at the Acute Phase and at Follow-up
(Yale Sample)

Sample	Acute Phase		Posthospital Phase		t
	N	M	N	M	(Acute vs. Posthospital)
Classical Schizophrenic	22	2.50	22	2.32	0.58
Nonschiz. Patients	30	1.37	30	1.67	−1.33
t (Schiz. versus Nonschiz.)	t = 3.65*		t = 1.56		

*P < .01

From Harrow, Harkavy, Bromet, & Tucker. *Archives of General Psychiatry*, 28, 179–182, 1973. Copyright 1973, by the American Medical Association, and reproduced by permission of the publisher.

sorting scores from our Chicago sample are not comparable in a precise way with those from the Yale setting. There are several advantageous features associated with the Chicago follow-up data; one is that it is based on a considerably larger sample of schizophrenics ($N = 46$). The Chicago sample was not only a larger sample, it also was assessed at an average of three years after the index hospitalization, which provides a more extended follow-up period, further from the original acute period during the index hospitalization. As can be seen in Table 5.5, the data from the Chicago setting showed significant schizophrenic-nonschizophrenic differences on bizarre-idiosyncratic behavior. The results from Table 5.5 indicate, however, that while the diagnostic comparisons were significant, they only just achieved significance at the $P < .05$ level.

The results from the Object Sorting Test on *changes* in bizarre speech from the acute phase to the follow-up period also are presented in Table 5.4, where it can be seen that the schizophrenic patients from the Yale sample did not show a significant decline in bizarre-idiosyncratic behavior at follow-up, as compared to their scores at the acute phase, on the Object Sorting Test. The Rorschach indices of bizarre-idiosyncratic thinking showed lower levels of this type of thought pathology at follow-up, and thus did suggest a significant decline from the most acute phase ($P < .05$). Although the group of schizophrenics from our Yale setting only involves a small sample of schizophrenics ($N = 22$), the mixed results from this population do not fit neatly with the other results we have noted earlier on samples of schizophrenics assessed at the phase of partial recovery. The samples we studied at the

TABLE 5.5
Percentage of Patients with Idiosyncratic Thinking on Object Sorting Test at Three-Year Follow-Up (Chicago Sample)*

Sample		*Level of Bizarre-Idiosyncratic Thinking*			
		None	*Mild*	*Severe*	*Very Severe*
Schizophrenics	($N = 46$)	41%	26%	22%	11%
Nonschizophrenic patients	($N = 29$)	52%	38%	10%	0%

*Schizophrenics versus nonschizophrenics: $t = 2.10$, $P < .05$.

From Harrow & Silverstein. Cognitive Processes During the Postacute Phase of Schizophrenia. In Human Functioning in Longitudinal Perspective, (Eds) Sells, Crandall, Roff, Strauss & Pollin. Williams & Wilkins: Baltimore/London, 1980. Reproduced by permission of the publisher.

phase of partial recovery showed significant declines from the acute phase on our measures of bizarre-idiosyncratic behavior. It is possible that a larger sample would have shown a significant decline on bizarre-idiosyncratic behavior during the follow-up period for all of the major indices, but this is still an open question. While the relatively small sample size may be one influence on the mixed results concerning whether there is a significant decline in bizarre thinking at follow-up, our data do suggest that in major acute treatment settings, the largest decline in bizarre-idiosyncratic behavior occurs immediately after the most acute phase, at the phase of partial recovery. Thereafter, until the next major psychotic episode (or major relapse), scores of bizarre-idiosyncratic behavior may show only slight increases or decreases during subsequent phases of the recovery period for most early, young, nonchronic schizophrenics. The disparity between the results on bizarre-idiosyncratic behavior at the follow-up period versus the phase of partial recovery indicates that there are a number of unresolved issues in this area that need to be subjected to further study and analysis.

At present we are unable to replicate, with certainty, these results on changes over time with our sample of patients from Chicago. Although the first patients in our follow-up sample from Chicago were studied intensively in other areas of functioning during the original index hospitalization (Harrow, Grinker, Holzman et al., 1977; Schwartz, Grinker, Harrow, et al., 1978), most of this particular sample of patients were not administered the Object Sorting Test to assess bizarre-idiosyncratic behavior at the acute phase. Thus, this sample could not be assessed directly in terms of changes in bizarre-idiosyncratic behavior from the acute phase to the posthospital phase. In our current study of several new samples of patients from Chicago, we are now collecting systematic data on large groups of schizophrenic and nonschizophrenic patients at several phases of their disorder, starting at the acute phase, and we intend to analyze their thinking over time. Our initial results are beginning to suggest a significant decline at follow-up for the schizophrenic sample.

Overall, the results on differences in positive types of thought disorder between schizophrenic and nonschizophrenic patients at follow-up, based on two separate samples from different geographic regions indicate some differences between the diagnostic groups. Thus, the data from the first sample show a near significant trend in the expected direction ($P < .15$), and the data from the second sample show significant, but not overwhelming, differences ($P < .05$). The trend toward more bizarre-idiosyncratic behavior for the schizophrenics at follow-up is clear: however, the diagnostic differences are modest in size. Probably the most important result that has emerged from this aspect of our research is our data indicating that *the majority of early, young schizophrenics are not very severely thought disordered at follow-up.* The differences between these young, early schizophrenic and non-schizophrenic patients were due to a small to moderate subgroup of schizophrenics who were high on bizarre verbalizations and thinking at follow-up. The answer to the question of whether or not bizarre-idiosyncratic verbalizations and thinking are characteristic features of early schizophrenics at follow-up would appear to be that it is characteristic, but that this only occurs for a subgroup of schizophrenic patients rather than for all of them. We intend to focus on this subsample of bizarre-idiosyncratic schizophrenics further in the future.

Our overall results on changes over time show a mixed trend in regard to whether there are less bizarre-idiosyncratic verbalizations and thinking as patients are assessed at follow-up and compared to their status at the earlier, more active phases of their disorder. The results were significant with some indices and samples, and nonsignificant with other indices and samples, indicating that the data in this area were not always uniform. The results we reported earlier showed a diminishing of bizarre-idiosyncratic thinking as schizophrenics emerged from the acute phase and entered a phase of partial recovery. Our most recent results with a new sample of patients in Chicago also suggest a just-significant reduction of this type of positive thought pathology at follow-up. It is possible that the amount of improvement in idiosyncratic verbalizations and thinking at follow-up depends partly on the particular task involved in assessment and the situation in which it is evaluated (e.g., verbal or motor behavior, social or nonsocial behavior). Another factor influencing results in this area may be whether the patients showed a severe level of thought pathology at the acute phase. Thus, those patients with very little thought pathology at the acute phase are not likely to show much reduction in thought pathology at follow-up, and a few show slight increases in thought pathology. Many of those schizophrenics with severe positive thought pathology at the acute phase tend to show some reduction after the acute phase. In an unselected sample of early schizophrenics, the mixture of the larger subgroup who have severe thought pathology at the acute phase with the smaller subgroup with little or no acute-phase thought pathology produces an overall sample of schizophrenics with a just-significant reduction in positive thought pathology at follow-up. Whether or not the overall reduction in thought pathology after the acute phase will be significant or only near significant depends in part on the size of the sample of schizophrenics evaluated, and on the sensitivity of the assessment techniques used.

IMPLICATIONS: RESULTS ON BIZARRE
VERBALIZATIONS AND THINKING AT FOLLOW-UP

In reviewing our data and attempting to answer questions about positive types of thought pathology from our results, we should note that the issues addressed by the follow-up results are ones that are central in conceptualizations about the role and importance of bizarre-idiosyncratic speech and positive types of thought disorder in schizophrenia. One of the major questions in this area concerns the issue: Is the postacute schizophrenic bizarre? A number of clinicians and theorists have assumed that major thought pathology persists throughout the course of schizophrenia, although some theorists such as Zubin have taken an alternate view (Zubin and Spring, 1977).

In response to this question about the persistence of positive thought disorder, when we contrasted the data obtained at the acute phase on schizophrenic-nonschizophrenic differences with that collected seven weeks later, during partial recovery, our initial results had begun to suggest that bizarre verbalizations and thinking are not a permanent feature for all schizophrenics. The results assessing patients at follow-up fit in with this conclusion.

Looked at from a broad perspective, the differences on bizarre verbalizations and thinking between schizophrenic and nonschizophrenic patients at follow-up just did achieve significance at the $P = .05$ level for our larger sample. There is some diagnostic effect, and a previous diagnosis of "schizophrenia" does carry *some* predictive weight in terms of later thought pathology. The data from our follow-up samples indicate that for a subgroup of early schizophrenics, major components of their disordered thinking persist past the acute phase, and are not just a function of acute pathology.

There is a general tendency for many schizophrenics high on bizarre-idiosyncratic thinking at the acute phase to show some signs of bizarre thinking at follow-up. On an overall basis, however, severe thought pathology is less frequent for young schizophrenics at the posthospital phase than usually has been hypothesized. Bizarre verbalizations and thinking are not invariant features of all schizophrenics, and do not persist in all early schizophrenics. The data on the level of bizarre-idiosyncratic thinking at the phase of partial recovery, and in the posthospital stage, support our earlier observations that schizophrenia is not a single-phase disorder with an invariant clinical picture. To some extent, these data indicating that the majority of schizophrenics do not show severe positive thought disorder at follow-up could fit the viewpoint of Zubin and Spring (1977), with their emphasis on schizophrenic vulnerability to episodes, as opposed to continuously present symptoms. However, we also found a subgroup of schizophrenics who were severely thought disordered at follow-up, and other data of ours indicate that a large percentage of schizophrenics show poor posthospital functioning.

Thus, difference in level of thought disorder between the diagnostic groups in the post hospital period is mainly accounted for by the subgroup of schizophrenics who show evidence of moderate to severe thought pathology at follow-up. Our initial data have suggested that from 20 to 35 percent of schizophrenics have severe levels of bizarre-idiosyncratic thinking at follow-up after the acute phase, with the exact rate of thought pathology dependent on the particular measure used to assess it and on other features. This group of thought-disordered patients could be considered an important group of schizophrenics. A question would be whether this subsample of patients with persistent bizarre-idiosyncratic thinking, or persistent positive thought pathology, are the "true" schizophrenics, who are likely to show significant declines in functioning and subsequent deterioration. This is a question we are beginning to study (Harrow, Silverstein, and Marengo, 1983). We are currently analyzing data on other characteristics of those schizophrenics with persistent bizarre-idiosyncratic thinking, including their premorbid adjustments, their posthospital functioning, their rates of rehospitalization, and their potential for other types of psychotic symptoms, such as delusions. Similarly, we are also analyzing whether a group of early, young schizophrenics with negative symptoms subsequently show characteristics that are associated with nuclear or true schizophrenia (Pogue-Geile and Harrow, 1984).

BIZARRE-IDIOSYNCRATIC VERBALIZATIONS AND THINKING DURING THE CHRONIC PHASE OF SCHIZOPHRENIA

In accord with our goal of studying disordered cognition at various phases of schizophrenia, we have assessed four samples of chronic hospitalized schizophrenics to obtain an estimate of bizarre language and thinking during the chronic phase. Some of this research, which is outlined in the current chapter, is described more fully in a series of reports (Harrow, Adler, and Hanf, 1974; Harrow, Tucker, Himmelhoch, and Putnam, 1972; Siegel, Harrow, Reilly, and Tucker, 1976).

All four of these samples of chronic schizophrenics were multiyear patients who had spent many consecutive years on the back wards of state hospitals. In this respect—having spent many years in continuous hospitalization—these patients were different from other chronic schizophrenic patients who have been rehospitalized a number of times for short to intermediate periods, but who have spent large amounts of time functioning on the outside between rehospitalizations. These latter types of patients who have spent many years of functioning outside of an institution, frequently interrupted by short rehospitalizations, have been labeled by some as "revolving-door" patients.

The first of the four chronic multiyear patient samples we assessed consisted of thirty-one female chronic schizophrenics, with their mean duration of continuous hospitalization at the time of assessment being 9.8 years. This sample was administered the Object Sorting Test to assess bizarre-idiosyncratic thinking, and the results were compared to those from several other samples. These results are presented in Table 5.6. This table also presents the results on a measure we call behavioral overinclusion (a measure based on the total number of objects selected by the patients during the seven sortings) (Bromet and Harrow, 1973). This measure of the total number of objects sorted has been used extensively by Payne in previous research (Payne, 1966; Payne and Friedlander, 1962; Payne and Hewlett, 1960). It is our belief that high scores on behavioral overinclusion can be influenced by factors such as excessive behavioral activity, and that lower scores can be influenced by a lack of excessive activity, with very low scores sometimes being produced by impoverished thinking and behavior. Factors such as impoverished thinking and behavior can be viewed as among the most important of the negative symptoms, with negative symptoms being seen by a number of theorists as a central type of schizophrenic psychopathology (Andreasen, 1979; Chapman and Chapman, 1973;

TABLE 5.6
Mean Scores of Chronic Schizophrenics on Indices of Thinking and Behavior from the Object Sorting Test

Diagnostic Group	Sample Size (N)	Biz.-Idios. Thinking	Behavioral Overinclusion
Chronic Schizophrenics	31	2.19	30.61
Schizophrenics, Acute Phase	28	3.00	41.81
Nonschizophrenics, Acute Phase	39	1.74	41.92

From Harrow, Tucker, Himmelhoch, & Putnam. *American Journal of Psychiatry, 128*, 824–829, 1972. Reproduced by permission of the publisher.

Fish, 1962; Strauss and Carpenter, 1974). The measure of behavioral overinclusion is presented because we believe that impoverished thinking and behavior and negative symptoms are important factors in considering cognition in chronic schizophrenics, as we shall note when we refer to it later in this chapter.

The object sorting results on bizarre verbalizations and thinking for this first sample of chronic schizophrenics were compared to those for a sample of acute schizophrenic and nonschizophrenic patients. These acute patients are the same sample whose results for the acute and partial recovery phases are reported earlier in Chapter 3 and earlier in the current chapter. The results showed at least a moderate to severe level of bizarre-idiosyncratic thinking for both schizophrenic groups, the acute and the chronic schizophrenics. There was, however, a trend for the scores on bizarre verbalizations and thinking of the acute schizophrenics to reflect more overt bizarre-idiosyncratic thinking than those of the chronic schizophrenics. The chronic schizophrenic sample did show more bizarre verbalizations than the nonschizophrenic patient sample. While this sample of chronic schizophrenics showed less bizarre verbalizations and thinking than the acute schizophrenics, the relatively severe scores of these chronic patients did suggest that bizarre verbalizations are characteristics of many chronic schizo-phrenics. It must be remembered that the comparison group of acute schizophrenics with which the chronic schizophrenics are being compared were assessed within two weeks of hospital admission. In practice, this means that the acute schizophrenic comparison group was preselected on the basis of being at or near to the height of their psychopathology at the time of evaluation.

The assessment of a second (and different) sample of chronic schizophrenics was conducted with different instruments than were used with the first sample; this time we employed the Proverbs and Comprehension Subtests to assess bizarre verbalizations and thinking. The results from this second sample of chronic schizophrenics, and from two samples of acute patients with whom they were compared, are presented in Table 5.7. This second sample of chronic schizophrenics, also from the back wards of a state hospital, consisted of thirty-two chronic female schizophrenics with a median length of hospitalization of fourteen years.

The results for the second sample of chronic schizophrenics that we assessed on bizarre-idiosyncratic verbalizations and thinking agreed in principle with those obtained for our first sample of chronic schizo-phrenics. Using different types of tests that are more heavily dependent on verbal skills than the tests employed with the first sample of chronic schizophrenics, we found results indicating that this sample of chronic schizophrenics showed approximately the same degree of bizarre language as a comparison sample of acute schizophrenics. They were significantly more thought disordered than the nonschizophrenic patient sample. In this case, the chronic schizophrenics were slightly less bizarre than the acute schizophrenics on the Comprehension Subtest, and slightly *more* bizarre on the Proverbs Test, with neither difference being close to significant. Overall, the results in Table 5.7 from these two verbal tests, comparing the chronic schizophrenics with the acute schizophrenic and nonschizophrenic patient samples, showed little difference on scores for bizarre-idiosyncratic thinking between the chronic and acute schizophrenics. However, both schizophrenic groups were significantly more bizarre than the nonschizophrenics ($P <$ .001).

The relatively high scores on bizarre verbalizations and thinking of this chronic schizophrenic sample raise the issue of whether these chronic schizophrenics were in an acute or active phase of their disorder, as were the acute schizophrenics. We cannot answer this question with certainty, but the data would suggest that a few of these patients were not in an active state of disorder, and not thought disordered, while the majority of these patients were in an active phase

TABLE 5.7
Results Comparing Chronic Schizophrenic Sample with
Acute Schizophrenic and Nonschizophrenic Samples on
Bizarre Verbalizations and Thinking Using the
Comprehension and Proverbs Tests

| | Bizarre Verbalizations and Thinking | | | |
| | Comprehension Test | | Proverbs Test | |
Sample	Mean	N	Mean	N
Chronic Schizophrenics	5.25	32	6.88	32
Acute Schizophrenics	6.24	25	5.56	25
Acute Nonschiz. Pts.	1.44	25	1.60	25

| | Comprehension Test | | | Proverbs Test | | |
	df	t	P	df	t	P
Chronic vs. Acute Schiz.	55	−0.68	NS	55	0.82	NS
Chronic Schiz. vs. Nonschiz.	55	3.32	.001	55	4.15	.001
Acute Schiz. vs. Nonschiz.	48	4.15	.001	48	3.30	.001

of their disorder. As we have noted earlier, chronic schizophrenics who have been hospitalized continuously for many years do not represent a complete sample of chronic schizophrenics. The majority of chronic schizophrenics are those who have been able to manage to function part or much of the time outside of the hospital, and thus had been screened out from this chronically hospitalized sample. In that respect, this type or sample of chronic schizophrenics who have been hospitalized for many years represents a select sample, constituting a very poor prognosis group.

Since the multiyear hospitalized chronic schizophrenic group already represents a poor outcome population of patients, the question arises as to whether to view them as more severely "ill." At present there are no absolute guidelines as to what type of criteria to use as measures for evaluating which schizophrenics are the most severely "ill." Thus, one could use as the criteria of severity of illness any of a number of factors, such as genetic loading for schizophrenia, or severity of psychotic symptom status, or earlier onset of disorder, or negative outcome. In many other disorders severity of symptom status is used as the criterion concerning the extent of "illness." In contrast, with schizophrenic patients we would view negative or poor outcome as the best criterion of who are the most severely "ill" schizophrenics. Measured along this dimension, the present sample of chronic schizophrenics, considered as a group, would rate as very disordered on a scale of severity of schizophrenic illness.

Interesting conclusions emerge when one applies to our data on bizarre-idiosyncratic thinking this criterion of negative outcome as an index of severity of the disorder. Thus, using this criterion, one would estimate that the more severly disordered schizophrenics (chronic, multiyear, hospitalized schizophrenics) are not necessarily the ones who are always the most pathological where bizarre-idiosyncratic thinking is concerned. These severely disordered schizophrenics do show bizarre-idiosyncratic thinking. Many, but not all, have very severe levels of it, some almost astronomic in severity, but other types of schizophrenics in active phases (e.g., acute schizophrenics) show severe bizarre-idiosyncratic thinking. In this respect, bizarre-idiosyncratic thinking during active phases would be a feature that is often present in severely disordered schizophrenics, but not an invariant feature that could be used to separate the most severely disordered schizophrenics from less severely disordered schizophrenics. Other evidence we have reported, suggesting that bizarre-idiosyncratic thinking at the acute phase does not predict subsequent outcome for early schizophrenics, would fit in with this conclusion (Harrow, Bromet, and Quinlan, 1974).

The third sample of chronic schizophrenics we assessed was administered a different type of technique to evaluate bizarre language and thinking—the fifteen-minute, tape recorded, free-verbalization interview, described in Chapter 3. The relevant results here are those that are based on our measure of overall deviant language and communication, essentially a measure of bizarre-idiosyncratic speech.

In this phase of our research we assessed fifteen chronic, multiyear, hospitalized schizophrenics, from a different hospital setting than the first two samples of chronically institutionalized schizophrenics. The minimum total hospitalization of these patients was four and a half years, and ten of the fifteen had been hospitalized for at least ten years. To assess questions about disordered thinking in multiyear, back-ward, chronic schizophrenics versus revolving-door, chronic schizophrenics, we compared the above hospitalized sample of chronic hospitalized schizophrenics to a sample of fifteen multiyear, chronic schizophrenics who had been living outside in the community (and functioning to some degree) for the previous year without hospitalization. These two chronic schizophrenic samples were compared to samples of twenty-six acute schizophrenics and twenty-five acute nonschizophrenic psychiatric patients assessed shortly after hospitalization.

The results with this third sample, using a different technique, suggested large significant differences between the multiyear, chronic schizophrenics and the disturbed nonschizophrenic sample, in terms of more bizarre verbalizations among the chronic schizophrenics ($P <$ .001). The long-term, chronic, hospitalized schizophrenics also showed more bizarre verbalizations than the chronic schizophrenics who had not been in the hospital for the past year, some of whom were at various stages of partial remission ($P < $.01). Despite the considerable degree of bizarre verbalizations of the long-term, hospitalized chronic schizophrenic sample, the acute schizophrenic sample tended to show about the same level of bizarre speech. Viewed in one way, if one were able to control precisely for thought impoverishment and their reduced rate of speech, the chronic schizophrenics might have shown even more bizarre verbalizations than the acute schizophrenic patients we assessed. During interviews with several chronic schizophrenics hospitalized for many years from this sample, and from our fourth sample, we have found extremely severe levels of bizarre thinking when we have been able to encourage the patients to verbalize their ideas more clearly.

Recently, we assessed a fourth sample of thirty-nine chronic, multiyear schizophrenics from a state hospital in the Chicago area, using our index of bizarre-idiosyncratic thinking derived from the Object Sorting, Proverbs, and Comprehension tests. We found that this sample of chronically hospitalized, multiyear schizophrenics was even more severely bizarre than an acute schizophrenic sample, even when the acute sample consisted of schizophrenics who were assessed during a medication-free period.

In addition, the chronic schizophrenics consistently showed more paucity of verbalizations, and more perseverations, with these results suggesting more thought impoverishment and more negative symptoms for the chronic schizophrenics. These characteristics were among the most prominent features we found in chronic schizophrenics who had been hospitalized for many years. Their many signs of thought impoverishment and evidence that they spoke less (used significantly fewer words) than acute schizophrenics may account for the less severe scores on bizarre-idiosyncratic speech for some of these samples. This potential thought impoverishment, or negative symptoms, of the chronic schizophrenics appears to be a major part of their cognitive disorder.

BIZARRE SPEECH AND THOUGHT IMPOVERISHMENT AS FACTORS IN CHRONIC SCHIZOPHRENIA

When we look at our overall results on these four samples of multiyear, hospitalized, chronic schizophrenics, with the samples assessed on different types of instruments, we can see that they showed both impoverished thinking or negative cognitive pathology, and a considerable degree of positive thought pathology. One question is: Are chronic schizophrenics as bizarre, or even more bizarre than samples of acute schizophrenics assessed at the height of their episode? Our results with four different samples of chronic schizophrenics indicate that many of these patients show severe levels of positive thought disorder. The data from our first sample of chronic schizophrenics, hospitalized for many years, suggest that these patients were not as bizarre as an acute schizophrenic sample. The results from the second and third samples suggested that they might be equally disordered in terms of bizarre-idiosyncratic speech. The results from our fourth and most recent chronic sample suggested that the chronic schizophrenics may be more bizarre than an acute schizophrenic sample. The issue of which type of schizophrenic has more bizarre-idiosyncratic thinking is one that we have not resolved with any assurance. We suspect that on balance, our preliminary results suggest in respect to bizarre *verbal-*

izations that multiyear, hospitalized, chronic schizophrenics are either equally bizarre or more bizarre than acute schizophrenics.

We should note that in general our data could fit in with the formulations held by both our own research group, and a number of other theorists (e.g., Andreasen, 1979; Fish, 1962), that one can find at least two important types of thought pathology in schizophrenia. One of these is bizarre-idiosyncratic verbalizations and thinking or positive types of thought pathology. This type of thought pathology is partly a consequence of factors related to schizophrenia and/or psychosis, and occurs during acute and *active* phases of schizophrenia, including active phases of chronic schizophrenia. It is also influenced by acute psychopathology and general distubance. The second type involves negative cognitive symptoms, with one of the key negative symptoms being impoverished thinking, often accompanied by concrete thinking. This type of cognitive pathology occurs partly as a function of general cognitive-intellectual deficit and/or decline in a subgroup of select patients, with many of those patients being chronic schizophrenics.

As we have noted, if the bizarreness of multiyear chronically hospitalized schizophrenics is looked at in terms of these patients being in an active phase of their schizophrenic disorder, we must analyze why their scores on bizarre verbalizations are sometimes slightly less severe than those of acute schizophrenics. Our interviews suggest that one factor that may influence these results could be that overt evidence of bizarre verbalizations appears less frequently in chronic schizophrenics because the patients are less active, less responsive, less vigorous, less productive, and *less verbal*. In addition, the bizarre-idiosyncratic thinking of some of these patients may not show, overtly, as much, because they are more withdrawn and *asocial*, and possibly attending less to the real world. Thus, it is harder to assess cognitive functioning in chronic schizophrenics. Even though these patients may have considerable idiosyncratic thinking, their lower level of responsivity, withdrawal, and possible *thought impoverishment* makes it difficult to evaluate their tendency toward idiosyncratic thinking or at least makes it more difficult to assess via verbal tasks.

Consistent with this thesis, a number of patients from the samples of chronic, multiyear schizophrenics we have assessed showed evidence of negative symptoms and of impoverishment. As can be seen in Table 5.6, the first sample we assessed showed extremely low scores on behavioral overinclusion, which can be influenced by impoverished thinking and behavior. The second sample of chronic, multiyear schizophrenics showed extremely pathological scores on measures of concrete thinking; these results are discussed in Chapter 7. The third sample of chronic, multiyear schizophrenics showed significantly more paucity of verbalizations than a sample of acute schizophrenics, again suggesting a lower level of responsivity and possible impoverishment.

Overall, to summarize our results, the data we have collected in this area suggest that the great majority of chronic, multiyear, hospitalized schizophrenics have positive thought disorder. A certain number of these chronic, multiyear, hospitalized schizophrenics show extremely severe bizarre speech. There are select other chronic schizophrenics, hospitalized at state institutions for many years, who are not thought disordered at all. However, there also are other chronic schizophrenics who have severe positive types of thought disorder, but who do not manifest this, overtly, due to low responsivity, withdrawal, impoverished thinking, attending less to the real world, and possibly, their thoughts having become more private and unreal. If this latter feature is the case, then they may have become more dependent on their fantasy lives, and are more likely to be utilizing private material. The private material may dominate their thoughts to a greater extent, with this being related to their increasing break with social reality, and their increasing social isolation.

WHAT KINDS OF FACTORS MIGHT LEAD TO, PRODUCE, OR INFLUENCE DISORDERED THINKING?

As we have noted earlier, it is our belief that a comprehensive program of research on disordered thinking in schizophrenia should be geared to finding out what are the most prominent types of thought pathology in schizophrenia, *and* in addition, what factors might lead to thought pathology or influence it. Our approach has been planned to answer the first series of questions about which type or types of thought pathology are prominent in schizophrenia, and during which phases of the disorder they play a role. Our research has also been planned to begin to approach the latter questions of what factors might influence thought pathology.

In relation to this latter goal of what factors might lead to or influence the appearance of thought pathology, several techniques or approaches have been tried. One popular, but naive, approach that is attempted quite frequently involves the determination of whether an aspect of functioning is impaired in schizophrenic patients (e.g., is there a short-term memory deficit, or some other impairment such as anhedonia?), without bothering to investigate whether this impairment covaries with the presence of thought pathology. The assumption here is that if the data indicate that this aspect of functioning is impaired in schizophrenic patients, then one can assume that this difficulty must be a factor leading to disordered thinking. This method has been widely adopted in projects in this area, with the belief at the end of the research report that the presence of this impairment in some or many schizophrenic patients is evidence that it causes thought pathology. Hence, this approach is utilized in a number of studies, even though no evidence is provided that schizophrenics with more of the impairment (e.g., short-term memory deficit) are more severely thought disordered.

Another slightly more sophisticated approach, which has also been attempted by others, involves *covariation* or a *correlational* approach. This approach is based on determining what specific factors are impaired in schizophrenia, and then investigating whether or not these factors covary with the presence or absence of thought pathology. Thus, using this approach, one would investigate whether a factor (such as a short-term memory deficit) was present in schizophrenics who are high on thought pathology, but not present in schizophrenics who are low on thought pathology. This is an approach based on inference, which only provides tentative information, but it still has some value for obtaining possible clues in the area. The limitations of this approach involve several potential difficulties. One of the major problems is that at times a third factor—such as general deficit, or general disturbance and upset, or an acute psychosis factor—may influence both variables and account for the seemingly high relationship. Even here, however, some information of possible value may be provided in this case, especially if one begins to investigate the common factors that may influence both of the variables being studied. Although this type of approach represents a considerable advance in sophistication over the previously noted technique, it has unfortunately been used only a limited number of times in this area.

The covariation or correlational approach can take other forms as well, some of which are even stronger that the original paradigm. As a first step, one can study specific schizophrenics who are high on a factor under investigation and see whether these particular patients also are high on thought pathology. As the second step, one can then study the same patients at a different phase of their disorder, or at a time when the patients are low on thought pathology, and see whether these same schizophrenics are also low on the factor under investigation at that time. This technique is a much stronger one. It is not a certain way of determining whether a factor influences thought pathology, but it does provide information with a slightly stronger foundation. It is still inferential and several possible interpretations could be made of the results. Thus, if the factor under investigation (such as short-term memory impairment) and thought pathology both covary together, one could hypothesize that (1) the factor under investigation influences or produces thought pathology, or it is possible that (2) thought pathology influences or produces impairment in the factor under investigation. It also is possible (as in the example noted in the previous paragraph) that (3) a third factor (e.g., general deficit) influences both variables, or that (4) some major underlying variable that produces thought pathology also influences or leads to the presence of the factor under investigation. In many types of research using this paradigm, the possibility that an underlying factor influences both variables is the most likely hypothesis or formulation. In this latter case, when a major underlying variable is responsible for the high correlations, the correlational findings can prove their value if they are used as a stimulus or clue to search for the major underlying variables that may be involved.

INFLUENCE OF ACUTE PSYCHOPATHOLOGY ON BIZARRE-IDIOSYNCRATIC SPEECH AND THINKING

One aspect of our research on some of the factors that might influence bizarre-idiosyncratic thinking, using a covariational approach, involves our studies over time of the influence of acute upset and general disturbance (Harrow, Grossman, Silverstein, and Meltzer, 1982; Harrow and Quinlan, 1977). Our studies of patients whose cognitive functioning we assessed at the acute phase and then reanalyzed at a subsequent phase of their disorder allow us to make inferences about the influence of acute upset, emotional turmoil, and general disturbance—all factors that are prominent at the acute phase.

Elsewhere in this book we have noted aspects of our research with *other* types of cognitive impairment at two phases of disturbance (e.g., concrete thinking, conceptual overinclusion, loose associations, stimulus overinclusion). In this other research we obtained results similar in principle to those described in the present chapter, studying patients in the midst of acute disturbance and then reassessing them six to eight weeks later as they emerged from this period of upset. During the course of the longitudinal research we have reported in this chapter we have analyzed data that bear on the potential influence of the acute upset, general disturbance, emotional intensity, and cognitive arousal found at the acute phase as factors influencing bizarre-idiosyncratic thinking and verbalizations. Our results suggest that bizarre thinking is influenced by acute disturbance and/or acute psychopathology, with higher levels of thought pathology occurring during such acute phases. We have found that there is some decrease in bizarre verbalizations when acute upset diminishes. These results occur for some non-schizophrenics also, which suggests that the mechanisms involved for this factor are not specific to schizophrenia.

How does the acute phase lead to or result in greater thought pathology? Our observation is that variables found at the acute phase, such as increased upset, acute turmoil, emotional intensity, and cognitive arousal, lead to a disruption of the patient's usual, habitual level of hierarchical skills and organization. The result is a lower level of organization and a disruption of a number of processes, with this including a disruption of central executive processes, and interference with the person's routine and usually successful mechanisms of coping. They often result in a lower level of organization and some dis-organization. Factors such as disorganization can be observed in many patients at the acute phase, and this has been written about extensively by a number of investigators. The disorganization, which involves a disruption of hierarchical skills and impairment in cognitive processes during the acute phase, occurs for schizophrenics, for manic patients, and for some other psychotic patients. Disorganization, arising as a consequence of acute disturbance and emotional intensity, is not the only underlying factor involved in the severe thought pathology found in schizophrenic and manic patients during the acute phase of disorder. Thus, other factors are involved in a major way also, since severe thought pathology is much more frequent and prominent in patients with certain specific diagnoses, such as in schizophrenic and manic patients, and in some other psychotic patients as well.

The data we reported earlier in this chapter, and our other more detailed data reports (Adler and Harrow, 1974; Harrow, Grossman, Silverstein, and Meltzer, 1982; Harrow, Tucker, Himmelhoch and Putnam, 1972), are in agreement with our conclusion that, as manic and schizophrenic patients, and some other psychotic patients, emerge from the acute phase of disturbance they become less disorganized, with a concomitant reduction in severity of thought pathology for many of these patients. This would tend to support the interpretation that in addition to diagnosis, variables associated with the acute phase of psychopathology, such as acute turmoil, general upset, emotional intensity, and cognitive arousal can lead to increased thought pathology (Harrow, Grossman, Silverstein, and Meltzer, 1982; Harrow and Quinlan, 1977).

The results on acute psychopathology as an important factor provide strong evidence that bizarre thinking is *not* just a function of whether the patient has a schizophrenic disorder or not. The more severe levels of bizarre verbalizations (and presumably of bizarre thinking) during periods of acute upset and disturbance for schizophrenic patients also must be viewed in the context of the total picture concerning disorganization and disruption of cognitive functioning during the acute phase. Thus, bizarre-idiosyncratic verbalizations is only one of several types of cognitive dysfunctioning during periods of acute disturbance.

INTERMINGLING OF MATERIAL FROM THE SCHIZOPHRENIC'S EXPERIENCE AS AN INFLUENCE ON HIS BIZARRE VERBALIZATIONS

Recently, our research group also explored a new, more direct technique to "get at" major factors that might lead to bizarre verbalizations and bizarre thinking in schizophrenics. The most direct manner of obtaining clues concerning possible reasons for bizarre schizophrenic speech (and thinking) would be to ask the patient directly about the reason why his language is so bizarre. Obviously, this will only be effective in rare instances, since the question is vague and it is likely to arouse hostile and/or defensive reactions by the patient. Further, it is likely that the patient is unable to answer such a general question, since it is not certain that he is even aware much of the time of how strange his verbalizations are.

The technique we did use involves a variation of the above: *specific* bizarre verbalizations were elicited from each schizophrenic to standardized questions. Following this, we were able to obtain estimates from the individual patients about the reasons for his own specific verbalizations, including his bizarre ones. A more detailed account of our research and the results we obtained using this technique can be found in a series of reports (Harrow, Lanin-Kettering, Prosen, and Miller, 1983; Harrow and Prosen, 1978, 1979).

The method we utilized involves three stages, with much of the value of the technique based on the stage in which the patient explores his reasons for his bizarre statements. While it might be difficult or impossible for many schizophrenics to verbalize why they often say strange things, it is much easier for them to discuss, in a matter-of-fact way, their reasons, associations, and thinking about the specific verbalizations they have given to specific questions, especially when some of their responses to the questions are good ones and others are not good ones. Our procedure was as follows:

1. In the first stage of this research, using our more direct technique, the Gorham Proverbs Test and the Social Comprehension Subtest of the WAIS were administered to each patient. Afterwards, eight of the patient's responses were selected for subsequent inquiry, with most of the material selected from the responses to the proverbs test. Three relatively "good" responses and five bizarre, strange, deviant, unusual, or incorrect responses were selected.
2. The following week, in an empathic, interested, and nonjudgmental manner, a senior clinician conducted a standardized, *taped* interview to find out the reasons for each of the eight responses selected.
3. After this interview, members of our research team rated the taped interviews. The ratings were scored on a number of dimensions theorized by others to be possible underlying reasons for schizophrenic patients' bizarre language. These included ratings on scales designed to score whether the bizarre responses were due to faulty logic, to primitive-drive-dominated thinking, to concrete thinking, to the use of a private language, and ratings of a number of other dimensions. As a result of our own observations, one of these other dimensions involved ratings on the frequency in a patient's responses of *intermingling* of aspects of his experiences, concerns, and conflicts into his overt verbalizations. We also asked about and rated how satisfied the patient was with his responses (both his good answers and his strange answers), to explore the schizophrenic's ability to maintain perspective about how inappropriate his own strange responses were and his degree of "insight" in this area.

Our research in this area is still in an early stage, but the initial findings, which we have recently reported, have led to a series of hypotheses about several factors involved in disordered thinking.

The results are based on looking at and rating a large number of possible variables that may play a role in bizarre schizophrenic verbalizations. The data suggested the presence of a variety of different types of factors that may be involved, rather than only one factor. While many different features appeared, some sporadically, some more frequently, one factor that appeared in the bizarre verbalizations of a large number of schizophrenic patients seemed particularly important. This factor, as noted above, is an intermingling into their verbalizations of material from their own experiences that reflects their concerns, needs, preoccupations and wishes.

Our ratings of intermingling were scored from the original responses to the proverbs test and from the material that emerged in the taped interviews concerning the reasons for each of the patient's specific responses. The ratings of the proverbs test responses and interviews were based on whether there was overt evidence of the patient's blending material from his own current or past experience into his responses, or whether the patient's responses were guided or influenced by these personal experiences from the very beginning of his verbalizations. Scores were assigned for intermingling only when the personal material that was blended into the response did *not* fit neatly with the typical consensual response to that particular proverb or question. Three examples of responses containing intermingled material from patients' personal lives follow:

1. *Q: "Don't cast pearls before swine."* A: "Don't give your good things to bad people. They might turn around and use your good things to make you sad. That's a good poem for this hospital cause people are depressed."
2. *Q: "A stream cannot rise higher than its source."* A: "A son is not greater than his father. Your father will be older and wiser than you."
3. *Q: "Shallow brooks are noisy."* A: "There's a lot of rocks in shallow brooks. It's sin and grief." [Later, when questioned during the interview, the patient explained.] . . . "The rocks kind of symbolize my sin and grief."

The results of our research, on possible reasons for schizophrenics' disordered speech, suggest that during active stages of the disorder, a tendency to blend or *intermingle* into their responses other related (but not completely appropriate) personal material is one immediate mechanism responsible for bizarre verbalizations. When patients were interviewed systematically about their correct and their bizarre responses, about 50 percent of the schizophrenics showed strong evidence (1) that their bizarre-idiosyncratic responses were influenced by an intermingling into these verbalizations of their concerns and preoccupations, or (2) that their responses to these neutral questions were directly guided by their personal concerns. Another 20 to 25 percent (depending on whether unequivocal evidence of at least two instances of intermingling was required as the criteria, or whether only one instance was required) showed weaker signs of such intermingling. This left an overall total of 70 to 75 percent of the schizophrenics (depending on the criteria used for rating) with a blending of their concerns and preoccupations into some or many of their bizarre responses, or a guiding of their bizarre-idiosyncratic responses by their personal concerns. Table 5.8 reports our early results on intermingling for a sample of schizophrenic and nonschizophrenic patients.

The schizophrenics' intermingling of their personal concerns and preoccupations into their language at an inappropriate point in the context of the session, making it appear strange and bizarre, was one factor influencing a large percentage of these patients' speech and behavior. It was not, however, the only factor that influenced their responses and made them appear bizarre and idiosyncratic; other factors also play either a major or a minor role. Thus, while most schizophrenics showed at least some signs of intermingling, many of these patients showed evidence of a combination of intermingling and other factors, as involved in their bizarre verbalizations, and there were other schizophrenics who did not show any overt evidence of intermingling at all. Overall, our evidence indicates that intermingling of schizophrenics' personal concerns and preoccupations is one factor, and an important one, entering into the overt appearance of most schizophrenics' thinking and speech at a point that is inappropriate to the context, making it appear bizarre, but that it is not the only factor involved. Bizarre thinking and bizarre speech in schizophrenia can appear as a consequence of confusion and disorganization, and as a result of other factors as well.

In addition, as can be seen in Table 5.8, our research has indicated that many disturbed nonschizophrenic patients also show some signs of intermingling on those occasions when they do show bizarre-idiosyncratic speech. However, since nonschizophrenics as a group show less thought pathology, they also showed slightly less intermingling.

TABLE 5.8
Percentage of Patients Showing Intermingling as an Influence on Their Bizarre Language

Sample	Very Clear Evidence of Intermingling as an Influence	Minor Evidence of Intermingling as an Influence	No Evidence of Intermingling as an Influence
Percentage of Schizophrenics ($N = 37$)	51	27	22
Percentage of Nonschizophrenics ($N = 16$)	38	25	38

Our suggestion here is that intermingling is not specific to schizophrenia, but rather that intermingling is one common factor that plays an overt role in the creation of much bizarre-idiosyncratic thinking and speech, regardless of the type of diagnosis. Closer analysis of the verbalizations of different types of patients who show greater degrees of bizarre-idiosyncratic thinking (and these will often be schizophrenics) will indicate that these patients frequently show intermingling as one of the prominent factors involved in making their language look bizarre. The view here is that *many of the major mechanisms involved in bizarre verbal behavior are the same for those nonschizophrenics who do show bizarre-idiosyncratic thinking as it is for schizophrenics,* although they are manifested more frequently by schizophrenics because of their more frequent and more severe thought pathology.

In addition to our research on the frequency of schizophrenics' intermingling of personal material into their speech, we have also conducted other types of analyses and reanalyses of the test material and taped interviews we collected in this phase of our research. Much of these additional analyses were designed to focus on a number of different aspects and features of intermingling, in order to determine their major characteristics.

In regard to the major characteristics of the intermingling, our detailed analysis has indicated that most of the time this personal material guides the patient's responses, or blends in with the responses from the very beginning of the verbalizations. Less frequently, it is first introduced into the responses in the middle of the patient's verbalizations (Harrow, Lanin-Kettering, Prosen, and Miller, 1983). The intermingled material is of interest and/or concern to the patient, it comes from the patient's experiences, and is related to his personal life, either in the past, or the present, or both. Usually the intermingled material is from concerns of the patient that are related overtly to his present experiences, or concerns based on his experiences during the last few years, rather than being centered, overtly, on childhood experiences. Our data suggest that the material that tends to be blended into the responses of the patient is typically *not* primitive-drive-dominated content, nor is it dreamlike material or grossly unacceptable unconscious material (Harrow and Prosen, 1978, 1979).

At first glance, the intermingled material appears to deviate grossly from the topic under discussion. When examined more closely with the patient later, at a time when he may have slightly better perspective, we have found that it does not deviate, consensually, as much as it first appeared to deviate from the topic under discussion. In addition, the patient usually has a "rationale" for the idiosyncratic verbalizations (Harrow, Lanin-Kettering, Prosen, and Miller, 1983).

DO THE SCHIZOPHRENIC'S BIZARRE VERBALIZATIONS MAKE SENSE TO HIM?

Our research on intermingling and other observations we have made have led us to propose that the material the schizophrenic intermingles, and his bizarre thinking and behavior in general, usually make internal sense to the patient, in terms of where he "is at" for that particular moment. An important factor here is the internal context of the patient. If we could get "inside" the patient and analyze his thinking at that particular moment, we would be able to see and understand that what the patient is saying or doing often makes sense from his point of view, even though the patient is saying and doing things that seem strange or bizarre to the outsider. All people, normals as well as schizophrenics, have an internal context. However, during a psychotic episode, the schizophrenic may have more difficulty preventing his internal context from dominating his perception of the external world. Thus, he will find it difficult to prevent this internal material from directing his real-world behavior, and in this situation he will not take proper account of the external demands of the situation. As a result, the schizophrenic may be unable to recognize when too great an adherence to his own internal context will make him appear socially inappropriate to others. The schizophrenic is still psychotic, even if one can explain some or much of his behavior in terms of his attending too much, overtly, to an internal context which, if we were aware of it, would make some sense to us and would make his behavior seem less strange to us. However, the usual standard for assessing whether a patient is psychotic does not depend on the appropriateness of his behavior from the point of view of his internal context; rather, it depends on his appropriateness in terms of the external "real-world" context or situation. There are, of course, times when the schizophrenic is very disorganized and confused, and at such times his behavior may make less sense, and it may be hard to link his behavior to an internal context even after a searching examination. Typically, however, what the psychotic patient says does make some sense when looked at from his framework. In recent research, using a word-association technique, we have begun to obtain evidence in support of our formulations in this area (Gordon, Silverstein, and Harrow, 1982).

One difference between the speech of the schizophrenic and that of the "normal" person (who also makes sense from his own internal framework) is that with the normal person, one generally does not need a special detailed analysis, or a translator, to understand what he is saying or why. The normal person adheres to the agreed-upon social conventions of attending more to the outside situation than to his own inner needs, and to other social conventions about what should and should not be said and done in a particular situation. Sometimes, even without a special analysis one can gain an idea of what the schizophrenic is saying by stopping to reflect on his verbalizations, and trying to understand where the patient "is at," and why he is saying seemingly strange things. In contrast, however, when the "normal" person says something, one typically does not need to stop to reflect on what he is saying, since his meaning is usually immediately apparent. The difference here between the normal person's speech and the schizophrenic's speech is an important one. Some of this difference is closely linked to the patient's adherence or lack of adherence to the background of social conventions used by the society of which he or she is a member. In this regard, adherence to the social and verbal conventions and agreed-upon types of behaviors in specific situations in our society is crucial for people to understand each other and to communicate successfully with each other in our, or *any*, society.

IMPAIRED PERSPECTIVE AS A MAJOR UNDERLYING FACTOR

A question of some importance is why the patient does not monitor and correct his own strange and inappropriate material. We have proposed that the patient's failure to adequately edit material that others would find embarrassing on a conscious level seems to be one of the major factors involved in his psychosis.

As we have noted, our formulation is that the schizophrenic's bizarre verbalizations seem to make sense to him at the moment, even though others cannot understand him and the verbalizations are obviously strange in terms of conventional social standards. Our hypothesis concerning difficulties in perspective and judgment about the social appropriateness of one's own language and behavior, which we have noted in Chapter 3, should be emphasized at this point. We have proposed that during active schizophrenic episodes, a major *underlying* factor involved in intermingling, and in most other aspects of bizarre language, is impairment in an important executive type of process. This process involves the schizophrenic's effective utilization of previously stored, or long-term, knowledge about what behavior is socially appropriate, or his ability to maintain perspective about the appropriateness of his own ideas and verbalizations (Harrow and Miller, 1980).

We should comment here that the approach about the importance of impaired perspective that we have taken includes utilizing constructs such as executive processes and metacognitive behavior. Metacognition in normals has been discussed extensively by Flavell (1979). Constructs of this type, however, have not been widely applied to pathological thinking, although some investigators have begun to use related constructs in their research. For instance, Cohen, Rosenberg, and associates have conducted research to find evidence linking disorders in communication by schizophrenics to problems in editing (Cohen, 1978; Cohen, Nachmani, and Rosenberg, 1974). Their views, which involve a two-stage stimulus-response process of "sampling" and "comparison" within an information-processing model, focus on a disorder in "editing," rather than a disorder in perspective. Holzman has studied "disinhibition" in normals (Holzman and Rousey, 1970, 1971) and in schizophrenics. In discussing what he believes is the schizophrenic's failure to disinhibit, he has used the construct of cognitive controls in a manner quite similar to the construct of executive processes (Holzman, 1978).

Impaired perspective as we view it may be accompanied by a decline in ability to monitor or edit out material that is not in tune with (a) the overall social situation (perspective-monitoring ability), or (b) more immediate aspects of the speech context (e.g., cognitive-semantic slips). This hypothesized difficulty of the schizophrenic in maintaining perspective about, and to a lesser extent difficulty in monitoring, his own bizarre behavior would fit in with the view that at the time of the *acute* schizophrenic's bizarre comments, he is unable to recognize how far from the consensual topic his personalized, inter-mingled material has led him.

The "normal" person is typically able to maintain reasonable perspective about his everyday language such that his preoccupations do not enter into his ongoing verbalizations in a gross, bizarre manner. At times, however, these personal preoccupations and concerns do appear in the normal person's thinking, language, and behavior in minor, partially disguised ways. When this becomes slightly more flagrant for the normal person, because of his better perspective about what is appropriate in the particular context, he recognizes it, finds it embarrassing, and uses his monitoring ability to adjust or "repair" his speech. In contrast, during periods of acute and/or active psychotic episodes, the schizophrenic may be unable to maintain perspective about and recognize the inappropriateness of mixing his own pre-occupations or concerns into his language and behavior (and he may be unable to monitor it in terms of his moment-by-moment speech behavior). Hence, at the time of his idiosyncratic language and strange behavior the schizophrenic may have temporarily lost the ability both (1) to maintain perspective about what is idiosyncratic to him versus what is appropriate in a social setting, and (2) to monitor his *own* everyday preoccupations, concerns, and wishes, so that they do not intermingle in a gross way with his routine, moment-by-moment, ongoing behavior.

We also have suggested that even if there is impairment in perspective about one's *own* verbalizations, the impairment is selective. We have proposed that this impairment in perspective occurs more in some areas of the schizophrenic's own behavior than in other areas. Thus, one can observe that the typical schizophrenic is not psychotic in every single area (e.g., even when hospitalized, he usually knows when relatives or friends are visiting him, and he usually knows when meals are being served and other patients have sat down to eat). In relation to the schizophrenic's impaired perspective, we have suggested that the difficulty concerns the patient's judgment about his own behavior more that it concerns his judgment about other people's behavior. Hence, we would expect that in an experimental situation the schizophrenic or thought-disordered patient would have better perspective about the adequacy, or social appropriateness, of other peoples' speech than he has about his own; later in this chapter we will discuss our exploratory research into this hypothesis. While much of our research has focused on impaired perspective as a factor closely involved in thought pathology, we also believe that impaired perspective plays a key role as one dimension of delusional ideation, although our early research in this area suggests that other factors may be even more important in the delusions seen in actively psychotic patients (Stoll, Harrow, and Rattenbury, in press).

Overall we regard perspective as a higher-level cognitive mechanism that is an integral part of routine thinking and serves central control functions in ongoing, moment-by-moment thinking. Since perspective is a higher-order control mechanism, it should be viewed as being at a different level of the cognitive process than some other factors involved in thought pathology, such as acute disturbance and emotional intensity, which can produce cognitive disruption, and the intermingling of personal material, which can produce interference with ongoing thinking. We have proposed that a prominent factor in schizophrenia (and in severely thought-disordered and psychotic patients in general) may be an impairment of that particular aspect of executive functioning that is involved in maintaining perspective about what type of behavior fits in with the social demands of the situation. If this occurred, then at the particular moment of the thought-disordered patient's bizarre verbalizations, he would have difficulty recognizing the inappropriateness of his verbalizations. Consequently, he would not perceive how far from the original topic his personalized, intermingled material has strayed. Nonschizophrenic patients and normals may also have some (but less) trouble monitoring their verbalizations, leading to small amounts of cognitive slippage, especially during periods of stress or upset.

It should be noted that at present the nature and range of executive functioning, and the monitoring process (or even the response-selection process), are not completely understood, and formulations about them remain speculative. Several investigators in the area of normal cognition have recently focused on select aspects of these processes (e.g., Deese, 1978; Jefferson, 1974; Schegloff et al., 1977).

Here we should reemphasize that this particular aspect of cognition, which we have proposed as being important in terms of playing a role in disordered schizophrenic verbalizations and schizophrenic delusions (and perhaps in the disordered verbalizations and delusions of many other types of psychotic patients) involves higher-level executive processes. These kinds of processes are not easily available for research, and have not been studied adequately, or clarified, or put into any completely satisfactory scheme for either "normals" or disturbed patients. One area that is potentially accessible to study involves the schizophrenic's ability to recognize whether his own and other peoples' speech and behavior are socially inappropriate or deviant. If it could be established that the schizophrenic lacks "insight" concerning the appropriateness of his own verbalizations, but has better perspective about the speech and behavior of others, this would provide one type of evidence to support formulations about difficulty in perspective as involved in disordered schizophrenic speech. Thus, if schizophrenic patients have better perspective about, or are better able to recognize, the pathological speech of other patients, it would suggest that even schizophrenics have the background *competence* to judge the adequacy of responses. However, factors in a particular speech situation (e.g., factors associated with a patient's overattention to his own internal context, possible factors associated with his misunderstanding of the total situation, and other factors associated with psychosis) may interfere with his ability to assess social norms. These social norms have been learned during childhood and adolescence, and continue to be acquired during adulthood. They are usually available from long-term memory storage and are usually available for routine use on a moment-by-moment, ongoing basis.

In the course of our research in this area we have conducted two related experiments to find evidence bearing on this formulation. In the first, mentioned earlier in this chapter, we explored this issue by inquiring in individual interviews how satisfied the patient was with a series of his own proverb interpretations. In this research, patients were asked about their previous disordered responses one at a time, and were also asked whether they wanted to change their responses. We found a moderate to large degree of insensitivity concerning the adequacy of their responses by many of the more thought-disordered patients.

The second and more important piece of supporting evidence involves a systematic experiment we conducted to provide evidence on the above formulations. In order to explore these hypotheses, we studied a group of schizophrenic and nonschizophrenic patients, some of whom were thought disordered, to evaluate their perspective. The task we used required them to assess or rate how "atypical" (or bizarre) were specific verbalizations of theirs and also to rate specific ver-balizations of other patients (Harrow and Miller, 1980). Again, proverbs questions and patients' responses were used as the main stimulus material. Perspective was assessed as the correlation between the patients' ratings of how "typical" or adequate their proverb responses were and the consensual ratings of how idiosyncratic these responses were in terms of their deviation from consensual standards. Higher correlations between the patients ratings and the consensual standards indicated good perspective and lower correlations indicated poorer perspective.

Among the series of findings we obtained, our data indicated that schizophrenics and thought-disordered patients showed significantly poorer *perspective* about how their own verbal behavior fit in with conventional social standards. Thus, they had lower correlations between their judgments about their own responses and the consensual social standards than nonschizophrenic patients had. In contrast, schizophrenics and other thought-disordered patients showed signifi-cantly higher correlations (and thus showed significantly better agree-ment) with conventional social standards in evaluating other patients' behavior than in judging their own behavior. These data would fit in with a formulation based on impaired perspective for schizophrenics, and to an even greater extent for thought-disordered patients, con-cerning the appropriateness of their own behavior.

In another aspect of our research in this area we studied whether thought-disordered patients and schizophrenic patients, in judging the adequacy of their own responses, showed poorer judgment in evalu-ating any *particular type of responses* (Miller, Harrow, Lanin, and Neiditz, 1981). The data indicated that *thought-disordered* patients showed significantly poorer judgment in rating their own *bizarre* responses than non-thought-disordered patients did in rating their own occasional bizarre responses. In particular, the thought-disordered patients tended to see their own bizarre responses as significantly more "typical" or less bizarre than non-thought-disordered patients did in judging their own occasionally bizarre responses. There was a similar but nonsignificant trend for schizophrenic and other psychotic patients to show poorer judgment in terms of rating their own bizarre responses in a more favorable light than did nonpsychotic patients in judging their own occasional bizarre responses. The data suggest that non-thought-disordered patients, upon rehearing their own occasionally bizarre responses will be more likely to recognize them as atypical or strange.

In this research, the thought-disordered and schizophrenic patients did not judge their own *non*bizarre responses in an unrealistically favorable light (and even tended to view a number of them as "atypical" responses). The results would support the view that thought-disordered and schizophrenic patients tend to show unrealistically favorable judgments about their *bizarre* responses in particular (Miller, Harrow, Lanin, and Neiditz, 1981). Taken as a whole, these data also would fit an interpretation suggesting poorer perspective about their own speech and behavior by thought-disordered and schizophrenic patients, with their poorest judgments occurring in evaluations of the adequacy of their own bizarre and psychotic behavior. Overall, our studies pursuing this line of research have seemed promising.

## PART III

CLASSICAL CONCEPTS OF DISORDERED THINKING

6

Primitive-Drive-Dominated Thinking and Schizophrenia

In the past three chapters we focused on one way of unifying a diverse range of disordered language under the label "bizarre-idiosyncratic thinking," and we summarized some of the major lines of our research in this area. As we have indicated, there are a number of other, perhaps more traditional, ways of looking at aspects of disordered language and thinking. These include focusing on such diverse aspects as "primitive-drive-dominated thinking," "loose associations," "abstract and concrete thinking," "boundary disorders," "conceptual overinclusion," and looking at various types of potential disorders of attention and perception. In each case some or many prominent theorists have focused on one of these aspects as a possible major factor in schizophrenia, in the belief that they hold the key to an understanding of schizophrenic thought pathology, and have produced at least some evidence for their outlook. These are respectable alternatives with solid traditions of inquiry behind them. Each one offers at least some promise for looking at or dealing with schizophrenic thought pathology. We have studied each aspect empirically, and in Chapters 6 through 12 we shall review our research on each of them.

A number of different theories of schizophrenia and of disordered thinking have been derived from psychoanalytic concepts, and several of them have been studied in the course of our research. One of these, based on concepts about a failure to develop adequate self-other boundaries during infancy, is discussed and examined in relation to cognition in schizophrenia in Chapter 9. Another important view of schizophrenia, based on psychoanalytic concepts, involves formulations about primary process thinking and about primitive-drive-dominated thinking. In general, the early importance of primary process thinking, and the later development of secondary process thinking, during the course of maturation occupies an important role in psychoanalytic theory concerning the nature and development of adult thinking. A number of psychoanalytically oriented thinkers have emphasized both the schizophrenic's difficulty in controlling primary process thinking, and also his problems in controlling one particular type of primary process material, namely primitive drive-dominated content (Bellak, 1966; Brenner, 1957; Freud, 1933, 1965).

Clinicians have been noting this phenomenon for many years. Thus, astute observers have reported that schizophrenic patients are unable to repress primitive oral, sexual, and aggressive drive content, and that this type of material emerges in their verbalizations at inappropriate times. Indeed, some have felt that the failure of repression with the emergence of primitive-drive-dominated thinking is one of the major features of schizophrenia. In addition, discussions about psychotherapy for schizophrenic patients have sometimes warned about the dangers of allowing the patient to bring up primitive drive material. This is based on the concern that the primitive drive material brought up by the schizophrenic patient can be almost unending in quantity, and will be difficult for the therapist to handle constructively.

Although both the comments by clinicians about the presence of primitive drive-dominated thinking, and the concerns about their emergence in psychotherapy are based on careful observations, a number of questions arise. Some of these are: How universal is the emergence of this type of material in schizophrenia? Does it occur in some or all schizophrenics? And, is it an essential factor in the genesis of schizophrenia? Thus, while hypotheses about primary process drive material and schizophrenia frequently group together all types of schizophrenic patients in uniform fashion, it is possible that the emergence of primitive drive-dominated thinking is not unique to schizophrenia, or that it is only characteristic of select subgroups of schizophrenic patients, such as chronic, desocialized, and deteriorated patients. Much of the previous research on schizophrenic thinking has involved studying patients at an advanced stage of their disorder (i.e., the chronic phase), when factors such as long-term institutionalization and secondary institutionalization may already have contaminated the clinical picture. To circumvent this problem, our research on drive-dominated content has focused on the acute stage. Two very specific questions in this area that we have attempted to deal with empirically are: (a) is the emergence of primitive drive-dominated thinking a characteristic of relatively young, acute schizophrenics? and (b) how unique is the emergence of this type of drive material to schizophrenia, or, does it also occur in other types of disturbed people?

We should note that aspects of our research in this area which are presented in this chapter have been described elsewhere in previous reports (Harrow and Prosen, 1978; Harrow, Quinlan, Wallington, and Pickett, 1976). In addition, in a separate review of the literature, we have provided a more complete review and description of work on drive-dominated thinking in areas other than schizophrenia (Lazar and Harrow, 1980).

Methodological issues in this area have always presented difficulties in studying these phenomena, since there is no ideal technique for "getting at" a concept such as primitive drive-dominated thinking. Fortunately, in an effort to facilitate the study of this type of material, Holt (1963; Holt and Havel, 1965) has developed an extensive scoring system for classification of Rorschach responses according to the type of drive material and the level of integration of the drive content. This technique of study has been used extensively by other investigators with a good deal of success (Lazar and Harrow, 1980). Thus, our research utilized Holt's scoring system and applied it to the responses of a large sample of schizophrenic patients during the acute phase of their disorder. Other measures of disordered thinking and perception were also used in our research to compare with the indices of primitive drive-dominated thinking to determine which is more important in the acute schizophrenic disorder.

Our research in this area attempted to focus on issues related to drive-dominated thinking and schizophrenia, since this is an area that has been the subject of extensive theoretical discussion. The question arises, however, as to whether other kinds of disorders show difficulty in controlling and directing drive material. In the current phase of our work we have explored this question by focusing on three other classes of people, in addition to schizophrenics.

The first of these additional foci concerns people with histories of rule-breaking behavior, or sociopathic trends. In the course of our own work in inpatient settings we have observed that overactive, seemingly high-energy, disturbed adolescents frequently get into trouble in relation to rule-breaking behavior (e.g., truancy, sexual promiscuity, or rebellious behavior toward parents and other authority figures). If a background of difficulty in handling drive-dominated material is one characteristic of these patients, it is possible that this background problem could be a factor that increases the likelihood of social difficulties in terms of rule-breaking behavior. Thus, it is possible that drive-dominated thinking could have important theoretical implications concerning the derivation of sociopathic behavior in some adolescents. Our research attempted to investigate this formulation with a sample of patients, to determine whether primitive-drive-dominated thinking and any specific type of drive content is associated with rule-breaking or sociopathic trends.

Another group that merits some attention is depressives. Some theories about depression discuss this disorder in terms of a relatively anergic state. In contrast, other theories view depressed patients as people with intense difficulty in handling primitive drive material, especially in relation to oral and aggressive drive content. More recent evidence on depression has provided data indicating that depression is not one uniform disorder, and suggested the possibility that the label "depression" is being applied to several different, possibly unrelated, types of disorders, with their major common feature being a common end state involving a "depressive" symptom complex. As a result of the different views on depression, particularly views relating to the prominence of oral drive content, it seemed worthwhile to examine whether this was a uniform feature in depression. One view would be that difficulty with oral drive content is uniform across all depressive patients. In contrast, an alternate view is that it is prominent in some but not all depressives, and a third possibility is that it is rare in any type of depression.

A third factor that may influence the emergence of primitive-drive-dominated thinking is the sex of the patient and this also was included as a variable for investigation. Sex-related differences in the expression of primitive drive content could conceivably occur as a result of a number of factors, such as possible differences between males and females in the strength of certain types of innate drives, or because of differences in social training and environmental expectations concerning drive-related behavior by the two sexes (e.g., in our society, drive-dominated behavior by females is discouraged, and frequently meets with more social disapproval than is the case with males).

In sum, our research on primitive-drive-dominated thinking and its emergence into consciousness attempted to assess the relative frequency of this phenomenon in schizophrenia and also attempted to focus on its role among several other types of people to answer the following specific questions:

1. Do schizophrenics show more primitive-drive-dominated thinking than nonschizophrenic patients during the acute phase of their

disorder, and is this type of primitive drive content an important characteristic of their thinking?

2. Do other types of diagnostic groups, such as depressives (for whom drive material has been proposed as an important factor), show strong indications of eruption of drive-dominated material?

3. Is difficulty in repressing primary process drive material only related to schizophrenia, or does it also relate to particular types of behavior, such as sociopathic or rule-breaking behavior, and does it occur more frequently in particular types of people (e.g., males)?

4. We also attempted to explore whether difficulties in handling *different types* of primary process drive material (such as oral, sexual, and aggressive drive material) are closely related, and hence whether they occur together in the same patients?

ASSESSMENT OF
PRIMITIVE DRIVE-DOMINATED THINKING

The major patient sample we studied to explore the relationship between schizophrenia and primitive-drive-dominated thinking involved 159 consecutive psychiatric inpatients from our Yale settings, with these patients comprising four major diagnostic groups. The four diagnostic groups were equated on major variables such as socio-economic class and educational level. On one major variable, age, the schizophrenics were significantly younger than the nonschizophrenics. However, several different types of analyses showed that within each diagnostic group, age was not related significantly to any of the indices of drive-dominated thinking, which suggested that age was not the major factor accounting for the diagnostic results.

To assess drive-dominated thinking, four major groupings of Holt's drive content categories were scored separately, using the Rorschach test, for primitive and also for more socialized drive content. These four are sexual (heterosexual only), oral, aggressive, and "miscellaneous" (e.g., anal, homosexual). We also used Holt's system to assess the degree to which a patient is able to control effectively or adapt successfully to the primary process elements in his thinking (Holt, 1963, 1970; Holt and Havel, 1965). This has been labeled by Holt as *defense effectiveness*, or *DE*. Details concerning the scoring of this system for assessing drive-dominated content and related concepts can be found in several of Holt's manuals (1963, 1970). The results we obtained using Holt's system are analyzed and presented in terms of the absolute number of each type of drive response on the Rorschach, and also in terms of the percentage of each type ((number of responses of each type/R) $\times$ 100).

The same test material was used to obtain scores on two other aspects of disordered thinking and perception. These two involve: (1) our Rorschach measure of deviant thought quality, which represents an index of bizarre-idiosyncratic thinking or positive thought disorder; and (2) an index of very poor form level, or F- (Quinlan, Harrow, and Carlson, 1973). This measure of poor form level is based on poor perception, or difficulties the subject may have in matching the percepts he reports to the actual qualities of the inkblot.

Satisfactory interrater reliability was obtained on these two indexes and on the measures of drive content, and defense effectiveness. The various indexes have been utilized and discussed previously (Lazar and Harrow, 1980; Quinlan, Harrow, and Carlson, 1973; Quinlan, Harrow, Tucker, and Carlson, 1972; Tucker, Quinlan, and Harrow, 1972). The Rorschach measure of bizarre-idiosyncratic thinking has been discussed in previous chapters, and is focused on further in Chapter 15.

To assess hypotheses about a relationship between drive-dominated thinking and potential sociopathic behavior, several personality tests were utilized. These included the OOH test, a test to assess various personality traits and patterns (Lazare, Klerman, and Armor, 1966), and the MMPI. Two scales were derived from the MMPI which are specifically related to a history of sociopathic or rule-breaking behavior: the Rule-Breaking Scale (Lowe, 1961), and a modified form of this scale developed by our own research team.

Schizophrenia and Drive-Dominated Thinking

The results from the overall index of primitive drive-dominated thinking suggest that its appearance is not an exclusively schizophrenic phenomenon and occurs to a limited extent in several different types of acutely disturbed patients. Tables 6.1 and 6.2 present the mean scores and tests of significance for the major diagnostic groups (using a two-way analysis of variance) on the overall index of primitive-drive-dominated thinking and for the individual measures of primitive drive content.

These results show that the total score for primitive drive material differed significantly among the diagnostic groups ($P <$ .01). The emergence of some socially unacceptable drive material was most frequent among the classical schizophrenics, but was also relatively common in the latent schizophrenic and borderline patients, and was

TABLE 6.1
Mean Scores[1] and Tests of Significance[2] for Schizophrenic and Nonschizophrenic Patients on Drive-Dominated Thinking

Means and Standard Deviations

	Classical Schizophrenics (N = 48)		Latent Schizophrenics (N = 35)		Personality Disorders (N = 38)		Depressives (N = 38)	
	M	SD	M	SD	M	SD	M	SD
Socially modulated drive content	5.92[3]	3.54	5.09[3]	3.37	5.61[3,4]	3.82	3.05[4]	2.71
Primitive drive content								
Overall primitive drive content	1.81[3]	1.83	1.57[3]	1.73	1.03[3,4]	1.31	0.50[4]	1.05
Primitive sexual drive content	0.58	1.30	0.51	1.05	0.08	0.35	0.16	0.49
Primitive aggressive drive content	1.13[3]	1.24	0.86[3,4]	1.22	0.84[3,4]	1.16	0.37[4]	0.81
Primitive oral drive content	0.10	0.47	0.17	0.45	0.08	0.27	0.03	0.16
Primitive drive content, miscellaneous	0.15	0.61	0.14	0.42	0.08	0.27	0.00	0.00
Other types of deviant thinking and perception								
Deviant thought quality (TQ)	21.90[3]	17.11	12.23[4]	12.72	9.55[4]	10.43	5.76[4]	9.54
Very poor form (F−)	2.25[3]	2.32	1.23[4]	1.48	0.92[4]	1.20	1.21[4]	1.30
Number of Responses	24.75[3]	8.47	22.80[3,4]	6.83	22.63[3,4]	5.54	20.05[4]	5.52

[1] The means are based on the absolute number of responses of each type.

[2] The tests of significance, to assess possible significant differences between the various diagnostic groups, are based on the percentage of each type of response (No. Resp. of Each Type/R) to control for number of responses. These tests of significance involved Newman Keuls Tests, derived from the anovas reported in Table 6.2

[3,4] Within each variable, diagnostic groups sharing the same superscript number are not significantly different from each other. Diagnostic groups not sharing the same number are significantly different ($P < .05$), according to the Newman-Keuls test.

From Harrow, Quinlan, Wallington, & Pickett, *Journal of Personality Assessment, 40,* 31–41, 1976. Reproduced by permission of the publisher.

found to a lesser extent in some patients with severe personality disorders.

Individual Newman-Keuls tests suggested that the significant overall results were influenced by the high scores of the schizophrenic patients, but this was not the major responsible factor (see Table 6.1). Rather, the data suggested that the low degree of primitive-drive-dominated thinking by the depressives was an even more prominent factor separating the diagnostic groups. The results on other aspects of the data related to issues concerning drive content and schizophrenia are reported below.

TABLE 6.2
Analyses of Variances[1] for Scores on Drive-Dominated Thinking

	Tests of Significance		
	Diagnosis (DX) F (df = 3/151)	Sex (S) F (df = 1/151)	Interaction (DX × S) F (df = 3/151)
Socially modulated drive content	3.96[3]	5.19[2]	0.91
Primitive drive content, overall	4.96[3]	3.18	3.83[2]
Primitive sexual drive content	2.19	2.80	2.27
Primitive aggressive drive content	2.60	1.21	1.75
Primitive oral drive content	1.20	0.28	0.48
Primitive drive content, miscellaneous	1.31	0.04	0.48
Other types of deviant thinking and perception			
Deviant thought quality (TQ)	11.29[4]	0.37	1.95
Very poor form (F−)	4.55[3]	1.23	1.77
Number of responses	2.67[2]	1.58	1.43

[1]Anovas are based on percentage of each type of response (No. Resp. of Each Type/R) to control for number of responses.
[2]$P < .05$.
[3]$P < .01$
[4]$P < .001$

From Harrow, Quinlan, Wallington, & Pickett, *Journal of Personality Assessment, 40*, 31–41, 1976. Reproduced by permission of the publisher.

Expression of Socialized Drive Content

Although the major questions posed involve the appearance of primitive-drive-dominated content, we also analyzed the test material in regard to the appearance of more socially acceptable drive content (Holt's drive level 2). The data on socialized drive content also are presented in Tables 6.1 and 6.2. The results on this type of drive content are similar to those on primitive-drive-dominated thinking. More socially acceptable drive material also differed significantly according to diagnosis ($P < .01$), with schizophrenics showing more of this type of socialized drive content. However, individual Newman-Keuls tests indicated that the most prominent factor responsible for the overall significant trends was differences between the depressives and each of the other three diagnostic groups, rather than the differences being due to uniquely high scores for the schizophrenics. In addition, the presence of more socially acceptable drive content appeared among all diagnostic groups, with the depressives showing the lowest scores. One important feature of the results on this aspect of drive content concerns the data suggesting a tendency for the diagnostic differences to be as large for socialized drive material as for primitive drive material. This suggests that if drive content is more characteristic of schizophrenia, then it is drive-dominated thinking at all levels, related to both primitive and social content, rather than only primitive drive content.

Type of Primitive Drive Material That Emerged

To facilitate the study of this type of material further, the appearance of both primitive drive content and more socialized drive material was broken down into the particular types of drive material that appeared. Our major focus will be on the appearance of primitive drive material (Tables 6.1 and 6.2). Primitive aggressive drive content was the most common type of drive material that emerged for the relatively young, acute patient sample. The overall F for diagnosis showed a trend ($P < .06$) for higher scores on primitive aggressive drive content among the classical schizophrenics (Table 6.2). The Newman-Keuls test indicated that the schizophrenics were significantly higher than the depressives ($P < .05$). At the same time, primitive aggressive content was also relatively frequent in latent schizophrenics and patients with character pathology. Thus, again while classical schizophrenics were highest on this characteristic they were not significantly higher than latent schizophrenics or personality disorders.

Primitive Sexual and Oral Drive Material

Primitive sexual drive material was not too frequent among these acute, upper-middle-class patients. When it did appear, it occurred almost exclusively among the classical schizophrenics and latent schizophrenic or borderline patients, although the overall F test only showed a nonsignificant trend ($P < .10$) toward differences between the diagnostic groups. Primitive oral drive material was quite rare among almost any of these acute patients.

Defense Effectiveness

Another type of analysis conducted concerned the scoring of "defense effectiveness." The study of defense effectiveness (DE) was directed toward the hypothesis, frequently made by clinicians, that when schizophrenics fail to repress drive material, they do so in a manner that is more poorly defended than when nonschizophrenics verbalize this type of material. The results did not support this formulation; there was no significant difference between the mean DE scores of schizophrenic and acute nonschizophrenic patients on responses involving primitive drive-dominated content. We regard this as an issue that is still open to question, and further data in this area would be valuable.

Comparison of Results on Primitive Drive-Dominated Thinking with Results on Other Indexes of Disordered Thinking and Perception

The scores on two other indexes of disturbed thinking and perception—(a) deviant thought quality, and (b) very poor form level, or F- —were analyzed for the same patient sample (Quinlan, Harrow, and Carlson, 1973). Again, the measure of deviant thought quality represents our Rorschach index of bizarre-idiosyncratic thinking. The measure of very poor form level, of F-, is commonly viewed as a Rorschach measure of distorted perception or poor reality testing. The utilization of these two indexes allowed us to assess the relative prominence and importance of drive-dominated thinking in comparison to other major types of potential deviant thinking and perception. The ANOVAs were significant for these two other measures of disordered thinking and perception which are not based on the appearance of primitive drive content. In contrast to the results on drive-dominated thinking, the individual Newman-Keuls tests indicated that the classical schizophrenics were significantly higher than all three of the other diagnostic groups on both deviant thought quality and very poor form level ($P < .001$).

Results Using Schizophrenia (Sc) Scale of the MMPI

Another measure we utilized to obtain an independent assessment of hypotheses in this area was the schizophrenia (Sc) Scale of the

MMPI. Scores of the indices of primitive drive content were related significantly to the Sc (schizophrenia) scale (see Table 6.3). The Sc score is frequently elevated in schizophrenic patients, although high scores on this scale are not exclusive to psychotic or schizophrenic patients. The Sc scale is composed of diverse kinds of items. These include questions tapping bizarre and unusual thoughts and behavior as well as items that assess isolation, dissatisfaction, alienation, and other dimensions. Thus, some nonschizophrenics, especially borderline patients who feel depressed and isolated, can obtain high scores on the Sc scale.

The Process-Reactive Dimension

Another type of analysis we conducted is associated with the process-reactive dimension in schizophrenia. Differences between process and reactive schizophrenics have been reported in a number of areas (Kantor and Herron, 1966), and we also have attempted to determine whether process or reactive schizophrenics are characterized by greater expression of primitive drive-dominated thinking. Our results indicated that while diagnosis influenced the extent of drive content, within a sample of *early* acute schizophrenics the process-reactive dimension did not differentiate the amount of drive material that appeared. Thus, among this acute schizophrenic sample, there were no significant differences in expression of drive content between process and reactive schizophrenics, using a modified version of the Phillips Scale (Bromet, Harrow, and Kasl, 1974) to assess this dimension.

Chronic Schizophrenia and Drive-Dominated Thinking

The research we conducted on primitive-drive-dominated thinking is based on a sample of relatively early schizophrenics. In regard to the relationship between schizophrenia and the scores for socially unacceptable drive content, it is possible that greater difficulty in repressing primitive drive material might be found among more desocialized and more deteriorated chronic schizophrenics. If primitive drive-dominated thinking is more common in chronic, multiyear schizophrenics (and as yet this possibility is undocumented), the question would arise as to whether or not it is a natural feature of deterioration over the course of the schizophrenic disorder, perhaps associated with a decline in social skills. One alternate possibility is that *if* it is more frequent in chronic schizophrenics, it is *not* intrinsic to the course of schizophrenia and is instead related to a lack of social prohibitions against the expression of primitive drives in some chronic hospital settings. Thus, one factor that could increase the appearance of

TABLE 6.3

Correlations between Primitive-Drive-Dominated Thinking and Rule-Breaking Behavior and Other Personality Variables

	Wrongdoing (N = 99)	Modified Wrongdoing (N = 99)	OOH dependency (N = 62)	Barron ego strength (N = 113)	Taylor anxiety (N = 67)	MMPI depression (N = 113)	MMPI Psych. Dev. (N = 113)	MMPI Schiz. (N = 113)	MMPI manic (N = 113)	OOH aggression (N = 62)
Overall primitive drive content	.46**	.49**	.06	−.23*	.13	.02	.29**	.40**	.42**	.20
Primitive sexual drive content	.27**	.27**	−.01	−.10	.03	−.09	.08	.12	.19*	−.12
Primitive aggressive drive content	.43**	.50**	.06	−.09	.16	.08	.26**	.32**	.34**	.31*
Primitive oral drive content	.23*	.24*	.09	−.22*	.23	.08	.17	.30**	.27**	.20
Primitive drive content, miscellaneous	.12	.07	.02	−.24*	.03	−.06	.08	.15	.18	−.01

*P < .05
**P < .01

From Harrow, Quinlan, Wallington, & Pickett, *Journal of Personality Assessment, 40,* 31–41, 1976. Reproduced by permission of the publisher.

primitive-drive-dominated content, could be the "permission" to express it, which could occur in certain subcultures and in selective situations. These might include the back wards of some state hospitals, and other select situations such as can be seen in mob actions and in certain wartime situations.

Further Research on Drive-Dominated Thinking in Schizophrenia

Recently our research team conducted a further study to determine whether drive is a major factor in schizophrenic thought pathology, using a new sample and a different technique: responses to a verbal task followed by extensive interviews about the responses. The results are in agreement with our earlier data. Again, we did not find evidence supporting formulations about the importance of the emergence of primitive drive-dominated thinking as a factor influencing thought pathology for most early schizophrenics (Harrow and Prosen, 1978).

Summary of Diagnostic Comparisons for Schizophrenics

The above information on drive-dominated thinking and schizophrenia provides preliminary answers to a number of questions in this area. The data indicate that the emergence of socially unacceptable drive material in patients' responses is not an exclusively schizophrenic phenomenon. It was more common in schizophrenics, with 71 per cent of the classical schizophrenics showing some (often weak) signs of primitive drive-dominated thinking. Other diagnostic groups, however, particularly latent schizophrenics, borderline patients, and acutely disturbed personality disorders, do show some emergence of primitive aggressive drive material. The data suggest that the significant differences among the diagnostic groups on drive-dominated content were influenced by the low scores by the depressed patients, although the higher scores by the schizophrenics also played some limited role.

In terms of the major question, separate scoring of the Rorschach for deviant thought quality or positive thought disorder, the score based on a comprehensive index of bizarre and idiosyncratic verbalizations, suggested that the schizophrenics were significantly more thought disordered in this particular area ($P < .001$). The significantly higher scores of the classical schizophrenics on the measure of bizarre-idiosyncratic thinking are in contrast to the less clear-cut differences on drive-dominated content.

Depression and Drive-Dominated Thinking

Hypotheses have been advanced concerning the importance of both oral and aggressive drive material in the dynamics of depression. The data in Tables 6.1 and 6.2 (especially the Newman-Keuls tests comparing the depressives with the personality disorders, with the borderline patients, and with the schizophrenics) suggest that the emergence of drive material is relatively rare in primary depressive disorders, and is significantly higher in other types of disturbed patients. Thus, our results did not support the forumulations that link oral and aggressive drive content to depression. Our research suggests that a characteristic of many patients with primary depressive disorders is a lack of drive-dominated thinking. In some respects, the data indicating a lack of drive-dominated thinking in depression may provide tentative support for older formulations that a key characteristic of some types of depressive disorders is an anergic state.

Since we did not systematically investigate all types of depression, it is possible that the hypotheses linking the presence of certain types of drive material to depressive syndromes may be accurate for select groups of depressives. As an example of one of many possibilities, some factor-analytic studies have reported evidence in some depressives of factors involving behavior that could be characterized as angry, demanding, and complaining (Grinker et al., 1961; Friedman et al., 1963). This behavior, however, is usually felt to be more characteristic of certain "neurotic" depressives and other milder and non-classical types of depressives. These are not the main types of depressives who formed the basis for the major formulations about oral and aggressive drive material and depression. While our results do not necessarily apply to every type of depressive, since our sample was limited, they do suggest that primitive drive material is not a prominent characteristic of all or most depressives.

It is still possible that some types of drive content are important at an unconscious level in depression, and that not even small traces of these emerge into consciousness. Before any assurance could be placed on this type of formulation, however, considerable documentation at some level would be needed. Overall, depressive patients may be "needy" because of their disorder, but simple straightforward hypotheses about primitive *oral* drive material emerging at conscious or preconscious levels in most types of depression have not been supported in our research.

Sociopathic Behavior and Drive-Dominated Thinking

The major focus of our research on drive-dominated thinking has been on its relation to schizophrenia. In addition, we have attempted to investigate its relevance to depression and to other types of disordered behavior. A type of behavior that our clinical observations of both inpatients and outpatients have led us to hypothesize may be related to drive-dominated thinking is sociopathic behavior. Table 6.3 presents our results on the relationships we found among our patients between primitive-drive-dominated thinking and rule-breaking behavior and other personality variables. The data in Table 6.3 suggest that socio-pathic behavior is related to primitive drive-dominated thinking. The correlations were significant between drive-dominated thinking and: (1) a history of rule-breaking behavior, as assessed on the MMPI Wrongdoing Scales (Lowe, 1961), and (2) high scores on the Ma scale of the MMPI. High Ma scores on the MMPI are often found in people who are hypomanic, overactive, impulsive, and relatively uninhibited.

The particular type of drive-dominated thinking was also examined more closely to determine which specific kind of drive content is most clearly associated with rule-breaking behavior. The results suggested that the strongest relationship is between aggressive drive material and rule-breaking behavior ($P < .01$) A similar pattern was found for the Ma scale. The relationship between sexual drive content and rule-breaking behavior was also significant, but not as strong as the one found for aggressive drive material.

Overview of Results of Relationship between Primitive-Drive Dominated Thinking and Sociopathic Tendencies

The data indicating that deviant acting-out behavior was related to the appearance of primitive-drive-dominated thinking support our hypothesis that rule-breaking or sociopathic behavior in disturbed adolescents and young adults is a frequent characteristic of more impulsive, drive-dominated individuals. One aspect of these data is that the results provide a link between a type of cognitive disturbance (the emergence of primitive drive-dominated thinking) and a type of social behavior (rule breaking). In another phase of our research, reported in Chapter 13, we have studied characteristics of disturbed hallucinogen users and found that high scores on drive-dominated thinking are a relatively frequent feature of disturbed hallucinogen users, regardless of diagnosis.

The positive relationship between primitive-drive-dominated think-ing and rule-breaking behavior (there was not as high a relationship with more socialized drive content) could provide clues concerning a factor influencing some sociopathic behavior. Obviously, sociopathic behavior does not represent a uniform phenomenon. Rather, diverse behaviors are involved, and they are related to and influenced by a variety of different types of factors. Our data provide evidence on one such variable that may influence it. Thus, we would propose that in some patients (and presumably in some "normals"), rule-breaking and antisocial behavior is difficult for the person to control completely, because of background physiological difficulties that are related to high energy levels, restlessness, and strong drives that the person cannot control or direct at will. These background drives, which are not completely under control, could manifest themselves in the form of primitive, drive-dominated thinking, and impulsive or "driven" sociopathic behavior.

Sex

Significant and near significant results concerning sex differences on three of the drive variables suggest that sex has some influence on the overt expression of drive content, although it is not a very powerful or dominant variable. Thus, the data on the sex of the patient as an influence on drive content (see Table 6.2) indicate that males had higher scores than females on modulated or socially acceptable expression of drive content (e.g., "a person eating ice cream," or "a man and woman kissing") ($P < .05$). Males also showed a nonsignificant tendency to be higher on overall primitive drive content ($P < .10$) and on primitive sexual drive content ($P < .10$).

Taken together, these results suggest that the sex of the subject may be a minor factor in terms of the emergence of drive content. The lack of a significant sex difference on primitive drive content was partly a function of relatively high scores on primitive drive content for a number of female patients with personality disorders and borderline states, and relatively low scores for a number of male personality disorders. This result was most prominent for overall primitive drive content where the interaction between sex and diagnosis was significant ($P < .05$) (see Table 6.2).

The influence that sex *does* exert could be related, in part, to differences in the strength of certain innate drives. The literature on innate sex differences in certain areas has always been controversial. Recently there have appeared a series of reports presenting further evidence to support formulations about biological differences between the sexes in temperament, activities, and on other dimensions. Regardless of whether or not these biological factors prove important, differences in the ways society treats males and females, and different standards set for them undoubtedly play a role. Hence the higher scores on the drive variables could be a product of the combination of (a) biological differences between the sexes in the strength of innate drives, and (b) differences in social training and expectations related to the greater discouragement for females of the overt expression of primitive aggressive (and other) drive material.

Relationship between Different Types of Drive-Dominated Thinking

Table 6.4 reports the correlations between the different types of primitive drive material. In the sample of patients we studied the relationships between the different types of drive-dominated thinking (e.g., sexual, oral, aggressive) were not significant in most cases. In particular, the relationship between the emergence of primitive sexual and aggressive material was relatively low ($r = .07$), providing some support for the usual distinction made between sexual (or libidinal) and aggressive drives. The only significant relationship between the various indices of primitive drive-dominated thinking was a significant correlation between oral and aggressive drive content ($P < .01$).

Additional support for the separation of the different types of drive-dominated thinking occurred with the significant relationships between the patients' scores for primitive, socially unacceptable drive-dominated thinking of each type, and the appearance of more socially acceptable drive content of the same type (e.g., primitive aggressive drive versus more socialized aggressive drive, $r = .32$, $df = 169$, $P < .01$; and primitive sexual drive versus more socialized sexual drive, $r = .33$, $df = 169$, $P < .01$). This would further suggest that the emergence of drive material, including primitive drive content, does not occur in a completely undifferentiated manner, even in such disorganized patients as many of the acute schizophrenics we studied. Rather, the particular

TABLE 6.4
Correlations between Different Types of
Primitive-Drive-Dominated Thinking (171 Subjects)

	Primitive aggressive drive content	Primitive oral drive content	Primitive drive content, miscellaneous
Primitive sexual drive content	.07	.11	.10
Primitive aggressive drive content		.45*	−.01
Primitive oral drive content			.01

*$P < .01$.

type of drive material seems to be an important factor, and shows some degree of specificity for the particular patient involved. Our results in this area are suggestive, but further information on this topic, using other types of samples (e.g., normals) and other types of data-collection techniques, would seem valuable to enable more definitive formulations on differences between the various types of primitive drive-dominated thinking (e.g., sexual versus aggressive) and the consequence of these differences.

ASSESSMENT OF THE CONSTRUCT OF DRIVE-DOMINATED THINKING

In looking at the overall results, issues arise concerning the nature of the construct of "drive," as well as the criteria to assess drive and drive-dominated thinking. In terms of the *concept* itself, as used in clinical work and in theoretical discussions, "drive" can best be viewed as a construct designed to integrate and "explain" a range of observations about human behavior, rather than as a visible entity. Although the focus in this chapter is on *primitive* drive content, over the years the concept of drive has been used in a variety of ways that are not linked to "primitive" material, with many of them focusing on the role of drive in normal human learning and personality. One major theory of schizophrenic disorganization and thought disorder, utilizing this latter type of drive concept, has been proposed by Broen (1968), and by Storms and Broen (1969, 1972). Their theory of thought disorder, influenced by Hull and Spence, emphasizes a breakdown in the hierarchical order of dominant and competing responses resulting from an interaction of high drive levels and low response strength ceilings.

Thus, drive has been a widely employed construct and has seemed useful. The concept is still on the construct level, although support for it can be found in a variety of easily observed overt behaviors that can be *interpreted* to fit the construct.

In terms of the *assessment* of drive and related constructs, our data suggest that primitive drive-dominated thinking is not a major factor in early schizophrenia. As we shall suggest shortly, we believe that impaired perspective and monitoring difficulties are factors that influence the data in this area.

In terms of a broader view of the construct of primitive-drive-dominated thinking, whether or not the overt and/or partially covert expressions of content that include drive-related themes are really expressions of primitive (and socialized) drive forces within people is still an open question. Since there is no absolute criterion of drive-dominated thinking, one possibility is that Holt's system is not a good method for assessing this construct; this possibility cannot be discounted completely. However, much formal research conducted by a number of investigators in a variety of settings would seem to provide support to Holt's technique for getting at drive-dominated content. Thus, the accumulation of research supporting Holt's technique of assessment provides some evidence that the present results bear on the relationship between schizophrenia and primitive drive content, rather than these results being due to an inadequate method of assessing the construct. The issue, however, is not a closed one at the present time.

OVERVIEW OF RESULTS ON DRIVE-DOMINATED THINKING IN SCHIZOPHRENIA

Our research on drive content was prompted by two major questions. One involved issues about primitive drive-dominated thinking as a key factor in early schizophrenia. The other, which we have also reported above, involved questions about the relationships between drive content and other key factors, such as select types of psychopathology (i.e., depression and sociopathic behavior), and select other variables such as sex.

In regard to the major question that prompted our research in this particular area—namely, the issue of the possible presence of drive-dominated thinking as a key factor in *early* schizophrenia—the overall results do not support theoretical views about its importance.

Our research in this area suggests that among relatively early schizophrenics, difficulty in preventing the emergence of drive-dominated thinking is not the major factor in accounting for their cognitive disorder, although it may have some minor influence. Looked at from another angle, our research data would seem to indicate that the emergence of socially unacceptable drive material is related to a number of factors. Schizophrenia is one of them. The trend toward primary process thinking of this type, however, was not exclusive to schizophrenics. Rather, the results suggest that it is found in a number of different types of disturbed patients, with the exception of the primary depressive disorders.

Considered in terms of a broader overall construct, *the concept of primary process thinking,* clear implications can be drawn from the significant differences between acute schizophrenics and all three significant differences between acute schizophrenics and all three nonschizophrenic groups on bizarre speech and poor reality testing (F-). They indicate that *some aspects* of what has usually been considered *primary process thinking* (factors such as bizarre-idiosyncratic thinking) are among the factors that are more characteristic or different about schizophrenia, and select other psychotic disorders (i.e., severe manic disorders). In contrast, the data on the appearance of primitive drive-dominated thinking suggest that this particular aspect of what has been regarded as primary process thinking does not strongly differentiate acute schizophrenic from disturbed nonschizophrenic patients, although it may account for a small percentage of the variance.

While the previous empirical literature in this area is relatively sparse, our research results on the relationship to schizophrenia of (1) drive-dominated thinking, and (2) other aspects of "primary process thinking" are in agreement with a study conducted by Silverman, Lapkin, and Rosenbaum (1962). Using a different type of sample (the young schizophrenic sample used by Silverman and colleagues was not at the acute stage and was from a long-term residential treatment center), they found no significant differences between their schizophrenic and nonschizophrenic patients for scores on primitive drive content. They also contrasted their measure of drive content with other "formal" measures of disordered thinking and found greater differences between the schizophrenics and nonschizophrenics among the other measures of disturbed thinking. Even the differences between their other measures of disordered thinking for the schizophrenics, as opposed to the nonschizophrenic patients, were barely significant and in a number of cases were nonsignificant. This may have been influenced by their samples being past the most acute stage usually found at the beginning of hospitalization. Overall, the present results on schizophrenic versus nonschizophrenic patients and Silverman's results form a relatively uniform set of findings: only little or no diagnostic differences in the appearance of primitive drive content and greater differences on other aspects of disordered thinking. This consistency occurred despite the fact that the two sets of findings are based on young schizophrenic samples from different types of institutions at different phases of their disorder.

DRIVE-DOMINATED THINKING AND IMPAIRMENT IN PERSPECTIVE AND MONITORING

In taking an overview of the results on the emergence of primitive drive-dominated thinking, our mixed data do suggest the possibility of a weak trend toward more drive-dominated thinking in some early schizophrenics. The trend, however, is too weak to lead us to believe that drive-dominated thinking is a major factor for all or most schizophrenics at this phase of their disorder. It is possible that drive-dominated thinking is a minor factor that emerges in select schizophrenics as a consequence of other more important factors.

One possibility that we would suggest and that would fit in with our view about the importance in schizophrenia of impaired perspective and monitoring difficulties is that the emergence of drive-dominated content sometimes seen in early schizophrenia may be influenced by two factors: (1) there may be some real difficulty in monitoring and adjusting one's speech on a moment-to moment basis, leading to the overt appearance of socially unacceptable verbalizations during periods of internal turmoil and extreme upset—with a tendency toward less adequate monitoring of many different types of material during such periods of extreme upset (e.g., a difficulty in monitoring both drive-dominated and non-drive-dominated material); and (2) there may be some difficulty in maintaining adequate perspective or judgment about what types of verbalizations and what types of conscious thinking are socially appropriate during early schizophrenia. This impaired perspective or impaired judgment about how inappropriate the emergence of this material would sound to a neutral observer could result in the seeming failure of some schizophrenics to repress drive-dominated content. Thus, at the time of its emergence, these patients would not even recognize how inappropriate its overt appearance is in terms of consensual social norms. Since the drive-dominated content would be only one of a number of different types of socially inappropriate material that could appear as a result of impaired perspective, it would not automatically be the most prominent disordered feature to be seen in the patients' speech. According to this view, one would expect, sometimes, to see primitive drive-dominated content as one of a number of possible disordered features of schizophrenic speech, and not necessarily as the most prominent one.

7

Abstract and Concrete Thinking

"Concreteness" is an aspect of thinking frequently linked to the schizophrenic thought disorder (Chapman and Chapman, 1973). In its most direct form, concrete thinking involves difficulty in rising above the immediate level of the stimulus. The patient who responds to the proverb, "Don't swap horses when crossing a stream," with "Don't trade horses when crossing a stream because you might get wet," displays concreteness. Increased concreteness is a feature sometimes found in brain-damaged individuals. The view that a disturbance in the abstract-concrete dimension is a prominent feature of disordered schizophrenic language and thinking is widely held.

The loss of abstract ability, or an increase in concrete thinking, can be viewed as a deficit symptom. As we have noted earlier, major theorists have grouped under the concept of negative symptoms various deficit symptoms and defect state symptoms that involve a deficit in, or an absense of, normal functioning (e.g., Chapman and Chapman, 1973). Among the cognitive symptoms that have been included under this concept are impoverished thinking, concrete thinking, poor intellectual functioning or intellectual deficits, and psychomotor retardation, although a number of other symptoms have been included as well.

Concrete thinking represents one of the more widely studied deficit or negative symptoms in schizophrenia. Some prominent theorists have considered concreteness as one of the essential features of schizophrenia (Arieti, 1974; Benjamin, 1944; Goldstein, 1944; Vigotsky, 1962). Thus, the presumed loss of ability to abstract successfully occupies a key place in theoretical conceptualizations about schizophrenia and has been used by some clinicians as an important diagnostic sign for this particular disorder. As a result of the widespread beliefs about its importance, and its key role as a deficit symptom, we chose to investigate the abstract-concrete dimension in our research on major theories of disordered schizophrenic cognition. Aspects of our research in this area, which are presented in this chapter, have been described in a series of reports (Harrow and Adler, 1974; Harrow, Adler, and Hanf, 1974; Harrow, Buckley-Marengo, Growe, and Grinker, 1979; Harrow, Marengo, Pogue-Geile, and Pawelski, in press; Harrow, Tucker, and Adler, 1972; Marengo and Harrow, 1979).

In terms of the original development of ideas about the importance of concreteness in the 1930s, Vigotsky viewed the essence of the schizophrenic thought disorder as the loss of ability to think in abstract concepts (Vigotsky, 1962). Kurt Goldstein developed parallel concepts of the categorical or the concrete attitude in patients with organic brain injuries and applied them to the problem of schizophrenic thinking (Goldstein, 1944; Goldstein and Scheerer, 1941). In later work, Goldstein emphasized that concrete thinking in schizophrenia is different from that found in many organic patients, noting that in schizophrenia its occurrence is selective. Although Goldstein at first seemed to regard concreteness as a basic factor in schizophrenia, in later writings he viewed concreteness as a protective mechanism against anxiety that originated in early stages of development (Goldstein, 1959). Among the early theorists in this area, Benjamin (1944) has also reported on the importance of concreteness, with his reports even suggesting that it is a more important feature in schizophrenia than it is in organic disorders.

Over the years several investigators who have developed multiple-choice, paper-and pencil tests to assess hypotheses concerning concrete thinking and related types of thinking in schizophrenia have reported positive results. These include both Gorham (1956) and L. Chapman (1960).

In many areas concerned with behavior disorders there has been considerable disagreement over how to define the basic concepts involved. There has been some variation in definitions about abstract and concrete thinking (this is discussed later in this chapter), but many recent investigators have been in rough agreement about these constructs. We view the constructs of abstract and concrete thinking as representing endpoints on a continuum marking the degree that one can go beyond the immediate specific stimulus situation or one's immediate specific experiences and shift one's thinking into less specific, more general, and more symbolic modes.

In the research we conducted, we utilized several techniques to assess the abstract-concrete dimension, including both verbal tests and sorting tests. In terms of the latter, we have used the Object Sorting test as one of the instruments to assess concrete thinking. Concreteness on the Object Sorting test is evaluated by assessing whether or not the patient has difficulty seeing or is unable to see more general dimensions associated with a stimulus object on the Sorting test. We also used a Proverbs test, and proverb interpretation, as another key technique to investigate the abstract-concrete dimension in schizophrenia. We regard the use of the Proverbs test as our most important method of assessing such deficit or negative symptoms as loss of abstract thinking. Concreteness on the Proverbs test refers to the tendency to use the key words and ideas in a phrase from a proverb in their original, nondecoded form. The patient tends not to translate the two units of the proverb into other phrases with more general or different meanings (e.g., "Shallow brooks are noisy" is interpreted concretely as "The water hits the rocks and makes noises").

While there have been earlier reports finding concrete thinking in schizophrenics, such as those of Benjamin (1944) and Goldstein (1944), the more recent literature on the importance of concrete thinking in schizophrenia has been mixed, with both positive and negative results (Brattemo, 1962; Cancro, 1969; Carson, 1962; L. Chapman, 1960; Maher, 1972; Oltmanns and Neale, 1978; Pavy, 1968; Payne and Hewlett, 1960; Reed, 1968; Saltzman, 1966; Watson, Wold, and Kucala, 1976; Wright, 1975).

Pishkin and Bourne have conducted sophisticated research in this general area, studying schizophrenic concept formation and problem solving. Their research suggests that schizophrenics can perform at certain levels of abstraction, but that they show deficits at other, more symbolic levels of abstraction (Pishkin and Bourne, 1981; Pishkin, Lovallo, Lenk, and Bourne, 1977). Shimkunas has used the mixed results on abstraction, along with the results of his own research (Shimkunas, 1970; Shimkunas, Gynther, and Smith, 1966; 1967), to propose a theory in which schizophrenics are seen as overgeneralizing and overabstract (Shimkunas, 1972).

The research we have conducted has been directed toward clarifying these disparate findings. Although much attention has been directed toward the abstract-concrete dimension, a number of factors that may

be important influences on the level of abstract thinking in schizophrenia have not been investigated systematically. Hence, a series of
questions remain unanswered about the role of concreteness in
schizophrenia.

If concreteness does play a role in schizophrenic thinking, is it a
central feature of all schizophrenic subjects, or of only chronic deteriorated schizophrenic patients? Much of the research reporting
concrete thinking as a prominent feature in schizophrenia is based on
work with chronic schizophrenic patients. It is quite conceivable that a
deficit or negative symptom such as a loss of abstract ability is a
characteristic of chronic schizophrenics, but (1) is only a product of the
"natural" downhill course of this type of schizophrenic patient, or (2) is
only a byproduct of factors not intrinsic to schizophrenia. These include
factors such as the institutionalization of chronically disordered people
(Wing and Brown, 1970), lack of social stimulation, and lack of verbal
demands on the patient. Although concrete thinking could be important
in institutionalized chronic schizophrenic patients, these patients may
represent the end-product of a select subgroup of schizophrenic
patients who originally had a more acute disorder (i.e., the subgroup
who later had continous hospitalization).

Another question related to these more general issues concerns
whether concrete thinking (and a deficit in abstract thinking) is a feature
of schizophrenic thought during the early stages of the disorder. If
concrete thinking is one of the primary symptoms of schizophrenia,
then this type of deficit or negative symptom should be present in the
early phases, such as during the acute phase.

The question of whether concrete thinking is present during the
acute stage is one of key theoretical importance. If concrete thinking is
not prominent during early phases, it would be hard to support
formulations that it is a *primary* factor leading to the disorder, or leading
to deficits in other areas, for the early schizophrenic patient.

Another key issue is related to cognitive deficits and negative
symptoms in schizophrenia as a function of the particular phase of the
disorder. If acute schizophrenic patients do show deficit in this area,
does their tendency toward concrete thinking then diminish as they
emerge from the acute or active phase and as their symptomatology in
other areas diminishes? In addition, if schizophrenic patients shift from
a concrete to a more abstract mode as they recover from the acute
phase, it becomes important to determine whether *nonschizophrenic*
patients also improve in this area as their general symptom level
diminishes. A similar improvement in nonschizophrenic patients might
provide clues about possible background mechanisms influencing the
level of concrete thinking. It might suggest that the deficit in abstract

thinking is a function of the acute or active phase of psychiatric disturbance and is not specific to schizophrenia.

Systematic investigations of the course of schizophrenic thinking in a longitudinal framework are relatively rare. Shimkunas, Gynther, and Smith (1966, 1967), while investigating the short-term course of abtract and concrete thinking, provided some data on changes in thinking during a five-week period for a series of schizophrenic patients recovering from an acute episode. Their data suggested decreasing concreteness during this five-week period for their average- and above-average-intelligence schizophrenics. Their research, however, did not include a control group of acutely disturbed nonschizophrenic patients. This type of research design makes it difficult to determine whether the schizophrenic patients are more concrete than nonschizophrenic patients at various phases, and whether any changes in concreteness are unique to the course of schizophrenia or are influenced by decreasing disturbances regardless of the type of disorder.

QUESTIONS POSED

The general plan of our research in this area was to investigate a number of samples of schizophrenic and nonschizophrenic patients on the abstract-concrete dimension during several phases of their disorder, using three key types of tests. These included two verbal tests, and one performance test (Object Sorting) which is less dependent on verbal skills. The plan involved studying one of the samples at the acute phase and then reassessing it at a second phase of disorder, as the sample began to emerge from the acute period into the phase of partial recovery. Another sample is currently being studied over a longer period at several phases of their disorder, with data having been collected on them at the acute phase, and early data available a year later at follow-up. In addition, we have studied and have data available on several samples of long-term, chronic, schizophrenics, who were studied in order to obtain a more complete picture of concreteness at different stages of the schizophrenic disorder.

Several important factors that may influence or even determine the level of concrete (and abstract) thinking in these samples have been studied. This led to a research design in which the following series of questions about possible influences on the level of concrete and abstract thinking in schizophrenia were posed:

1. Are all schizophrenics concrete? Is diagnosis (in terms of *schizophrenia*) an important influence on the abstract-concrete dimension?
2. Does acute disturbance or acute upset influence the level of abstract thinking, independent of diagnosis?
3. Is the phase of the schizophrenic disorder an influence or a determinant of the level of concrete and abstract thinking?
4. Are chronic schizophrenics more concrete than acute schizophrenics?
5. Is the level of concrete thinking in schizophrenics related to the type of schizophrenic disorder, in terms of process or reactive schizophrenia?
6. Is the level of concrete thinking related to idiosyncratic thinking or bizarre thinking in schizophrenic and in nonschizophrenic patients?
7. Does intelligence influence the level of concrete thinking in schizophrenic and nonschizophrenic patients?
8. How does potential concrete thinking and a deficit in abstract ability fit into an overall view of thought pathology?

SAMPLES STUDIED

To answer the above questions about the role played by a deficit in abstract thinking in schizophrenia, three samples of patients were studied, with the investigation covering four different phases of the schizophrenic disorder. These three samples include the following:

A. Sample 7A included sixty-four psychiatric patients (thirty-two schizophrenic and thirty-two nonschizophrenic patients). From the Chicago Followup Study (Harrow, Grinker, et al., 1978; Harrow, Silverstein and Marengo, 1983; Pogue-Geile and Harrow, 1984). Half of each of these samples was from Michael Reese Hospital and Medical Center, and half from the Illinois State Psychiatric Institute. These relatively young patients (mean age = 23 years at the time of their index hospitalizations) were studied for concrete thinking using the Object Sorting test, during the first three weeks of hospitalization (the acute phase) and then followed up a little over a year later.
B. Sample 7B included 121 young psychiatric patients from Yale-New Haven Hospital. All 121 of these patients were studied during the

first ten days of acute hospitalization (acute phase), with the Proverbs and Similarities tests. Ninety-five of these patients were reassessed with the same instruments six to eight weeks later, during the period of partial recovery. These ninety-five patients, studied at two phases of their disorder, included twenty-five relatively young classical schizophrenics (mean age = 21 years), twenty-three latent schizophrenics, and forty-seven disturbed non-schizophrenic patients.

C. Sample 7C included thirty-two multiyear, chronic schizophrenics from a state hospital. The median length of hospitalization of these thirty-two chronic schizophrenics was fourteen years (chronic phase). These patients were assessed on the abstract-concrete dimension with the Proverbs and Similarities tests.

ASSESSMENT OF THE ABSTRACT-CONCRETE DIMENSION

Proverbs and Similarities Tests

To assess abstract and concrete thinking, and changes in them over time, two of the three patient samples (samples 7B and 7C) were administered thirteen proverbs from the Benjamin Proverbs Test, and a test of Similarities. We view proverbs tests, in general, as ranking among the best methods of evaluating performance on the abstract-concrete dimension. Several standard scoring systems were used to assess the abstract-concrete dimension, as well as several new ones that we developed specifically for our research.

Scales can be derived from the Proverbs test to assess both abstract and concrete thinking. Three scales that we used from the Proverbs test to assess abstract thinking involve: (1) a standard measure of abstract thinking previously constructed and used successfully by Meadow and and Greenblatt (Meadow, Greenblatt, and Funkenstein, 1953; Meadow, Greenblatt, Solomon, and Funkenstein, 1953); (2) a scale constructed by our research team, based on the number of correct abstract responses; and (3) a scale we derived based on all abstract responses, regardless of whether or not they were correct, incorrect, or bizarre. These three measures are described briefly in a previous report (Harrow, Adler, and Hanf, 1974), and more fully in a detailed manual (Marengo, Harrow, and Rogers, 1980).

Two indexes derived from the *Similarities Scale* of the WAIS (Wechsler, 1955) were utilized. The Similarities Scale, which has often been used as a measure of abstract ability, consists of thirteen pairs of words for which a similarity must be found (e.g., orange-banana, both are fruit). One of the two scales (the Total Score) was the standard scoring system described in the WAIS manual (Wechsler, 1955). The other score derived from the Similarities Scale involved the absolute number of correct (abstract) responses by a subject. In this latter system, each correct abstract response was assigned a point, and partially correct answers were not given credit.

Object Sorting Test

One of the three patient samples (sample 7A), which included patients studied at two different phases of their disorder, was administered Part I of the Goldstein-Scheerer Object Sorting Test and scored for concrete thinking. The Object Sorting Test permitted the use of an instrument that is less dependent on verbal learning or verbal skills. Scores for sorting objects in a concrete way on the Object Sorting Test are measured by whether the patient has difficulty seeing, or is unable to see, more general dimensions associated with a stimulus object on the sorting test. A more complete description of this scoring system is described in our manual on the Object Sorting Test (Himmelhoch, Harrow, Tucker, and Hersh, 1973).

We have discussed in detail in a recent report the type of conceptual behavior required by the structure of the Proverbs and Object Sorting tests. We have also discussed in detail issues concerning similarities and differences between the type of abstract and concrete performance assessed with the Proverbs and Object Sorting tests (Harrow, Marengo, Pogue-Geile, and Pawelski, in press).

DO SCHIZOPHRENICS SHOW A DEFICIT
IN ABSTRACT THINKING?

The Abstract-Concrete Dimension

A short discussion would seem appropriate on the issue of whether or not abstract and concrete thinking belong on the same dimension, and if they do, whether they represent opposite ends of a continuum.

It has usually been assumed that abstract and concrete thinking do belong on the same dimension, with some theorists stating this explicitly, and others apparently assuming it without explicitly stating it, using such terms as "concrete" to represent nonabstract thinking, or using the term "abstract" to represent nonconcrete thinking.

Some theorists, however, have put other types of thinking on this dimension, and/or have assumed that abstract and concrete are *not opposite* ends of the dimension.

Classical theorists such as Vigotsky (1962) have contrasted abstract thinking with thinking in "complexes," with this being one type of concrete thinking. Vigotsky felt that the major characteristic of schizophrenic thought pathology is "a regression to a more primitive level called thinking in concrete complexes" (Vigotsky, 1962).

Other theorists, such as Kurt Goldstein (1944), have considered bizarre and idiosyncratic thinking as "concrete," and contrasted this type of thinking with abstract thinking. A problem with this latter type of classification system involves the point or place on this dimension where one could place thinking that is *both* abstract and idiosyncratic. As can be seen from the material presented in Chapter 3, in our own research we have come across a number of examples of abstract idiosyncratic responses.

A second tendency is to consider abstract and concrete thinking as belonging on the same dimension, but not to consider abstract and concrete as opposite ends of the continuum. As we have noted earlier, this can be seen in a recent analysis by Shimkunas, who hypothesizes that concrete thinking or *under*generalization (or underinclusion) represents the low end of a continuum, and autistic responses or *over*generalizing (or overinclusion or insufficient discrimination) represents the opposite end of the continuum. In this formulation, abstract thinking represents a point somewhere inbetween these two ends of the continuum (Shimkunas, 1972).

In our own analysis we have assumed that abstract and concrete thinking belong on the same dimension, and can be placed at the opposite ends of the continuum. We believe, however, that there are many responses that are neither extremely abstract nor extremely concrete, and thus fall somewhere in the middle, perhaps leaning slightly toward one or the other end of the continuum.

Since there are many responses that illustrate some middle points, we believe scores on abstract and concrete thinking may not move perfectly together in reciprocal fashion, as the absence of a concrete response may be an abstract response, or it may be a response somewhere in the middle of the continuum, with this response not being quite concrete, and yet not being completely abstract either. The dimension is not a perfect one. The first step in defining a continuum such as the abstract-concrete one is to define how, or at what point on the continuum, various types of responses will be placed. After the definition has been established, then it is an empirical matter as to whether or not abstract and concrete thinking move perfectly together (at the opposite ends of the continuum) and whether or not scores on abstract and concrete thinking move in exact reciprocal fashion.

Since, as we have noted earlier, we do not understand normal thinking well at the present time (normal thinking on both the abstract-concrete dimension and other aspects of normal thinking also), caution should be exercised in any formulations made in this area.

In general, our research suggests that for reasonably intelligent people, at the middle and upper ends of the ability level, scores on correct abstract thinking often will discriminate better than scores on concrete thinking, as far as possible cognitive deficits in schizophrenia are concerned. This is because for people of high ability levels, even with deficits in their ability, usually only a limited reduction in performance can be expected, rather than a complete inability to function at all. Thus, for people at a medium or high level of ability, the cognitive impairment due to psychopathology leads to deficits in abstract performance or reduced levels of abstract ability, rather than totally concrete behavior. The work of some others would seem to support this.

Information from the Object Sorting Test on Concrete Thinking at the Acute Phase

Table 7.1 presents the results on concrete thinking at the acute phase for sample 7A, a group of sixty-four relatively young schizophrenic and nonschizophrenic patients from our Chicago settings, using their data from the Object Sorting test. The results reported in Table 7.1 on concrete thinking for these sixty-four patients showed significant differences between the schizophrenic and the nonschizophrenic patients ($P < .05$). These results from the Object Sorting test do suggest more concreteness for the schizophrenics, even in early stages of their disorder.

Perhaps of greater importance concerning formulations in this area, the data also were analyzed in terms of the individual scores for concreteness within each of the patient samples. When this type of analysis was conducted, it was found that the raw scores for concreteness for most of these early schizophrenic patients were not high, indicating only a limited amount of concreteness among the schizophrenics.

Although we have focused on an analysis of the results from the Object Sorting test for this particular sample of schizophrenics, they also were assessed on the abstract-concrete dimension using the Proverbs test. These schizophrenics also showed significantly more concreteness than the nonschizophrenic patients on the Proverbs test, with slightly greater schizophrenic-nonschizophrenic differences on this verbal test, and with minor indications from this sample that the Proverbs test may be a slightly more sensitive index of patients' performance on the abstract-concrete dimension than the Object Sorting test. However, the raw scores for concreteness of most of the schizophrenic patients on the Proverbs test also did not show extremely concrete behavior by this relatively young sample.

We believe that any potential differences that emerge when the Object Sorting test is used, in contrast to potential results from the Proverbs test, should be viewed in light of the type of behavior that the Object Sorting test evaluates (Harrow, Marengo, Pogue-Geile, and Pawelski, in press). The Object Sorting test is less dependent on previous verbal learning and verbal skills. This provides an important contrast to the more verbal forms of behavior assessed by the Proverbs test. The use of the Object Sorting test in combination with the use of more purely verbal tests (such as a set of proverbs) allows the evaluation of concrete behavior to be more general, more complete, and less dependent on one specific technique, index, or specific type of behavior.

Overall, the raw scores of the patients that we obtained from both the Object Sorting test and the Proverbs test suggest that, in relatively young schizophrenics studied at the acute phase, concrete thinking, a type of negative symptom, is not the most prominent factor, although a clear deficit in this area was found for the schizophrenics.

TABLE 7.1
Mean Scores on Concrete Thinking at the Acute Phase for Sample 7A (Object Sorting Test)

	Mean	S.D.	N	t	P
Schizophrenic patients	2.75	2.85	32	2.47	< .05
Nonschizophrenic patients	1.34	1.49	32		

Information from the Proverbs Test

Tables 7.2, 7.3, and 7.4 present the results on the abstract-concrete dimension for sample 7B, a larger sample of acute patients from our Yale setting who were administered a series of verbal tests, including the Proverbs test, and a test of similarities. These verbal tests were administered to the sample at two early phases of their disorder, the acute phase and the phase of partial recovery about seven weeks later.

In general, the data from the Proverbs test in Tables 7.2 and 7.3 support the results presented in Table 7.1 from the sample of patients who were studied using the Object Sorting test at the acute stage. They also suggest that an impairment in abstraction is not the most important factor in early schizophrenia, although it could play a more important role in later chronic stages of the disorder.

In Tables 7.2 and 7.3, the data on deficits in abstract performance indicate that there were trends for the schizophrenic subjects to show

TABLE 7.2
Mean Scores on Indexes of Abstract Thinking and Intelligence at the Acute Phase for Sample 7B

	Classical Schiz. Mean (N = 25)	Latent Schiz. Mean (N = 23)	Nonschiz. Mean (N = 47)	Classical Schiz. versus Nonschiz. t (df = 70)
Abstract Thinking (Proverbs Test)				
1. M-G correct abstract responses	15.52	17.52	18.36	1.68*
2. A-H all correct abstract responses	14.96	17.39	18.02	1.89*
3. A-H all abstract responses	17.52	19.70	20.11	1.73*
Intelligence (WAIS)				
4. Comprehension Scale	20.04	20.26	20.53	0.48

*P < .10

more impaired abstract performance during the two early phases of their disorder that were studied. These trends were found at both the acute phase and the phase of partial recovery. Perhaps of most importance, however, the absolute scores from this sample indicate that despite the decrement, both schizophrenic and nonschizophrenic psychiatric patients were relatively *low* on concreteness during the acute phase of their disorder and shortly thereafter. For sample 7B, there was an average of only one complete proverb (or two halves) interpreted concretely from the thirteen proverbs presented. This sample was an upper-middle-class group of above-average intelligence, and we believe that this is an important influence on their performance. Thus, the results indicated only limited deficits on the abstract-concrete dimension during early phases of their disorder for this type of sample.

When we looked at the data more closely, we found that the results showed a consistent trend for at least some deficits in abstraction by the schizophrenic patients. Thus, using the system devised by Meadow and

TABLE 7.3
Mean Scores on Indexes of Abstract Thinking and Intelligence at the Phase of Partial Recovery for Sample 7B

	Classical Schiz. Mean (N = 25)	Latent Schiz. Mean (N = 23)	Nonschiz. Mean (N = 47)	Classical Schiz. versus Nonschiz. t (df = 70)
Abstract Thinking (Proverbs Test)				
1. M-G correct abstract responses	17.76	18.78	21.23	2.68**
2. A-H all correct abstract responses	17.68	18.83	20.38	2.32*
3. A-H all abstract responses	20.36	21.65	21.98	1.52
Intelligence (WAIS)				
4. Comprehension Scale	21.12	21.39	21.70	0.54
5. Information Scale	19.20	20.43	19.70	0.68

*P < .05
**P < .01

TABLE 7.4
Mean Scores on Indexes of Abstract Thinking from the Similarities Tests at the Acute Phase and Phase of Partial Recovery (Sample 7B)

	Acute Phase		Partial Recovery Phase	
	6 Similarities: Total Score	7 Similarities: No. Correct (Abstract Resp.)	6 Similarities: Total Score	7 Similarities: No. Correct (Abstract Resp.)
Classical schiz.: mean (N = 25)	18.28	8.00	18.32	7.92
Latent schiz.: mean (N = 23)	19.57	8.30	21.04	9.22
Nonschizophrenic: mean (N = 47)	17.55	7.62	19.38	8.49
t test: Classical schiz. versus nonschizophrenics (df = 70)	0.61	0.58	1.11	1.00

From Harrow, Adler & Hanf. Archives of General Psychiatry, 31, 27–33, 1974. Copyright 1974, by the American Medical Association, and reproduced by permission of the publisher.

Greenbatt (Meadow, Greenblatt, and Funkenstein, 1953; Meadow, Greenblatt, Solomon, and Funkenstein, 1953) for scoring the Proverbs test for *correct abstract* responses (Table 7.2, Index 1), the schizophrenic patients tended to score lower on abstract thinking at the acute phase ($P = .01$), and were significantly lower during the phase of partial recovery ($P < .01$). The results were similar to these when we employed the other more refined system that we constructed for scoring correct abstract responses, which combines all types of correct abstract responses, including correct, but idiosyncratic, abstract answers (Table 7.2, Index 2). The data indicate that among relatively intelligent patients, during the nonchronic stages, the schizophrenic disorder may interfere with, or lead to some decrement in ability to assume an abstract attitude correctly. However, the interference or decrement is apparently not extreme, since most patients were able to give a relatively high number of correct abstract responses.

When the score for all abstract responses (regardless of whether they were correct, incorrect, or bizarre) was utilized (Table 7.2, Index 3), the schizophrenic patients again tended to give less abstract responses, although the results were not significant at either phase of the disorder. The results suggest that while the ability of schizophrenic patients to abstract *correctly* may show some decrement during non-chronic stages, their tendency to assume an abstract attitude (even if it is sometimes incorrect) does not show as large a decrement in comparison to nonschizophrenic patients.

Tests of Similarities and Relation to Intellectual Ability

When we used the two indices from the Similarities subtest to assess deficits in abstract ability in sample 7B (presented in Table 7.4), there were no significant differences between diagnostic groups at either phase of disorder. In addition, employing a separate analysis, the performance of the schizophrenic subgroup was not poorer on the Similarities test than on the other intellectual tests such as the WAIS Information and Comprehension tests, when age-corrected norms derived by Wechsler were utilized (Wechsler, 1955).

The Similarities subtest has been used by many clinicians as an index of abstract ability in schizophrenic patients, and the present results cast some doubt on formulations in this area derived from the clinical use of this test. Performance on the Similarities test showed significant, but not high, correlations with the other indices of abstraction (ranging from $r = .26$ to $r = .33$). In contrast, analysis of the relationship between the Similarities test and the two other tests of verbal intelligence (the WAIS Information and Comprehension tests) showed high correlations (all above $r = .50$). The data clearly suggest that although the Similarities subtest may tap aspects of abstract ability in schizophrenia, it is a less sensitive test for possible schizophrenic pathology than other indices such as the Proverbs test.

As we have noted earlier, other research of ours has suggested that schizophrenic psychopathology does not appear under all types of stimulus situations. Schizophrenic psychopathology is more likely to appear when the patient is presented with unstructured stimuli, or in nonstructured situations. However, it will also frequently appear in response to structured stimuli, providing that the response or behavior is not automatic, stereotyped, sharply limited (as in a multiple-choice situation), or a well-practiced type of behavior. In the case of the Similarities test, the briefer responses (frequently two or three words) and the more structured responses required on this test may be factors that make it less sensitive to schizophrenic psychopatholy. Also, while intelligence is a confounding factor in any test of abstraction, this may be true to an even greater extent for the Similarities test, which is primarily an intelligence test.

The lack of differences between groups on the Similarities test raised the issue of differences on overall intelligence. Control data on possible intellectual differences between the various groups studied are important when any type of ability is being assessed. Since intellectual ability is so closely linked to cognitive ability, it is of crucial importance when cognitive abilities are being evaluated. In addition, since there was evidence suggesting a relationship between the abstract-concrete dimension and intellectual ability, it became even more important to assess possible differences between the groups in intellectual functioning in areas not as disturbed by the psychotic process, in evaluating the questions currently being studied.

The results reported in Tables 7.2 and 7.3 on possible intellectual differences using two different measures suggested that there were no significant differences between the schizophrenic and the nonschizophrenic patients at either the acute phase, or the phase of partial recovery. This suggests that any possible differences between the diagnostic groups that did emerge on the abstract-concrete dimension, at the early phases, is not principally a result of differences in intellectual ability.

Summary of Data at Early Phases of Schizophrenia

The results on the presence of deficits in abstraction, one type of negative symptom in early phases of schizophrenia, were relatively straightforward. Based on data collected at two time periods in the nonchronic stages of the schizophrenic disorder (the acute phase and partial recovery), the results indicate that there is a deficit in abstract ability in relatively intelligent, early schizophrenic patients, although the deficit is circumscribed. The limited nature of the impairment was accentuated by the results being mixed concerning significant schizo-phrenic-nonschizophrenic differences, with the magnitude of the differences depending on the type of test and index used. The relatively limited deficit on the abstract-concrete dimension for all diagnostic groups suggest that, during early phases, concreteness is not the major factor associated with their psychopathology.

SUBTYPES OF EARLY SCHIZOPHRENIA AND THE ABSTRACT-CONCRETE DIMENSION

The next step we undertook was to assess various subtypes of early schizophrenics on the abstract-concrete dimension, as a result of the lack of a prominent degree of concreteness among most early schizophrenics. This becomes more important because of the possibility that formulations about the central position of concrete thinking in schizophrenia might apply to select subtypes of schizophrenia, even though our evidence indicates that they do not apply to early schizophrenics as an overall group.

The first of the systems of categorizing schizophrenics into subtypes that we examined was the paranoid-nonparanoid dimension. Our results did not show significant differences between young paranoid and nonparanoid schizophrenics in ability to abstract during early phases of their disorder.

The other major dimension for categorizing these early schizophrenics is the process-reactive dimension, based on patient's level of competence in the social-sexual area (Phillips, 1966). The issue of whether process schizophrenics are more concrete than reactive schizophrenics has been the subject of a number of studies (Eliseo, 1963; Tutko and Spence, 1962; Watson, 1973), although it has been difficult to investigate this question in early, young schizophrenics with chronicity controlled (Cancro, 1969). To obtain scores on the process-reactive dimension, we utilized our version of the Phillips Scale (Phillips, 1953), which we had previously modified to allow assessment of females and of younger patients (Bromet, Harrow, and Kasl, 1974). We have analyzed the scores on the abstract-concrete dimension of two large groups of process and reactive schizophrenics: (1) the sample of patients from our Yale inpatient setting (sample 7B), and (2) a large sample of schizophrenic patients from our Chicago inpatient setting.

Our subgroup analysis on the abstract-concrete dimension for our population of New Haven inpatients included samples of process schizophrenics, reactive schizophrenics, and nonschizophrenic patients. The results of our analysis indicated that reactive schizophrenics did not differ significantly from the nonschizophrenics on the scales of abstractness or concreteness at either phase studied. However, the process schizophrenics tended to differ from the other schizophrenic group. During the acute phase, the process schizophrenics were significantly less abstract ($P < .05$) than both the reactive schizophrenics and the nonschizophrenics. There also were trends (nonsignificant) for process schizophrenics to be more concrete than reactive schizophrenics and nonschizophrenics. During partial recovery the process schizophrenics were significantly less abstract ($P < .05$) than the nonschizophrenics, but were only slightly less abstract than the reactive schizophrenics ($P > .20$). The overall results from our Yale inpatient setting on differences on abstracting ability between process and reactive schizophrenics suggest the following:

1. Reactive schizophrenics did not differ significantly on the abstract-concrete dimension from nonschizophrenic patients.
2. During relatively early phases of their disorder there was a tendency for process schizophrenics to be more concrete than both reactive schizophrenics and nonschizophrenics. This trend was significant on some indexes and near significant on others.
3. During the pre-chronic phases, among the relatively high-ability schizophrenics from our Yale inpatient setting even process schizophrenics only showed a limited deficit on the abstract-concrete dimension.

In contrast to these results from our sample of patients from New Haven, when the large sample of patients from our Chicago inpatient setting was studied, the differences on concrete and abstract thinking between process and reactive schizophrenics were not significant (Marengo and Harrow, 1979).

From the above two samples of patients several possible conclusions can be drawn. (a) One of these possibilities is that some of the process schizophrenics represent a slightly different type of patient, a few of whom started their disorder at an earlier age and thus have progressed further along in the course of their disorder, and this accounts for some of the differences. (b) A second possibility is that the process-reactive dimension represents a continuum of severity, with more "severe" schizophrenics more likely to fit into the process category, despite at least some overlap in severity. (c) A third possibility is that the process schizophrenics represent a completely different type or category of patient.

Our evidence is incomplete in this area, although our earlier analysis would suggest some combination of the first two possibilities, which tends to place process and reactive schizophrenics on a continuum of severity, with the possibility that some of the process schizophrenics started their disorder at a younger age, and were further along in the course of their disorder, at the time of their assessment. Other analyses of ours suggest that chronicity of schizophrenia may influence results on potential differences that sometimes appear between process and reactive schizophrenics. Age and potential chronicity were better controlled in our sample of patients from Chicago, for whom there were no process-reactive differences.

DOES THE LEVEL OF ABSTRACT AND CONCRETE THINKING REMAIN CONSTANT AS PATIENTS' CLINICAL CONDITIONS CHANGE?

Table 7.5 reports the results (from Sample 7B) of the tests of significance associated with changes in the level of abstract and concrete thinking seven weeks later as patients showed signs of clinical recovery. These results in Table 7.5, based on the raw scores summarized in Tables 7.2, 7.3, and 7.4, indicate a strong tendency for improvement in abstraction as patients emerged from the acute stage and entered into partial recovery. The improvement was significant or near significant for all types of patients. A beginning hypothesis in this area would be that the improvement is associated with a decrease in acute psycho-pathology and occurs concomitantly with improvement in other symptoms.

The results showing a significant improvement in abstraction for these relatively highly intelligent schizophrenic patients, as they moved into the stage of partial recovery, are similar to the results reported by Shimkunas on a somewhat more chronic sample of schizophrenics (Shimkunas, Gynther, and Smith, 1966). As we have noted earlier, Shimkunas did not study a comparison group of disturbed nonschizo-phrenic patients. In the present research, the addition of an acute nonschizophrenic group, and the other results noted below showing some improvement in general intellectual functioning, provided further information. They suggest that in the pre-chronic phases, the improvement in abstract thinking (and conversely the decrement during the more acute phase) is not unique to schizophrenia, but rather occurs in disturbed patients of all diagnostic types.

The background information from data on intelligence and symptom level shows that in order to appraise the role of abstract and concrete thinking accurately, data in this area should not be looked at in isolation. They must be considered in conjunction with data from other areas. In the present case, to appraise data on changes in the abstract-concrete level in schizophrenia, it is important to consider parallel changes in intellectual efficiency in general, parallel changes in the level of psychopathology (e.g., psychotic symptoms and idiosyncratic thinking), and parallel changes in nonschizophrenic patients emerging from the acute phase of their disorders.

TABLE 7.5
Tests of Significance for Changes Over Time on Indexes of Abstract and Concrete Thinking and Intelligence (Sample 7B)

	Classical Schiz. t-test (df = 24)	Latent Schiz. t-test (df = 22)	Nonschiz. t-test (df = 46)	Total Sample t-test (df = 94)
Abstract Thinking (Proverbs Test)				
1. M.G. correct abstract responses	2.01	1.13	3.43**	4.04**
2. A-H all correct abstract responses	2.42*	1.72	3.01**	4.25**
3. A-H all abstract responses	2.91**	2.13*	2.54*	4.34**
Intelligence (WAIS)				
4. Comprehension Test	1.71	2.05	2.28*	3.46**
Abstract Thinking (Similarities Test)				
5. Total Score	0.09	3.17**	3.79**	4.29**
6. No. Correct abstract responses	0.28	3.18**	3.14**	3.60**

*P < .05
**P < .01

The results on the change scores from the index of intelligence that was administered at both time periods (WAIS Comprehension subtest, Table 7.5, Index 4) did indicate a near-significant improvement for the schizophrenic and borderline patients ($P < .10$); and significant improvements for the nonschizophrenic patients ($P < .05$) and for the overall sample ($P < .001$). These results indicate that during the acute period of their disorder, there is at least some general impairment in overall comprehension for the patients, with this applying to patients of all diagnostic types. The change scores suggest that some of the improvement in abstraction is related to a more general increase in intellectual efficiency during the phase of partial recovery.

In addition to the cognitive data, background data also were obtained on parallel changes in patients' level of psychotic symptoms and other types of symptoms and disordered behavior during partial recovery, when abstract and concrete thinking were being studied. They are discussed at the beginning of Chapter 5, and Table 5.1, based on data from the same ninety-five patients currently being discussed, shows a significant improvement in psychotic symptoms for the present sample of schizophrenics as they emerged from the acute phase. These results, involving considerable improvement in other areas of psycho-pathology at the same time, indicate that the reduction in concrete thinking during partial recovery should be viewed as part of a more general picture involving improvement in a number of areas.

In summary, the data on changes over time on abstract and concrete thinking for the current patients of average and above-average in-telligence showed that some improvement occurred for both schizo-phrenic and nonschizophrenic patients as they emerged from the acute phase. The results suggest that there was a deficit in these areas during the acute phase that was not just a function of schizophrenia, but was related, at least in part, to acute disturbance in general. The data also indicated that as acute pathology diminished, there was some improve-ment in other intellectual areas as well.

THE LEVEL OF CONCRETE THINKING DURING THE POSTHOSPITAL PHASE OF SCHIZOPHRENIA

Table 7.6 presents the major results on concrete thinking at the posthospital or follow-up phase for the thirty-two schizophrenic and thirty-two nonschizophrenic patients from our Chicago inpatient settings (Sample 7A), studied slightly over a year after discharge from their acute hospitalization. The results from this sample permit cognitive assessment at a different phase of their disorder, when the effects of acute psychopathology and of residing in a hospital had diminished.

The following results emerged from this follow-up sample, whose acute-phase results are presented in Table 7.1.

1. There were no significant differences between the schizophrenic and nonschizophrenic patients on concrete thinking during the post-hospital phase, although there was a trend for more concreteness in the schizophrenic sample ($P = .11$).

2. The relationship between scores for concrete thinking on the Object Sorting test, and scores for intelligence on a different test (the WAIS Information Scale) were significant.

The current results were obtained during a third phase of the schizophrenic disorder, when the effects of acute psychopathology and of the hospital setting were controlled, by assessing patients at the follow-up period. These results indicated that both schizophrenic and nonschizophrenic patients showed some improvement on the abstract-concrete dimension, and the differences between schizophrenic and nonschizophrenic patients had diminished, although schizophrenics still tended to show some limited deficits on the abstract-concrete dimension.

It should be noted that the current results, collected over a year after acute hospitalization, represent data from a relatively young schizophrenic sample. Hence, the evidence noted above applies to patients in a pre-chronic stage of their disorder, rather then to chronic schizophrenic patients who have been hospitalized for many years.

While the schizophrenic sample could be considered as being in a stage of partial recovery, other data of ours on this sample of sixty-four patients provide clues as to their functioning in noncognitive areas. These data indicate that the schizophrenics, at the time of their assessment for cognitive functioning, were performing significantly

TABLE 7.6
Mean Scores on Concrete Thinking at the Posthospital Phase for Sample 7A (Object Sorting Test)

	Mean	S.D.	N	t	P
Schizophrenic patients	1.75	2.38	32	1.62	0.11
Nonschizophrenic patients	0.97	1.33	32		

more poorly than the nonschizophrenic patients in social and interpersonal areas, in work performance, and in other symptomatic areas. Thus, the results indicating that the schizophrenics were only slightly more concrete than the nonschizophrenics during the posthospital period occurred at a time when the schizophrenic patients were functioning much more poorly in noncognitive areas. The overall results provide support for our hypothesis that a deficit in abstract thinking, one type of negative symptom, is not the major characteristic of schizophrenic cognition during the early phases of their disorder. The overall results cited earlier also provide further evidence of some relationship (in this case a significant relationship) between scores on the abstract-concrete dimension and intelligence.

THE RELATIONSHIP BETWEEN ABSTRACT THINKING AND IDIOSYNCRATIC THINKING

The tendency to engage in abstract thinking and the ability to abstract successfully involve complex cognitive processes, and it is possible that they may be sensitive to and disrupted by a number of factors. One such factor that we investigated concerns some degree of disruption from the underlying factors responsible for bizarre-idiosyncratic thinking.

To provide inferential evidence on whether or not a deficit in abstract performance might be influenced by idiosyncratic thinking, or factors that produce it, the results on our sample from our New Haven inpatient setting (Sample 7B) concerning the abstract-concrete dimension were compared to other data on idiosyncratic thinking by these patients. The relationship at both early phases (acute phase, and phase of partial recovery) between idiosyncratic thinking (as assessed by an index from the Comprehension subtest) and various indices of abstract thinking derived from the Proverbs test were all significant, with the six correlations ranging from $r = .33$ to $R = .44$. Similarly, the correlations between idiosyncratic thinking and behavior, as assessed by the psychiatrists' ratings, and various indices of abstract thinking derived from the Proverbs test ranged from $r = .34$ to $r = .45$. Thus, patients (both schizophrenic and nonschizophrenic) who showed evidence of bizarre-idiosyncratic thinking tended to score lower on abstraction and to be more concrete. These results showing a relationship between positive thought disorder (bizarre-idiosyncratic thinking) and a deficit in level of abstraction, a type of negative symptom occurred on indices from several different tests, and from behavioral observations as well, with the similar results occurring when different techniques were used.

Conclusive evidence as to whether or not idiosyncratic thinking or underlying factors that determine it interfere with, disrupt, or lead to a deficit in ability to abstract successfully cannot be provided by correlational data alone, although clues in this area can be obtained from these results. The significant correlations between idiosyncratic thinking and level of abstraction at both phases of the patients' disorders can be interpreted in a number of ways. Two of the more important possibilities are as follows: (1) these data provide some clues suggesting that idiosyncratic thinking may have interfered with abstract ability; or (2) a second possibility is that some of the background mechanisms that influence or lead to positive thought disorder (e.g, acute confusion-disorganization, interference from personal material or intermingling, etc) also lead to some deficit in abstract thinking, and thus can increase the levels of some types of negative symptoms. It should be noted that idiosyncratic thinking was not uniformly related to all intellectual abilities assessed, since the scores on abstraction showed a higher relationship to idiosyncratic thinking than did the indices of intelligence from the Comprehension and the Information subtests.

INTELLECTUAL ABILITY AND ITS RELATIONSHIP TO THE ABSTRACT-CONCRETE DIMENSION

An understanding of the relationship between the abstract-concrete dimension and intellectual ability is of key importance in any assessment of abstract thinking and possible deficits in this area. As we have suggested in several preceding sections, data on the relationship between abstract thinking and psychopathology or other features are difficult to interpret without knowledge of parallel data concerning intellectual ability, and whether any deficits that occure are unique to the abstract-concrete dimension, or extend to other types of intellectual functioning as well.

In order to study this relationship we analyzed the data from the Information and Comprehension subtests of the Wechsler Intelligence Scales (Wechsler, 1955) from our New Haven inpatient sample. Both of these indices of intelligence showed high positive relationships to abstract thinking, and moderate to high negative relationships with other indexes of concrete thinking. The relationships between these variables were assessed at both of the two early phases of the patients' disorders: the acute phase and the phase of partial recovery. The results on the relationship between abstraction and the various indices of intelligence were all significant, and ranged from $r = .45$ to $r = .48$ at the acute phase, and $r = .34$ to $r = .43$ at the phase of partial recovery.

These data on intelligence are in agreement with reports by others. They indicate a relatively high relationship between intelligence and abstract ability. These results could suggest that abstraction is either a component of intelligence (depending on how one defines intelligence), or is a closely related function. However, while the diagnostic groups did not differ on the two standard indices of intelligence used, they did tend to differ on abstraction. Thus, there were significant differences between schizophrenic and nonschizophrenic patients on abstract performance, and this stands in contrast to the similar scores of these diagnostic groups on the two indices of intelligence used. We have suggested that abstract performance in early schizophrenics may be influenced by the cognitive impairment and idiosyncratic thinking associated with schizophrenic disorders because it is a complex and demanding cognitive function, involving symbolic manipulation and demanding greater effort. This would imply that abstract performance is linked to cognitive ability and general intelligence, but that other potentially disruptive factors can influence or interfere with abstract performance more easily than they interfere with simple types of intellectual performance.

CONCRETE THINKING AND ITS IMPORTANCE IN CHRONIC SCHIZOPHRENIA

Much of the focus of our studies on abstract and concrete thinking has been on schizophrenics during the early phases of the disorder, as we were looking for clues as to what factors are important prior to potential influences such as chronic institutionalization, a possible deteriorating clinical course, secondary gain, and the effect of factors such as social withdrawal.

Since a deficit in abstract thinking has been hypothesized to be prominent in schizophrenics, and its occurrence was not the major factor during early phases of the disorder, it seemed appropriate to analyze its possible presence during later chronic phases. It was hoped that this would provide some idea about the natural course of the schizophrenic disorder and provide clues on possible deterioration in certain types of schizophrenics.

We have studied three samples of multiyear, chronic schizophrenics from different state hospitals in Connecticut and Illinois. Similar results have emerged from these three samples, and thus we will focus our discussion on the first of these samples—a group of thirty-two multiyear, chronic schizophrenics from a Connecticut state hospital. Data on these patients were collected by D. Adler as part of a medical-student thesis at Yale University (Adler, 1972; Adler and Harrow, 1974; Harrow, Adler, and Hanf, 1974). These patients had a median length of hospitalization of fourteen years. The data from this sample of schizophrenics in the chronic phases indicate that these patients had significantly more deficits in abstract thinking ($P < .001$) and engaged in more concrete thinking ($P < .001$) than the schizophrenics we have assessed at the acute phase.

While the multiyear, chronic schizophrenics showed considerably more concreteness (one type of negative symptom) than acute schizophrenics, they were not significantly higher than the acutely disturbed schizophrenic patients on scores for idiosyncratic thinking or positive thought disorder, derived from the Proverbs and Comprehension tests. Viewed as a group, the chronically disturbed schizophrenic subjects were also significantly lower in intelligence ($P < .001$) than the acutely disturbed sample. The extremely poor performance of the chronic schizophrenics on the abstract-concrete dimension and their generally lower intellectual performance were very prominent characteristics of this group.

When the chronic schizophrenics were looked at more closely, however, it became clear that a small subgroup of six of these patients did not show the same pattern. These six patients showed more adequate intellectual performance on our tests of intelligence. There was little difference in abstract performance between our acute-phase schizophrenic patients and this subsample of six chronic schizophrenics who could be matched with the acute sample on intelligence. Thus, we have a picture of extremely poor performance on the abstract-concrete dimension for the great majority of chronic, multiyear, state hospital schizophrenics, coupled with poor performance on intellectual tasks in general, but without necessarily more *overt* bizarreness among these patients than among acute schizophrenics. We have found this pattern across samples from several different state hospitals. We have also been able to find small subsamples of chronic hospitalized schizophrenics in each chronic setting who do not show this pattern of apparently severe deficits. A number of inferences about abstract and concrete thinking in chronic, multiyear schizophrenics can be made from these data.

1. While concrete thinking is not a crucial factor in the relatively early acute phase, among many chronic, multiyear, hospitalized schizophrenics, this type of negative symptom is a very prominent feature. The significantly lower scores on abstraction (and higher concreteness scores) probably represent a combination of a severe deficit in abstraction for many of these chronic patients, and an initial low level of ability for others of these patients. However, this coexists along with an extremely low level of intellectual performance that cuts across performance in a wide number of cognitive areas. Only a small subsample of them did not show this low level of overall intellectual performance, and the scores of this small subsample of patients on abstraction were also adequate. The strikingly poor abstract performance for the great majority of multiyear, chronic schizophrenic patients would seem to be a product of limited native ability in the cognitive area and/or overall intellectual deficits and deterioration associated with the natural course of the schizophrenic disorder. Other variables that could contribute are: (a) some deterioration that could be associated with long-term institutionalization and a lack of social stimulation; and (b) motivational problems that are frequently more prominent in patients with chronic than with acute schizophrenia (Detre and Jarecki, 1971).

2. Another implication of these data concerns the disparity between the level of bizarre-idiosyncratic thinking and performance on the abstract-concrete dimension. One hypothesis would be that concreteness and deficit in abstraction are *only* due to interference from processes associated with bizarre-idiosyncratic thinking, which have presumably led to a deficit on the abstract-concrete dimension. However, while there is a significant correlation between these two factors, our data do not indicate a uniform relationship between bizarre-idiosyncratic thinking, a measure of positive thought disorder on the one hand, and abstract-concrete performance, a type of negative symptom. Thus, our results indicate that patients with acute and chronic schizophrenia had similar relatively high scores on bizarre-idiosyncratic thinking, or on positive thought disorder, but despite this differed sharply on concrete thinking, a type of negative symptom. These data do not support the above hypothesis. They suggest that other factors in addition to idiosyncratic thinking play a major role in the deficit in abstract thinking, and in the negative symptoms found among chronic schizophrenic patients (i.e., variables associated with impoverished thinking and other types of negative symptoms, and also the possibility that a large percentage of chronic, back-ward schizophrenics could have been people of limited intellectual ability to begin with). The data referred to above, with the many unanswered questions that emerge

from them, highlight the importance of longitudinal research on schizophrenic thinking to study factors associated with and responsible for possible deterioration over time (Strauss, M., 1973).

OVERVIEW—ABSTRACT AND CONCRETE THINKING IN SCHIZOPHRENIA

The present research on deficits in abstraction, one type of negative symptom, produced evidence that it is not the major factor in the psychopathology of *early* schizophrenia. Our results were obtained employing three major, and several supplemental, samples of patients, studied at four phases of the schizophrenic disorder. Our investigations used three techniques to assess the abstract-concrete dimension, including two that rely heavily on verbal responses (the Proverbs and the Similarities tests) and a method that places much less emphasis on verbal skills (Object Sorting). The data comparing schizophrenics with other disturbed patients at various phases of the disorder did find some deficits in abstraction during early phases of the schizophrenic disorder. A number of variables, however, seem to play a role. Thus, abstract and concrete thinking may represent end-points on a continuum, but deficits on this dimension can be determined by a variety of factors, any of which can tend to lower the level of performance of the patients. Some of these factors are more important than others.

Factors associated with schizophrenia did play some role in deficits in abstraction, even during early phases of the disorder. When our young schizophrenic samples were studied in more detail, our first wave of data suggested that process schizophrenics may show a greater deficit on the abstract-concrete dimension. The phase of the disorder was of considerable importance for schizophrenia. Acute psychopathology was a factor, and during active or acutely disturbed phases of disruption, patients of all types, including nonschizophrenics, were less abstract. The single most powerful influence on abstraction is intelligence, intellectual level, or cognitive ability, with our evidence, and that of others, supporting a thesis that abstract ability should be considered a component of intelligence, although it may tap aspects of intelligence related to complex problem solving and concept formation. Factors involved in or associated with idiosyncratic thinking also may interfere with the ability to abstract successfully; this is discussed further later in this chapter.

The results on the abstract-concrete dimension for schizophrenics stand in contrast to those obtained on other cognitive dimensions, such as the data indicating that idiosyncratic thinking or positive thought disorder is a more central factor in early schizophrenic behavior. Thus, a deficit in abstract thinking was not the most prominent factor associated with the schizophrenic patients' cognitive disorder in the early phases. This was indicated by a number of factors: (1) There were much larger differences during early phases of disorder between diagnostic groups on psychotic symptoms, a major type of positive symptom, both in the present research and in other research of ours (using clinicians' ratings, ratings from patients' charts, and using extensive interview schedules to assess delusions and other psychotic features). (2) There were scores indicating severe bizarre-idiosyncratic thinking, or positive thought disorder, at the acute phase for both the present and similar schizo-phrenic samples we have studied. (3) The present evidence indicated that during the acute phase, nonschizophrenic patients also show some limited degree of impairment in abstraction. At the same time, the deficit in abstract thinking cannot be totally ignored in relation to differences between schizophrenic and nonschizophrenic patients, and this also is discussed in greater detail in the next section of this chapter.

The evidence suggesting that *abstraction should be considered a component of overall intellectual ability* has been given less than adequate attention by some clinicians in their theoretical views on deficits in abstraction in schizophrenia. Recently, however, there has been an increasing number of reports by investigators in the clinical area noting the closeness of the relationship between abstraction and intelligence. The evidence in our research supporting this position includes (a) high correlations between these two factors at three different phases of the patients' disorders; (b) intelligence and abstraction moving together in the sense of both showing a deficit during the most acute period, followed by some recovery in both of them seven weeks later; and (c) the data indicating that the chronic, multiyear schizophrenics who were extremely concrete also showed considerable intellectual deficit in other areas.

The positive relationship found in the current research between impaired abstraction and idiosyncratic thinking is of some theoretical interest. Although abstraction is a component of intelligence, abstract performance on the Proverbs test seems to be affected by bizarre ideation and schizophrenic cognitive difficulties to a slightly greater extent than some other aspects of intellectual functioning. One factor that may help account for this is that abstraction is a relatively complex component, involving symbolic manipulation. Further, the Proverbs test allows, and even facilitates, a high degree of idiosyncratic thinking, which might interfere with abstraction. The Proverbs test tends to elicit idiosyncratic verbalizations because it does not structure the patients' responses, in contrast to multiple-choice problems which structure responses and thus make idiosyncratic thinking and verbalizations less likely. The combination of (1) the complexity of the task, together with (2) the nonstereotyped nature of the responses, may be the major reasons why abstraction on the Proverbs test tends to be slightly more susceptible to interference from schizophrenic psychopathology and bizarre ideation. Evidence showing this slightly greater influence of schizophrenic psychopathology on abstract performance on the Proverbs test than on many other components of intelligence included (1) high correlations between bizarreness and abstraction, in contrast to the relatively lower associations between bizarre responses and performance on other intellectual tasks; and (2) the tendency toward some diagnostic differences on abstraction, in contrast to the other intellectual tasks that showed even smaller diagnostic differences.

In light of our evidence on concrete thinking, and that of other recent investigators, one may ask what the basis was for the original positive reports about the importance of concrete thinking in schizophrenia by others. Most of the previous positive reports about its importance were based on studies of chronic schizophrenics, or were based on comparisons of schizophrenics with nondisturbed "normals." When normals were compared with schizophrenic patients, any differences found might have been due to the schizophrenics being *disturbed* people or their being *hospitalized psychiatric patients*, regardless of whether or not they are psychotic and/or schizophrenic. In a research design comparing schizophrenic patients with normals without a control sample of disturbed nonschizophrenic patients, all of the above factors are confounded with the schizophrenic factor.

Equal or more serious problems arise when one compares *chronic schizophrenics* with normals. Long-term chronic schizophrenics, hospitalized for many years, represent a select subgroup of patients, most of whom have shown severe deficits and/or deterioration. These chronic schizophrenics represent those patients with the worst outcome or most severe disorder. Differences in cognitive functioning at various phases of the schizophrenic disorder, however, may be important for theories about schizophrenia, and as we shall discuss shortly, our results on the abstract-concrete dimension in the chronic schizophrenics exemplify this point.

Overall, it appears that if there is a primary or single essential symptom in schizophrenia, the abstract-concrete dimension is not the answer, since a deficit in this area is not the most prominent factor during early stages of the disorder, and is not likely to be an important influence or determinant of other early features of the disorder. There is, however, a limited decrement in abstraction in early young schizophrenics, and concreteness is more prominent at a later phase in the select group of chronic schizophrenics who later show deterioration.

A TWO-FACTOR MODEL OF COGNITIVE IMPAIRMENT IN SCHIZOPHRENIA

In regard to how a deficit in abstraction and increased concreteness fit into our overall view of cognitive disorders, we have reported earlier that one way of viewing disordered thinking in schizophrenia is in terms of a model of two major types of symptoms, positive and negative symptoms. Included in the first of these is positive thought disorder, which involves unusual, strange, and bizarre thinking and can be assessed with our comprehensive index of bizarre-idiosyncratic thinking. The second type, negative symptoms, can involve a variety of features, among which are cognitive impoverishment, involving a decline or deficit in intellectual abilities and efficiency. Severe deficits in abstract ability and concreteness are most closely tied in with the second type of cognitive impairment, namely cognitive deficits in intellectual abilities and efficiency, and can be viewed as a negative symptom. Our data also suggest that the ability to abstract successfully can be impaired when there is an occurrence of the first type of cognitive difficulty, namely bizarre-idiosyncratic thinking, although we view this type of impairment in abstract performance as a side-effect of the cognitive interference that can be associated with bizarre-idiosyncratic thinking and positive symptoms.

Although some theorists have viewed the presence of positive symptoms as implying the absence of negative symptoms, and vice versa, our research has suggested that these two types of symptoms do not necessarily show a negative relationship. We have found a large number of chronic "backward" schizophrenics who are severely delusional and also show strong negative symptoms and severe deficits. In addition, other patient groups frequently show positive correlations between positive and negative symptoms, since the underlying factors that lead to positive symptoms in some areas may also lead to deficits in other areas.

1. In regard to these two major types of cognitive impairment, we would propose that the first type, severe bizarre-idiosyncratic thinking, is related to psychotic behavior in schizophrenia. In this respect, it is closely tied in with one of the most dramatic features of schizo-

phrenia, namely strange and delusional ideas and behavior. Our evidence indicates that bizarre-idiosyncratic thinking is especially prominent in the acute phase of schizophrenia, and in the acute phase of some other types of psychoses as well, such as acute manic disorders, but is also present in active chronic phases of schizophrenia. Our suggestion here is that in early young schizophrenics there is an *acute psychosis factor* that interacts with, and is one influence on, the level of (a) bizarre-idiosyncratic thinking, as well as (b) other psychotic reality distortions such as delusions, hallucinations, and strange experiences. Our early evidence suggests that this constellation of delusions accompanied by bizarre-idiosyncratic thinking can be found in some other psychotic patients. However, the combination of both positive thought disorder and delusions as two closely linked variables (with a potentially high correlation to each other) is less frequent in these latter types of disorders than it is in schizophrenia.

In respect to positive thought disorder and the concept of bizarre-idiosyncratic thinking, we have in general discussed this concept in Chapters 3 through 5, where we outlined some of our empirical results in this area. We proposed in Chapter 5 that impaired perspective, which involves the effective utilization of long-term, stored knowledge about the social appropriateness of one's own planned speech and behavior, and the intermingling of personal concerns and needs are closely tied in with this type of cognitive disorder and malfunctioning.

We have noted and discussed above, in relation to this first major factor, positive thought disorder or bizarre-idiosyncratic thinking, that ability to abstract successfully is also influenced by this type of positive thought disorder. At the same time, severe deficits in ability to abstract seem to be even more closely associated with the second major type of cognitive impairment.

2. The second major type of symptoms, negative symptoms, includes, among others, *impoverished cognition* and a *deficit in intellectual abilities*. Concreteness, or a deficit in abstraction, is viewed as a negative symptom and could be regarded as a type of intellectual decline or deficit. In contrast, many of the other types of cognitive impairments we discuss in this book are closely related to or a component of the first of these two types of cognitive impairments, positive symptoms and bizarre-idiosyncratic thinking. Thus, unlike some of the other cognitive features studied in this book, our data indicate that concreteness, a negative symptom, is much more common in chronic, seemingly impoverished and deteriorated, back-ward schizophrenics.

Is intellectual *deterioration* a uniform feature of these back-ward schizophrenics? An alternate possibility is that some of these severely deficited back-ward schizophrenics *always* showed a low level of intellectual ability, even prior to the onset of their disorder. This could involve the possibility that a moderate to high percentage of the seemingly deteriorated back-ward schizophrenics are from the segment of the population with initial low levels of ability. If this were the case, then, among schizophrenics, those with lower levels of ability and lower intellectual potential have a greater chance of ending up as back-ward schizophrenics. In this possibility some or many of these seemingly deteriorated back-ward schizophrenics would not be showing a drastic decline, but rather would always have been people with low ability levels.

Seventy years ago many schizophrenics eventually became chronic schizophrenics, spending most of their adult lives on the back wards of state hospitals. Apparently, many or most of these schizophrenics showed considerable deterioration. In modern times it is a *select* subsample of schizophrenics who wind up as multiyear, chronic schizophrenics with many years of hospitalization on the "continuous treatment services" (back wards) of state hospitals. It is conceivable that schizophrenics with low native intelligence and low native ability are more likely than higher-ability schizophrenics to be among the select sample who will end up spending many years on the continuous treatment services of state hospitals. If this is the case, then one would expect fewer of the patients on the back wards of Veterans Administration Neuropsychiatric hospitals to show what appears to be extreme deterioration, since these patients had to pass examinations demonstrating some initial level of competency before being inducted into the armed services.

If our formulation here is correct, then the extremely poor performance of a very large percentage of multiyear, chronically hospitalized schizophrenics in today's state hospitals could be due to both (1) low native ability to begin with, for some of these patients, and (2) intellectual deterioration as part of the course of their disorder for other back-ward state-hospital schizophrenics. Our preliminary detailed analysis of data collected from back-ward schizophrenics suggests that some of them have shown declines in ability during the course of their disorder and others were low-ability and low-potential patients to begin with.

To return to the issue of how concrete thinking and impaired abstraction fit into the overall picture of cognitive disorders in schizophrenia, a major point here is that concreteness is related to both types of cognitive impairment: (a) negative symptoms, especially intellectual declines and deficits, and (b) positive symptoms and bizarre-idiosyncratic thinking. Thus, concrete thinking is a negative symptom, and represents a deficit or low level of intellectual efficiency and ability, and is *very* prominent in severely deficited chronic schizophrenics. However, it is also found, to a lesser extent, in early acute schizophrenics, with factors associated with positive thought disorder and bizarre-idiosyncratic thinking leading to some limited deficits in abstraction for acute young schizophrenics.

8

Looseness of Associations

W ell ... I do like to cook sometimes ... It seems like I'm not cooperative with anybody anymore. It seems like everybody runs on one track and one's on another; it seems to me like everybody's running around. I think I'm making myself this nervous because I eat too much. I don't know how much to eat or anything, and that's just it—I don't know what I want to do all day long and I have to ask people and then one girl—well, they keep switching back and forth—like one will be on monitor and one will be a buddy or something—I'm still confused about that—and ... going out for a walk yesterday—I wanted to get out—but it was kind of cold outside, and I ... um ... a lot of times I worry about my parents—if they've gotten home or not or if they've been tied up somewhere. And ... I don't feel like I'm crying to people—the way I act I feel like I'm kind of bold, and hurting them. And, uh ... that's just it—I don't know what I want to do. I'm all confused. And, uh ... I'll talk to one person about one thing—and I'll talk to another person about something else—and maybe I'll get them all confused that way. And, uh ... like I have no sense of direction—somebody's got to lead me by the hand.

The patient who spoke in the above monologue had been asked to talk about any topic concerned with her hospitalization. She had recently been admitted to the psychiatric unit suffering from acute disorganization, overwhelming anxiety, and severe disruption of her thinking—an acute schizophrenic break. Her words exemplify many aspects of psychotic disorganization, but one of the most prominent features is how her topics shift willy-nilly between sentences and sometimes even within the same sentence. An idea in one sentence appears to touch off associations that appear in the next without a logical connection between them; for example, she goes from talking about a person on "buddy" status (able to go for walks with another patient) to going out for a walk (in her case, with a staff member). This passage exemplifies a feature of schizophrenic speech that has long impressed investigators—the apparent looseness of associations.

Bleuler (1950) attempted to identify the single basic underlying disorder in schizophrenia that would account for all of the deficits of the syndrome. He settled on the "breaking of associative threads." In normal speech, according to Bleuler, the person plans what he is going to say and excludes other ideas by forming "associative threads" among the planned topics. These underlying "threads" normally are purposeful and reality oriented, unlike the associative connections presumed to operate in primary-process thinking. They are not, therefore, the type of association studied in the word association test, but rather they are to be found in speech.

In a recent theory of schizophrenic disturbance, Chapman and Chapman (1973) review a series of studies, and conclude that disordered thinking in schizophrenics can be understood to reflect "excessive yielding to normal biases." For example, Chapman, Chapman, and Miller (1964) studied the errors of schizophrenics and normals in a vocabulary test in which the correct use of the word was "nonpreferred," or the less common use of the word. In the sentence "He likes *rare* meat," the word "rare" has a preferred meaning (not common) and a nonpreferred one (uncooked). Schizophrenics, in contrast to normals of equal tested intelligence, more often make the error of selecting the preferred or dominant meaning ("not common" for "rare"), a type of error that is infrequent in normal subjects. Loose associations, according to the Chapmans, are those in which the normal error bias is exaggerated.

Maher (1972) reviewed another aspect of schizophrenic disruption, in written communications by schizophrenics. Of interest was *where* the looseness occurs in the sentence. In normal speech, it is often possible to delete some words without totally losing the communication, since so much of normal language is redundant. Between sentences, however, there is less redundancy, so that deletion of the last word in a sentence raises the ambiguity. Thus, according to some theorists, in schizophrenics' written communications, the "loose" association occurs most often at the point of greatest ambiguity, between sentences.

Other aspects of schizophrenic speech

Looseness of association, which is a type of positive thought disorder and probably one of the most important, is one of the more emphasized qualities of schizophrenic speech. However, it is by no means the only one. Others have commented on the appearance of *blocking*, or the inability to complete a sentence, possibly because of conflicting associations or anxiety. Another important characteristic of speech not necessarily limited to schizophrenics is *vagueness*, or the incomplete and ambiguous communication. Related to vagueness, but more severe, are gaps in communication, in which the speaker leaves out important words that the listener must fill in.

Accordingly, we decided to study these aspects of the speech of schizophrenics and other patients to determine whether these are distinguishing features of schizophrenic speech, and also to see how stable these features are over the course of hospitalization. Given the central role that Bleuler ascribed to looseness of association, it was thought desirable to find some way to quantify the types and frequencies of loose associations. By comparing looseness with other forms of speech disruption, the question of how unique or central looseness is to schizophrenia might be assessed.

PROCEDURES

In this aspect of our research, a series of patients were given a standard fifteen-minute "free-verbalization" interview, which has been described in Chapter 3. The sample of patients we have studied using this free-verbalization technique was collected by Drs. Frank Reilly and Andrew Siegel. The patients studied in this research were given one of two sets of instructions.

All patients were directed to speak for seven and a half minutes on each of two topics: (a) a mental-health topic and the events leading to the hospitalization, and (b) non-mental-health events. The order of topics was varied systematically across patients. After the introduction, the interviewer spoke only when he found it necessary to encourage the patient to continue talking, and his comments were limited to that goal (e.g., "Could you please go on"; "Could you say more?"; etc.).

Drs. Reilly and Siegel, along with Dr. Gary Tucker and the present two investigators, conducted this research with the goal of studying loose associations more closely. Major aspects of our research using this method, along with various methodological procedures we used for these investigations, have been described in greater detail in a series of reports (Reilly, Harrow, Tucker, Quinlan, and Siegel, 1975; Reilly, Harrow, and Tucker, 1973; Reilly, Quinlan, Harrow, and Tucker, 1975; Siegel, Harrow, Reilly, and Tucker, 1976, 1978; Siegel, Reilly, Harrow, and Tucker, 1973).

ASSESSMENT OF LOOSE ASSOCIATIONS AND OTHER TYPES OF DEVIANT VERBALIZATIONS

All interviews were taped, transcribed, and then rated with satisfactory reliability by experienced clinicians on ten variables. For scoring purposes, the non-mental-health section and the mental-health section of each transcript were divided into two equal parts: these four sections of each tape were scored separately. Since the transcripts varied in length to some degree, the length of each section of the transcript was noted to correct for sparse records that give little opportunity for looseness of associations to appear. The final looseness-of-associations scores were divided by the number of words in that section of the particular patient's record.

The variables scored incorporated a number of the characteristics of schizophrenic speech described by Bleuler and other theorists, as well as some additional ones thought to be theoretically relevant and worthy of analysis. These variables are:

1. *Looseness of associations.* This was defined as a lack of connection between ideas so that the reason for a shift in thought is questionable or at times even incomprehensible to a listener; continuity of thought and the hierarchical logical development of concepts are lacking to a greater or lesser degree. Six variants of looseness were defined depending on whether the shift in thought occurred within or between sentences, was slight or drastic, or involved a change in subject. These six variants were scored separately, according to the following criteria:

Level 1: Mild shift within a sentence (e.g., "I was going along the street with Carol, . . . she likes walking").
Level 2: Mild shift from one sentence to the next, same topic (e.g., "I related to him, you know that I had in the past been under psychiatric treatment. I feel that I'm about ready to terminate").
Level 3: Drastic shift from one sentence to the next, same topic

(e.g., "I came here to Connecticut . . . it was so strange . . . such tough luck we had . . . oh, I miss my stepmother").

Level 4: Mild shift from one sentence to the next, different topic (e.g., "I was on medication and I asked him if he would take my pressure. He says it was fine. That is all well and good. Well in the office I had a nice acquaintance with a fellow that knows my family well").

Level 5: Drastic shift from one sentence to the next, different topic (e.g., "I studied hair . . . as a hairdresser in Hartford . . . I got my license . . . and/uh I think my sister went under a different name . . . ").

Level 6: Drastic shift within a sentence (e.g., "So . . . that didn't make matters, let's see . . . I think if she didn't know better . . . ").

Thus, the distinction suggested by Maher of loose associations between sentences as contrasted to loose associations within a sentence is made, as well as whether the shift results in a change of topic or not.

2. *Gap in communication.* Essential information is missing; the reader or listener *may*, with more or less accuracy, be able to guess at or supply this information, but the speaker behaves as if he were unaware of the defect in the communication.

3. *Private meaning.* Here words, phrases, or ideas are put forth that are somehow unique to the speaker, only fully meaningful to and completely comprehensible by him. Neologism would be an extreme example of this deviance.

4. *Blocking.* There is an abrupt pause or cessation of the train of thought or associative pattern, so that the speaker does not immediately proceed. When the speaker does proceed, there is minimal or no connection with what he had been talking about before.

5. *Delusional thinking.* Here the speaker's spontaneous verbalizations cue the listener in to the fact that (a) he is presently delusional, or (b) he talks of past delusions. (Present and past delusions were scored separately.)

6. *Vagueness of ideas.* Statements are grammatically complete, but words, phrases, and sentences are so imprecise and/or abstract that it is difficult for the listener to follow or comprehend what the speaker is conveying, in terms of meaning.

7. *Abrupt shifts in time.* The speaker passes rapidly from time period to time period without a clear logic for his shifts.

8. *Repetition.* The speaker actually repeats the same group of words, phrases, or interjections.

9. *Perseveration.* The same basic idea (not necessarily the same words) is reiterated or reworked with a lack of movement or direction to the train of thought.

10. *A global score* was given by the rater for each section as to the overall severity of the speech pathology, which took into account variables 2 through 9.

11. *Productivity.* The number of words in each of the four sections was counted, both to correct the looseness scores for length of protocol and to assess paucity versus fluency of speech.

The score for each type of looseness for each of the four sections was a direct sum of the number of elements fitting that particular category of looseness. Individual and sum scores for looseness of associations were calculated, according to a weighting system that alloted levels 3,5, and 6 higher scores for deviance. For all other categories of deviant verbalizations, at the end of each of the four sections in each transcript the rater gave a numerical rating from zero (indicating no pathology) to four (indicating maximum pathology) for each of the categories. This numerical rating was based on the frequency and the severity of each characteristic in that portion of the transcript.

Samples

Two samples were studied in order to compare (1) acutely psychotic hospitalized schizophrenics with other acute psychiatric inpatients both at the height of their illness and later in partial remission, and (2) groups of hospitalized and nonhospitalized chronic schizophrenic patients, to assess the effects of severity of disorder, and of social deprivation, on communication.

Acute Patients

The subjects were twenty-six schizophrenic patients and twenty-five nonschizophrenic patients interviewed during their first week of hospitalization at the psychiatric inpatient division of the Yale-New Haven Hospital. The schizophrenic sample consisted of relatively young acute schizophrenics who had not been chronically hospitalized. Of the twenty-six schizophrenics in the sample, eighteen had not been hospitalized before. Of the twenty-five nonschizophrenics, twenty-one had not been hospitalized before. The difference in frequency of previous hospitalization was not statistically significant. All twenty-six schizophrenics also met the criteria for a schizophrenic diagnosis on the *NHSI*. The comparison population was made up of eleven patients with neurotic or psychotic depression and fourteen patients with personality disorders or nondepressed neurosis admitted over the same time period. One of the schizophrenic patients was mute throughout the initial interview and her protocol was not used in the analyses. A second interview, six to eight weeks later, was obtained for twenty-three of the schizophrenics and nineteen of the nonschizophrenics who continued to be hospitalized. (There were no significant differences on any of the variables scored in the first interview between patients discharged in less than six weeks and those remaining in the sample after six weeks.)

The median age of the entire sample was twenty-three years. There was a nonsignificant trend for the schizophrenics to be younger than the nonschizophrenics. However, a younger age among the schizophrenic sample would not account for these patients' higher scores on disordered verbalizations at the acute phase, since there were no significant correlations with age, either overall or within schizophrenics. The schizophrenic and nonschizophrenic samples did not differ significantly in IQ, or in years of education (mean years of education for schizophrenics = 13.33; for nonschizophrenics = 13.43). A larger proportion of schizophrenics were on phenothiazines; this should tend to reduce the schizophrenics' scores on the measures of deviant verbalizations (and thus work against the hypotheses). These patients were not used in our other investigations.

Chronic Schizophrenic Patients

Two samples of chronic schizophrenic patients were studied: nonhospitalized and hospitalized. The sample classified as chronic schizophrenic, nonhospitalized, consisted of fifteen schizophrenics, all of whom were enrolled in an outpatient program for chronic patients at the Connecticut Mental Health Center. Each had been hospitalized at least two times for psychiatric reasons, and had been hospitalized for at least twelve months, but each had been functioning in the community for at least twelve months prior to the interview.

The sample classified as chronic schizophrenic, hospitalized, was a group of fifteen schizophrenics, all of whom were currently hospitalized at a state hospital in Connecticut. At the time of the interview, every patient had been hospitalized continuously for at least two years and the minimum total length of hospitalization for any one of these fifteen subjects was fifty-four months. Ten had been hospitalized more than ten years.

The mean age and mean age of onset of the chronic hospitalized sample were 42.8 and 25.4 years, respectively, and of chronic non-hospitalized sample were 38.9 and 28.2 years (the differences are nonsignificant). Eight of the hospitalized schizophrenics and ten of the nonhospitalized schizophrenics were females. Each of the two samples had eight patients who had never been married and seven patients currently married or once married. All thirty subjects had been on phenothiazines for many years.

All patients spoke during the interview to at least a limited extent; however, the hospitalized patients spoke significantly fewer words than the nonhospitalized chronic schizophrenics. No patients' data were discarded.

The data we collected will be considered from several perspectives; first, the acute patients at the start of their hospitalization will be explored, followed by the changes that occurred over the period of hospitalization in which partial symptomatic relief was generally attained. Next, the comparison of the two chronic schizophrenic subsamples will treat the question of whether looseness, a type of positive thought disorder, and other aspects of disrupted speech remain after several years of the condition. Then the differences in types of speech disruption as a function of the topic will be treated. Finally, we will examine the degree to which disrupted speech constitutes a unitary or multifaceted entity.

Schizophrenics and nonschizophrenics with acute symptoms

The data comparing the schizophrenic and nonschizophrenic patients on looseness of associations are presented in Table 8.1. There were clear differences between the schizophrenic and the nonschizophrenic groups. Looseness of associations was present in both the schizophrenic and the comparison sample. However, whereas both samples showed some evidence of the milder forms of looseness (e.g., level 2 and level 4 in the rating system), the schizophrenic population was significantly higher than the comparison population in all types of looseness except mild within-sentence, same-topic looseness (see Table 8.1). On our ratings for the more severe manifestations of looseness (levels 3, 5, and 6), we found that approximately 80 per cent of our schizophrenics showed at least a fair amount of severe looseness and that such severe looseness was rare in our control population of acute psychiatric patients.

The data for the remaining speech variables are presented in Table 8.2. The overall results indicate that there were significant differences on all variables examined. The variable that most highly discriminated between the two groups was the global Overt Deviant Verbalizations.

"Gaps in communication" might be viewed as a partial measure of the speaker's ability to gauge the amount of knowledge he can expect the listener to have of him and of his situation. This phenomenon occurred in almost all schizophrenics. It was approximately three times more frequent in schizophrenics than in nonschizophrenics ($P < .001$).

Private meaning included what Bleuler would have called neologisms, as well as private ideas and phrases. Private meanings were extremely rare in our control group, and were significantly more frequent in the schizophrenic population ($P < .001$).

TABLE 8.1
Loose Associations: Mean Scores for Acute Schizophrenic and Nonschizophrenic Patients

Degree of Loose Associations	Loose Associations Incidence/1,000 words		t-test
	Schizophrenic (N = 26)	Nonschiz. (N = 25)	Schiz. versus Nonschiz. t
Level 1 Mild, within-sentence	0.26	0.13	1.27
Level 2 Mild, between-sentence	4.44	1.78	2.75[1]
Level 3 Drastic, between, same topic	3.43	0.17	4.18[1]
Level 4 Mild, between, different topic	1.31	0.43	3.30[1]
Level 5 Drastic, between, different topic	3.88	0.35	3.30[1]
Level 6 Drastic, within-sentence	0.76	0.00	3.34[1]
Total looseness (weighted)[3]	32.45	3.90	4.80[2]

[1]$P < .01$.
[2]$P < .001$.
[3]The weights assigned were: levels 1, 2, 4 = 1; levels 3, 5 = 3; level 6 = 6.

From Reilly, Harrow, Tucker, Quinlan & Siegel. *British Journal of Psychiatry, 127*, 240–246, 1975. Reproduced by permission of the publisher.

Blocking, long looked upon as a hallmark of schizophrenic speech, was by no means a universal characteristic of our schizophrenic sample. Only 50 percent of our schizophrenics showed even mild evidence of this phenomenon, and there was little evidence of it (8 percent) in our control group.

Vagueness of ideas was present to a mild degree in 20 percent of the control group, but was of a much more pronounced character in the schizophrenic population, 80 percent of which had at least one instance.

Repetition and perseveration were found to a mild degree in more than one-half, and abrupt shifts in time in close to one-third, of these acute schizophrenics; all of these were extremely rare in the control group.

A summary measure, overall global rating of overt deviant verbalizations, is also presented in Table 8.2. There is a high degree of consistency with which the schizophrenic speech samples can be

TABLE 8.2
Types of Deviant Verbalizations: Mean Scores per Segment for Acute Schizophrenic and Nonschizophrenic Patients

Types of Deviant Verbalizations	Mean Scores (potential range = 0–8)		t-test Schiz. versus Nonschiz. (t)
	Schizophrenic (N = 26)	Nonschiz. (N = 25)	
Gaps in communication	3.81	1.14	5.31[3]
Private meanings	3.36	0.36	6.83[3]
Blocking	2.69	0.82	4.13[3]
Present delusions	3.37	0.00	5.84[3]
Past delusions	0.50	0.00	2.43[1]
Vagueness of ideas	4.94	2.00	4.82[3]
Abrupt time shifts	0.79	0.24	2.52[1]
Repetition	1.54	0.36	3.01[2]
Perservations	1.84	0.52	3.23[2]
Global rating of overt deviant verbalization:	5.90	1.56	8.33[3]

[1]$P < .05.$
[2]$P < .01.$
[3]$P < .001.$

From Reilly, Harrow, Tucker, Quinlan & Siegel. *British Journal of Psychiatry, 127,* 240–246, 1975. Reproduced by permission of the publisher.

identified on the global measure as well as on many of the individual measures. The correlation of the two summary measures, weighted looseness and global overt speech deviation are presented in Table 8.3. In examining the intercorrelation of the measures, it is clear that the scores are highly related to one another (except for past delusions), and may constitute one or only a few factors.

Looseness was significantly associated with the sex of the subject (males had more severe loosening of associations) and the sum of overt deviation was correlated with marital status (married patients had less overt deviation), but these correlations were only moderate in degree and were not consistent, although more extensive study may be needed before they can be totally dismissed

TABLE 8.3
Total Loose Associations and Overt Deviant Verbalization
Rating: Correlation with Other Variables

Variable	Total Looseness	Global Overt Deviant Verbalizations
Marital status	−.14	−.33[1]
Sex	.31[1]	.11
Age	−.02	−.20
Gaps in communication	.76[3]	.82[3]
Private meanings	.61[3]	.82[3]
Blocking	.56[3]	.69[3]
Present delusions	.65[3]	.67[3]
Past delusions	.05	.25
Vagueness of ideas	.58[3]	.81[3]
Abrupt time shifts	.37[2]	.47[3]
Repetition	.52[3]	.48[3]
Perseveration	.49[3]	.56[3]
Global rating of overt deviant verbalizations	.77[3]	

[1] $P < .05$.
[2] $P < .01$.
[3] $P < .001$.

COMMENT

The findings lead to a number of possible conclusions about schizophrenic language and thinking. Some aspects of overt deviation, such as present and past delusions, were absent from the protocols of nonschizophrenics. This would be expected, since the nonschizophrenic sample was essentially a population of nonpsychotic patients. Other forms of overt deviation and looseness, however, did occur in the speech samples of the nonschizophrenics.

Looseness, a type of positive thought disorder, is by no means a unique or isolated finding in the spontaneous verbalizations of schizophrenics, and is usually found in combination with vagueness of ideas and gaps in communication, that is, with other measures of careless, imprecise, and disorganized communication. These traits were also found in the speech of some acutely hospitalized nonschizophrenic patients, but to a much milder degree. In other words, when milder forms of looseness, vagueness, and precision are carefully looked for, they appear to be present to some extent in the spoken verbalizations of most hospitalized patients.

The overall results can be looked at from several viewpoints.

1. During the acute schizophrenic episode, some aspects of the clinical picture are influenced by confusion and disorganization; we have discussed this in greater detail in Chapter 5. One consequence of this confusion might be a drastic, albeit transient, social breakdown in which interpersonal, externally directed communication becomes difficult for a while. There would then be in the acute schizophrenic episode, for many of these patients, a temporary incapacity to be in a state of consistent, coherent, and effective verbal and interpersonal contact.

2. The breakdown of coherent communication also could be influenced by intermingling of personal material and a withdrawal into one's self, in which egocentric, inner-directed, highly personalized concerns are paramount.

3. Perhaps the data might be conceptualized in terms of a continuum between schizophrenic patients on the one hand, and other disturbed patients and normals on the other hand. This view would incorporate the following possibilities:

a. Almost all people, including nonhospitalized "normals," show looseness of associations to some degree (i.e., our impression is that if looseness were carefully looked for in "normals," mild forms of it would clearly be present to a limited degree in many normals).

Serious or flagrant forms of looseness, however, would be very rare under most circumstances. It is possible that under conditions of extreme stress more flagrant examples of looseness might occur slightly more frequently in some normals.

b. A certain portion of the schizophrenic patients who show marked looseness during the acute phase may have always been somewhat vague, imprecise, and elusive in their speech (as in their relationships).

c. During the stress of the acute illness, whatever its basis or precipitant, this chronic predisposition to looseness and vagueness becomes much more overt. In the nonschizophrenic the difficulty in communication may become more pronounced but usually remains mild in severity; for the subgroup of the schizophrenics, what would be seen as mild looseness or vagueness during remission becomes drastic and readily apparent looseness during the acute episode.

Change over the course of hospitalization

While loose associations and other evidence of disrupted speech were common and severe during the acute phase of illness, the question arises as to whether looseness is a stable feature of the schizophrenic's speech or whether it is a byproduct of the acute symptomatology that diminishes as the acute disruption subsides. If loose and disrupted speech is a persisting characteristic of the schizophrenic, it is worth noting whether it is the mild or severe levels of looseness and disruption that remains. After six weeks of hospitalization, the more acute symptoms (e.g., hallucinations, extreme anxiety) have usually diminished in intensity (see Table 8.1), but the schizophrenics show sufficient psychopathology to make further hospital treatment advisable.

As we have noted, twenty-three of the twenty-six schizophrenics and nineteen of the twenty-five nonschizophrenics assessed during the acute phase of hospitalization were in the hospital six weeks later for a second free-verbalization interview using the same procedures as in the first interview. A comparison of patients discharged before the second time period with those patients remaining in the sample showed no significant differences in any of the variables studied at the beginning of hospitalization. The different rate of early discharge (three of twenty-six, versus six of twenty-five) was not statistically significant. Two questions were assessed in the analysis: (1) was there a significant change over the six weeks? and (2) was there a continuing significant difference between schizophrenics and nonschizophrenics during partial remission six to eight weeks later?

Findings

The evaluation of change over the six-week period was assessed by a repeated-measures Analysis of Variance, while the significance of the difference remaining between the diagnostic groups was assessed by *t*-tests for variables from the second period only. The data for looseness levels appear in Table 8.4 and for the overt deviant verbalization scores in Table 8.5.

The overall difference between schizophrenics and nonschizophrenics on looseness, a type of positive thought disorder, remain highly significant. Only the *F*-ratios for level 1 (a very infrequent form) and number of words were not statistically significant. The two sets of *F*-ratios of particular interest are those for time period or phase of disorder, reflecting the degree of change, and for the interaction of time period by diagnosis. For looseness, level 5 (drastic shift from one sentence to the next, different topic), and the summary score for drastic (but not for mild) looseness, and the weighted sum of looseness, showed both a significant drop from the first to the second time period, and a significant interaction of diagnosis by time period. In each case, the significant drop in the looseness score was found to be determined primarily by a larger drop in the score for schizophrenics than for nonschizophrenics. In Table 8.5, a similar pattern was found for gaps, private meaning, present delusions, and global overt deviations, and a similar but not quite significant trend was found for blocking, vagueness, and repetition. In accord with other data that we presented in Chapter 5, the striking frequency of deviant verbalizations of schizophrenics at the acute phase diminished in partial remission. This rapid and striking improvement corresponded to the clinical impressions about these patients as they recovered from the acute episode.

If schizophrenics show recovery in looseness and deviant speech, do they become indistinguishable from other, nonschizophrenic patients? A look at the column on the far right-hand edge of Tables 8.4 and 8.5 suggests that the free verbalizations of schizophrenics remained quite distinguishable from nonschizophrenics even in this more benign phase. Significant differences occurred between groups for two of the separate looseness levels and for mild looseness, and for all of the deviant verbalization categories except present delusions and repetition. Even for the nonsignificant categories, near-significant trends frequently appeared. The speech of schizophrenics was a distinctly looser and more disrupted feature of their clinical appearance than was true of their nonschizophrenic counterparts.

TABLE 8.4
Looseness of Associations at Two Phases of Disorder: Means, Analyses of Variance, and t-Test[1]

Categories of Looseness of Associations	Mean Incidence of Looseness per 1000 Words				Analysis of Variance[2]			t-Test
	Nonschizophrenics (N = 19)		Schizophrenics (N = 23)		Diagnosis (D)	Time Period (T)	Interaction (D × T)	Time 2 Only df = 40
	Time 1	Time 2	Time 1	Time 2				
Level 1	0.07	0.09	0.28	0.10	2.68	1.45	2.26	0.08
Level 2	1.49	1.49	4.66	3.54	13.82[6]	1.41	1.37	2.96[5]
Level 3	0.14	0.11	3.24	1.76	8.69[5]	2.97	2.73	1.81
Level 4	0.43	0.98	1.37	1.38	4.74[4]	1.02	0.98	0.71
Level 5	0.33	0.08	4.09	0.93	9.48[5]	8.00[5]	5.78[4]	2.13[4]
Level 6	0.00	0.00	0.73	0.29	7.78[5]	2.56	2.56	1.42
Mild looseness	1.84	2.48	5.91	4.89	15.32[6]	0.11	2.18	2.84[5]
Drastic looseness	0.48	0.18	7.22	2.59	11.25[5]	7.32[5]	5.66[5]	1.94
Weighted sum[3]	3.34	3.12	32.64	14.68	14.35[6]	6.82[4]	6.49[4]	2.03[4]
Mean number of words per 7-minute segment	793.55	736.50	924.31	855.04	2.83	2.25	0.02	1.54

[1]This table only includes data from the forty-two patients who were available at both time periods, and does not include data from the additional nine patients (used in Table 8.1) who were only assessed at the acute phase.
[2]F ratios, $df = 1, 40$.
[3]Weights used were: L1, L2, L4 = 1; L3, L5 = 3; L6 = 6.
[4]$P < .05$.
[5]$P < .01$.
[6]$P < .001$.

TABLE 8.5
Overt Deviant Verbalizations at Two Phases of Disorder: Analyses of Variance and t-Test[1]

Variable	Nonschizophrenics (N = 19)		Schizophrenics (N = 23)		Analysis of Variance[2]			Time 2 t-Test df = 40
	Time 1	Time 2	Time 1	Time 2	Diagnosis (D)	Time (T)	Interaction (D×T)	
Gaps	1.05	0.82	3.81	1.79	18.91[5]	13.77[5]	8.60[4]	2.07[3]
Private meaning	0.26	0.26	3.08	2.08	37.82[5]	4.12[3]	4.12[3]	4.13[5]
Blocking	0.58	0.40	2.73	1.81	23.34[5]	5.04[3]	2.23	3.74[5]
Present delusions	0.00	0.00	2.90	0.56	19.08[5]	18.66[5]	18.66[5]	1.93
Past delusions	0.00	0.00	0.54	0.73	6.88[3]	1.72	1.72	2.80[4]
Vagueness	1.68	1.68	4.75	3.46	20.23[5]	3.92	3.92	2.72[4]
Abrupt time shifts	0.21	0.05	0.85	0.27	8.89[4]	9.42[4]	3.10	2.16[3]
Repetition	0.42	0.45	1.67	0.87	7.45[4]	3.28	3.74	1.61
Perseveration	0.45	0.63	1.73	1.60	9.46[4]	0.16	0.45	2.40[3]
Global overt deviation	1.29	1.08	5.79	3.48	62.60[5]	16.87[5]	11.71[4]	4.88[5]

[1] This table only includes data from forty-two patients who were available at both time periods, and does not include data from the additional nine patients (used in Table 8.2) who were only assessed at the acute phase.

[2] F ratios, $df = 1, 40$

[3] $p < .05$.

[4] $p < .01$.

[5] $p < .001$.

An examination of the scores for schizophrenics offers some suggestions about the nature of the change and the nature of the residual disorder. Level 2 (mild shift between sentences, same topic) and *mild* looseness remain relatively high, while the more drastic and bizarre forms (level 5, drastic looseness) showed a considerably greater decline in absolute frequency. Private meanings and vagueness remained above a mean score of 2.0, and gaps, blocking, and perseveration remained above 1.5, while other scores dropped below 1.0. These scores suggest a pattern of speech marked by a vague indefiniteness, mild changes that the listener may be able to fill in on his or her own, some gaps and perseveration of topics, but without the grossly bizarre qualities found during the acute phase.

As in other aspects of our research reported elsewhere in this book, the residual speech patterns of schizophrenics suggest what these patients may be like in partial remission. One can follow them more readily. The gaps they leave are easier to fill in, but such patients come across without clarity or conviction. The vague, elusive quality of speech is reflected in some of their adoptions of phrases from the counterculture—they are "sort of, like" in their descriptions of others, they go "into" things without well-defined criteria of participation. If their speech reflects their pattern of interpersonal relationships, for some schizophrenics vagueness and lack of definition may serve as protective but more culturally accepted barriers between themselves and others, reducing the potential for either intimacy or hostility. This subgroup of schizophrenics may become engaged in "talking without speaking, hearing without listening,"

Chronic Schizophrenics

The findings with schizophrenics in partial remission raise the question about what characterizes schizophrenic speech in chronic patients. Two types of "chronic" patients are of interest: those who have been able to maintain themselves, however marginally or adequately, in the community ("ambulatory"), and those who for one reason or another have required hospitalization for an extended period of time. There are a wide variety of reasons why one patient remains in the hospital while another is able to live outside, but two influences may be a more severe schizophrenic disorder, and a difficulty in thinking effectively and in communicating effectively with others. From a different point of view, persons who interact on a day-to-day basis in situations that do not treat them as patients may retain or develop communication skills that are not always required of patients in hospital settings. Regardless of which is cause and which is effect, the comparison of hospitalized and nonhospitalized schizophrenic patients allows an assessment of the differences in speech of these two populations.

In addition, a direct comparison of multiyear, chronic schizophrenics with acute schizophrenics would be desirable. However, the great differences in background of the patients, the settings in which the speech samples were gathered, and other differences make a strict comparison impossible. Thus, a precisely controlled comparison of early acute schizophrenics and multiyear hospitalized schizophrenics cannot be conducted. Attempts to match these two types of schizophrenic samples would also involve selecting out atypical acute schizophrenics and comparing them to atypical chronic schizophrenics. Despite the absence of precisely matched samples, however, some overall trends can be used to suggest similarities and differences.

Findings

The results from the two chronic patient samples are presented in Tables 8.6 and 8.7. A striking feature that characterizes the difference between the two samples is found in the last item in Table 8.7; non-hospitalized patients said almost twice as much as hospitalized patients on both mental-health and non-mental-health topics. Whether this type of negative symptom (impoverishment) is a consequence of severity of the schizophrenic disorder or the effect of institutionalization is unclear, although recent research of ours would suggest that it is not just a consequence of long-term institutionalization (Harrow, Marengo, Pogue-Geile, and Pawelski, in press). The rate of speech for non-hospitalized chronic patients is approximately at the level of our acute schizophrenics, so chronicity per se would not accout for the paucity of speech.

In both of these populations of chronic schizophrenics, looseness of associations did not appear to be the most prominent characteristic. *Severe* looseness was not frequent in both samples. Mild forms of looseness (level 1 and level 2) did occur to a considerably greater extent in both samples. The only significant differences between the two groups lay in the direction of a tendency for mild looseness (level 1 and level 2) to be more prominent (per unit of speech) in the hospitalized than in the nonhospitalized patients. Overall, there was less looseness among these chronic schizophrenics than might have been anticipated.

There was a moderate amount of vagueness in both samples, although there was little difference in the degree shown by the two

TABLE 8.6
Mean Scores for Chronic Schizophrenics on Various Types of Loose Associations

Different degrees of Loose Associations[1]	Non-Mental-Health Topic			Mental-Health Topic		
	Hospitalized	Nonhospitalized	Test of Significance *t*	Hospitalized	Nonhospitalized	Test of Significance *t*
Level 1	5.53	1.85	2.14[2]	4.98	4.03	0.38
Level 2	10.36	7.03	0.91	11.28	5.17	2.40[2]
Level 3	1.40	3.01	1.04	4.48	1.49	1.59
Level 4	0.00	0.27	1.47	0.32	0.13	0.56
Level 5	1.27	0.66	0.77	1.52	0.16	1.69
Level 6	0.32	0.61	0.43	0.29	0.09	0.92

[1]Final scores for various categories of loose associations represent incidence of loose associations per 1,000 words.

[2]$p < .05$.

From Siegel, Harrow, Reilly, and Tucker. *Journal of Nervous and Mental Disease*, 162, 105–112, 1976. The Williams and Wilkins Co., Baltimore, MD. Reproduced by permission of the publisher.

TABLE 8.7
Mean Scores for Chronic Schizophrenics on Measures of Deviant Speech Patterns
(Possible Range = 0-8)

	Non-Mental-Health Topic			Mental-Health Topic		
	Hospitalized	Nonhospitalized	Test of Significance t	Hospitalized	Nonhospitalized	Test of Significance t
Gaps in communication	0.13	0.53	2.12*	0.27	0.27	0.00
Private meaning	0.47	0.53	0.12	0.40	0.20	0.68
Blocking	1.40	0.53	1.75	0.93	1.33	0.71
Delusional, present	1.60	1.07	0.56	1.20	0.47	1.23
Delusional, past	0.00	0.40	1.19	0.33	0.33	0.00
Vagueness	1.67	1.60	0.09	1.87	2.13	0.34
Abrupt time shifts	0.20	0.13	0.48	0.00	0.07	1.00
Repetition	1.32	0.33	1.51	1.20	0.00	2.55*
Perseveration	4.20	2.53	1.91	3.53	1.40	3.31*
Overall deviance	4.40	2.20	2.68*	4.07	1.93	2.92*
Number of words	367.87	733.48	3.80**	350.53	734.60	4.23*

*P < .05.
**P < .01.

From Siegel, Harrow, Reilly, and Tucker. Journal of Nervous and Mental Disease, 162, 105–112, 1976. The Williams and Wilkins Co., Baltimore, MD. Reproduced by permission of the publisher.

types of samples. Relatively high scores occurred for perseveration in both groups of chronic schizophrenics. There was significantly more perseveration and repetition among the hospitalized schizophrenics than among the nonhospitalized schizophrenics.

Ratings for overall deviant verbalization were relatively high in both samples of chronic schizophrenics. This was especially true of the hospitalized patients, who were significantly higher on this variable. Thus, fourteen of the fifteen hospitalized schizophrenics showed a considerable degree of overall deviant verbalizations (a score of "2" or higher on this 0–4-point scale) for at least one of the four segments rated. Even among the ambulatory chronic schizophrenics who are living outside of a hospital, seven of the fifteen showed at least one score of "2" on one of the four segments on which they were rated for overall deviant verbalizations.

Despite the high scores on overall deviant verbalizations, there were relatively low scores on many of the specific categories of deviance. No one type of category accounted entirely for the high scores on overall deviant verbalizations. It appears that while select types of deviant verbalizations showed high scores in the sample, there was considerable variation in the type of deviance shown by the different patients.

The Foulds scale (Foulds, Hope, McPherson, and Mayo, 1967a) for delusions was obtained on each of the patients. Scores showed marked variations. The scores of the hospitalized chronic schizophrenics ranged from 0 to 11 with a mean of 6.0. There were no trends to support a strong relationship between the Foulds scores and speech variables in this population. The scores for the nonhospitalized chronic schizophrenics ranged from 0 to 11 with a mean of 4.5. Here it was evident that those nonhospitalized patients who scored higher on the Foulds scale scored correspondingly higher on private meanings, delusional thinking, vagueness, abrupt time shifts, repetition, and overall deviant verbalization. No significant correlations were found between the measure of overall deviant verbalizations and sex, or age, or total length of hospitalization.

From the present research it is evident that the hospitalized chronic schizophrenic patients showed more evidence of language and speech disturbance in select areas and on an overall index than did the nonhospitalized chronic schizophrenics. This finding might be interpreted in a number of ways: (1) the differences could presumably be related to premorbid development or personality; (2) the differences might possibly be related to the effects of institutionalization; (3) the differences could be influenced by clinicians' criteria for discharge, or their stereotypes of the health-sickness dimension and of what constitutes severe psychopathology; or (4) most important, the differences might actually be a measure of the severity of illness. On review of the patient hospital charts in each population, most of the patients would be classified as poor premorbid schizophrenics. In addition, the differences were probably not attributable only to the effects of chronic institutionalization, since there was not a significant relationship between length of hospitalization and overall deviant verbalization. Consequently, most of the differences noted are probably more related to the discharge criteria and severity. Some support of the findings for speech patterns being a measure of the severity of illness in the data indicating that the more delusional nonhospitalized schizophrenics (Foulds scale) scored correspondingly higher on most of the speech patterns measured.

The data suggested that perseveration and impoverishment, two negative symptoms, are important features, relatively high among chronic schizophrenics. A major way that the outpatient chronic schizophrenic patients (who function to some degree in society) differed from long-term hospitalized chronic schizophrenics concerns variables related to paucity of verbalization and impoverished thinking. It is probable that impoverished thinking and negative symptoms are one key aspect of the course of deterioration for the select group of very poor prognosis, chronic, schizophrenics who remain hospitalized for many years, or permanently.

Further suggestive evidence on the role of paucity of speech was obtained when the mean number of words spoken by each of the two samples of chronic schizophrenics was compared with those of our acute schizophrenics and our acutely disturbed nonschizophrenic sample. The chronic hospitalized schizophrenics gave significantly fewer words than both the acute schizophrenics and the acutely disturbed nonschizophrenic patients ($P < .001$). Even the sample of nonhospitalized, chronic schizophrenics showed a nonsignificant trend toward more paucity than the acute schizophrenics ($P < .10$), and than the acutely disturbed nonschizophrenics sample ($P < 0.15$). These data fit in with results we have collected on concrete thinking in other schizophrenic samples (see Chapter 7) and suggest that paucity and possibly impoverished thinking, and negative symptoms in general, are not uniform for all schizophrenics but are more a function of severe chronic schizophrenia.

The fact the overt looseness of association is not the most prominent element in the populations studied is noteworthy. This may, in part, be explained in that we have narrowed the definition of looseness from its customary broad clinical application. However, it is precisely this type of clarification and standardization that would seem helpful in delineating differences in varying subgroups of the schizophrenic syndrome.

There are several other considerations of importance in relation to the lack of high absolute scores on loose associations for the current sample of chronic schizophrenics. The present results do not provide complete evidence on the issue of a weakening of the *underlying* associative process, as formulated by Bleuler, since such an underlying weakness could conceivably manifest itself in various ways other than just overt loose associations (such as by other types of disordered speech and behavior).

As we have noted, a precisely matched sample of early schizophrenics, to be used as a comparison group, was not obtained, although our sample of acute patients provides a rough baseline. The rough indications, comparing the two samples, suggest that there were somewhat fewer overt loose associations in the present chronic patients than in a sample of younger acute schizophrenics.

Another related factor bearing on the overall issue is that overt signs of loose associations were not more prominent in the present two samples of chronic schizophrenics than were some of the other overt signs of speech disturbance that were rated, especially negative symptoms, such as perseverations.

Overall, overt signs of loose associations were not extremely frequent in these chronic schizophrenics (although a few very striking instances of loose associations and other signs of positive symptoms did appear). The speech impoverishment found in these chronic schizophrenics may have contributed to the infrequency of overt signs of loose associations in the current sample.

The results indicating that statistically significant differences between the two chronic subpopulations studied were found on some of the same patterns of speech (paucity, perseveration, and repetition) that characterize them collectively as a group are noteworthy. Our findings of statistically greater degrees of paucity, perseveration, repetition, and overall deviant verbalization in hospitalized versus nonhospitalized chronic schizophrenics might be useful in beginning to predict which chronic patients, newly admitted or otherwise, are likely to function in an ambulatory capacity in the future. This could be an important issue at a time when so great an emphasis is placed on discharging patients from state hospitals.

OVERVIEW

The findings for the looseness and overt deviation variables indicate that the scoring of free verbalizations can be done reliably and with a great deal of sensitivity to the differences in the speech of different patient populations and to the changes within patients over time, and on different topics. In comparison to other variables examined elsewhere, the scoring of speech samples provides unusually clear and consistent findings.

The results indicating that the speech of the acute schizophrenic is distinctly loose fits in with the data we have presented in other chapters on positive types of thought disorder in schizophrenia. Speech is the most essential tool for ongoing daily social interaction. For whatever reasons that speech becomes loose and disordered, the loss of ability to communicate in an undisrupted fashion probably increases the already alienated state of the incipient psychotic patients, and may intensify anxiety by reducing the effectiveness of the patient's effort to obtain relief. Loose and disrupted speech can thus be seen as a contributor to the painful state of the acutely disturbed schizophrenic.

Is looseness of associations the central process in the thought disorder of schizophrenics? The more drastic forms of looseness are found most prominently in acute phases of schizophrenia and are somewhat less frequent in partial remission or in more chronic patients. Even mild forms of looseness are found more often in the speech of schizophrenic patients than in that of nonschizophrenics, and more often in hospitalized chronic schizophrenics than in nonhospitalized schizophrenics. But looseness per se did not show a sharply different picture from other aspects of disorderd speech.

Of course, Bleuler's initial hypothesis about schizophrenic looseness was not directly tested. Bleuler believed that the looseness of association was prominent in the schizophrenic's underlying thought formation. Looseness of overt speech is one of the more likely aspects of the behavior of the schizophrenic to provide clues about an underlying loosening of associative threads. While the overt speech of the schizophrenic shows loosening of associations, it also displays many other facets.

The free-verbalization scores also illustrate a point that is relevant to the question of whether one utilizes structured or unstructured responses for eliciting evidence of thought disorder. The free-verbalization interview presents one of the more unstructured formats for eliciting evidence of disordered thinking, and is also a situation that displays some of the clearest differences between acute schizophrenics and other acutely disturbed patients, and between hospitalized and nonhospitalized chronic patients. It may be that one of the schizophrenics' distinctive features is disorganization in the absence of structure, or, put in other words, the schizophrenic may not effectively utilize his internalized controls to guide his thinking and speech in the absence of routine cues. Less structured situations, while more difficult to quantify, may come closer to the source of the ongoing or the acute situation that elicits the schizophrenic's disordered and bizarre behavior or allows it to occur.

Perspective monitoring and looseness of associations

The findings from the study of schizophrenic speech lend support to the concept of faulty perspective monitoring. To a greater or lesser degree, coherent speech requires that the speaker organize his own ideas and their attendant associations in a way that the listener can follow. Loose associations, gaps, private meaning, vagueness, delusions, abrupt time shifts—all make it more difficult to follow the meaning of the speaker; in these forms, the speaker fails to monitor his own verbal production from the perspective of the listener. Blocking, repetition, and perseveration suggest a related but not equivalent process. Blocking, or abrupt stopping of a train of thought, represents a monitoring of speech that prevents the emergence of an idea at the expense of coherence to the listener. Repetition and perseveration, on the other hand, suggest a faulty monitoring or recall of one's own speech, possibly because internal concerns override the goal of communication.

Certainly, the adage that "to be a good clinician one must be a good listener" is supported by the findings.

Impaired perspective and looseness of associations

Our results using the free verbalization technique could fit in with a view about impaired perspective in schizophrenia. To a greater or lesser degree, coherent conversation requires that the speaker be able to attend less to his or her private concerns and that, using long-term stored knowledge about what is socially appropriate, attend to the external context. There was almost no evidence in the taped interviews to indicate that the thought-disordered schizophrenics were embarrassed, upset, or aware of their loose speech. Loose associations, gaps, private meanings, vagueness, and abrupt time shifts all make the schizophrenics harder to understand and make them look odd and bizarre. We have interpreted the material from the taped transcripts of the fifteen-minute interviews, including the patient's lack of embarrassment about verbal behavior, as being consistent with a picture of the schizophrenic as having difficulty in using effectively stored knowledge about what behavior is socially appropriate. In this type of situation the pataient's internal concerns will frequently override the goal of communication, and the patient will not recognize how inappropriate his or her speech and behavior appear to others.

## PART IV

BOUNDARY-RELATED PHENOMENA

9

Boundaries in Schizophrenia

The concept of a psychological boundary disturbance has received a great deal of attention in the literature on schizophrenia (Blatt and Wild, 1976; Blatt and Ritzler, 1974; Quinlan and Harrow, 1974; Johnson and Quinlan, 1980). What are "boundaries" in the psychological sense? As with any ideas that rely on analogies to physical objects, the term "boundary" is often used as if its definition were readily apparent. In fact, most treatments of psychological boundaries treat the construct as a given. For our purposes, a working definition of boundary can be, "a region in space or time at which an entity is deemed to begin and/or end." This definition is extended to apply to intrapsychic boundaries since "intrapsychic space" is a symbolic analogy to physical space. The difficulty in defining boundaries stems from the very basic nature of boundaries: to assert that object exists implies that such an object is limited and bounded. It is this very basic nature of "boundary" that leads theoreticians to conceptualize the very basic disturbance in schizophrenia as a boundary disturbance (e.g., Blatt and Wild, 1976). Within our framework of shared social perspective, maintaining boundaries between ideas, representations, and psychological systems is a strongly held assumption. Where violations of boundaries occur, such as with mythological creatures, the results are generally treated as unusual or fantastic. Playful use of fabulized combinations occurs in such areas as cartoons and fantasy-oriented films. Artistic works presenting fused images are not uncommon. In each case, the blurred or fused boundaries rely on the nonveridical violation of "reality" for their effect. The use of boundary violations in artistic and fantasy representations for the effect produced attests to the consensual expectation that objects are separate; violation of boundaries is unexpected and "unreal."

Psychological boundaries have been a subject of psychological interest for some time. Freud (1965) first conceptualized the primitive ego as a stimulus barrier that reduced the intense external forces on the psyche. In more developed conceptualizations of the ego (Freud, 1927, 1977), an important function of the ego is to regulate the psychic systems. Thus, two types of boundaries can already be distinguished: (1) boundaries between psychological systems usually in the analytic sense of ego, id, and superego, and (2) boundaries between the person and the outside, especially other persons or interpersonal boundaries. We will examine two other types of boundaries: (3) boundaries between objects or the representations of objects, and (4) an emphasis on either the barrier aspects of a physical boundary or the penetrability of a physical boundary as in the barrier and penetration responses.

In his paper on the "influencing machine," Tausk (1948) introduced the concept of boundary to the study of schizophrenia. Federn (1952) extended the emphasis on boundaries, viewing psychosis as a withdrawal of cathexis in the ego boundary. Blatt and Wild (1976) have summarized the literature on boundary disturbances in extending the hypothesis that boundary disturbances are the fundamental phenomena of schizophrenia.

A disturbance of intrapsychic boundaries is presumably observed in the intrusion of id-related or drive-dominated thinking, which is treated in Chapter 6. Conceptually, the disturbance arises from the failure of the ego to regulate id impulses. Such a boundary "disturbance" is not restricted to psychiatric disturbances, however, and may emerge under stress, reduced consciousness, or in drive-induced states. Nonetheless, significant and persistent intrusions of drive-dominated material may be much more likely in schizophrenia, according to the boundary hypothesis.

"Interpersonal boundary" disturbance is a form of disruption more frequently attributed exclusively to pathological states. The most frequently cited form is "fusion" in which the distinction between two persons is lost either momentarily or for sustained periods. Mahler (1968), among others, describes the very earliest state of the infant's thinking process as a fused state in which the mother and infant are one.

Blatt and Wild (1976) postulate that the earliest cognition of the infant is an awareness of boundary, for example, between hunger and satiation, and most important, between self and not self. Disturbance in the very early mother-child relationships, Blatt and Wild propose, results in the inability to maintain boundary distinctions in later life, and an attempt to fuse psychologically with others or a fear of such fusion. Such fusion experiences are frequently noted in the clinical experience with schizophrenics (Jacobsen, 1964; Federn, 1952; Searles, 1965) in which the child or parent talks "as if" the parents and child were one. For example, "We are feeling anxious about leaving the hospital," might be said by a patient's parent without discussion with the patient who may, in fact, be eager rather than anxious to leave. Tendencies to fuse with others are seen as the core of psychopathology in some systems, such as Kaiser's (Fierman, 1965).

Measurement of psychological boundary disturbance poses a number of problems. The proposed disturbance is intrapsychic and not readily accessible to observation either by the person or by an outside observer. Multiple techniques are needed to establish at least construct validity for this concept.

Zucker (1958) used three techniques: the Mosaic test, the figure-drawing technique, and the Rorschach. The Mosaic test involves construction of a form or picture using various tiles; a boundary disturbance is indicated when the subject uses areas surrounding the tray for his design, indicating difficulty in maintaining the boundaries of a task. The second aspect, Fluid Contours, is seen in the Mosaic when the design has broken contours suggesting "a lack of firmly protecting boundaries between an ego and a non-ego." The figure-drawing test used by Zucker allows for a number of scorings for boundary disturbance. The signs of boundary disturbance on the Rorschach will be described in detail later.

Landis (1970) devised a number of validating tests for his dimensions of boundary permeability and impermeability. These tests assessed various aspects of expressive and representational behavior such as the thickness of a frame a subject drew around a picture, the distance that the subject placed between figures and a spontaneously constructed social scene, the breadth of grouping on a color-sorting task and various copying and drawing tasks for which the thickness of boundaries and the separation of figures were assessed. Landis reports a number of correlations between boundary properties on these tests with the permeability or impermeability of boundaries scored on the Rorschach. While each of the construction, drawing, and naming tests used by Zucker and Landis represent an innovative and interesting approach to the assessment of boundaries, none of the tests has the kind of consensus of use as the Rorschach measures of boundaries.

The most common measure of disturbed boundaries has been the *contamination* response on the Rorschach. In the contamination response, two incompatible or incongruous percepts are portrayed as inextricably linked together. For example, a red detail may be seen as "Fire Island" because it was perceived as an island and was red, suggestive of fire. Here, the percept of fire is blended with and not distinguished from the percept of an island. A second example was given: "It looks like a bear-skin rug, and it looks like a bat, it's a bat-skin rug." While it is remotely conceivable that someone may have preserved a bat skin to serve as a rug, such a purpose or rationalization was not suggested by the subject's further description: "It must have been preserved for scientific reasons." This response shows the steps in the occurrence of a contamination. Two percepts are perceived: a bat and a bear-skin rug. Both are plausible interpretations, but they lose their distinctiveness and become collapsed into one percept, a bat-skin rug.

The nature of the boundary disturbance presented in the contamination response is somewhat different from the intrapsychic or interpersonal boundary disturbances described above. The contamination is a loss of boundaries between two concepts, or perceived objects. A boundary disturbance in the *representation* of objects, argue some theorists (e.g., Blatt and Wild, 1976) occurs because of the inadequate establishment of other boundaries. Blatt and Ritzler (1974), for example, maintain that there is a causal relationship between the schizophrenic person's confusion of himself, of his environment, and a resulting confusion when he attempts to reason in abstract or figurative terms.

While the rationale behind the importance of contamination responses is not universally agreed upon, investigators employing the Rorschach as a measure of thought disorder are in accord in placing the contamination as a consistent indicator of pathological thinking. The response, for example, receives heavy weighting in the delta index (Watkins and Stauffacher, 1952), and in the Phillip's revision of the developmental level scoring system (Phillips, Kaden and Waldman, 1959). Weiner (1966) reports a highly significant discrimination of schizophrenics from nonschizophrenics on the basis of contamination responses. Very few patients or normal subjects produce even one contamination response, although a number of schizophrenics also do not.

Blatt and Ritzler (1974) grouped the records of psychiatric inpatients in a long-term hospital on the basis of relatively "pure" types containing: (a) contaminations, (b) confabulations, (c) both contaminations and confabulations, (d) fabulized combinations, or (e) none of the indexed responses. (Fabulized combinations will be discussed below; confabulations are discussed below and in Chapter 15.) Blatt and Ritzler found that, within this relatively homogeneous group of severely disturbed patients, those groups with contamination, with or without confabulations, tended to have the most severe disorders, to be the least socially adjusted, and to have the poorest outcome in the course of psychiatric treatment.

The fabulized combination response is, in some systems for scoring the Rorschach, also an indicator of potentially pathological disturbance potentially related to boundary. In the fabulized combination, two incongruous percepts are arbitrarily combined in an unrealistic fashion. For example, a centaur, a horse's body with a human head and trunk, or Pegasus, the winged horse, are fabulized combinations that have occurred in mythology. The distinction between a fabulized combination and contamination is that in the fabulized combination, the distinctions between the two percepts are kept distinct, whereas in the contamination they are blurred. For example, a subject saw a contamination response in the Card X of the Rorschach: "A lady moth because it had a moth's head and lady's hair." Had the subject said, "a moth with lady's hair," thereby keeping the moth and lady distinct, the response would instead be a fabulized combination. Rapaport, Gill, and Schafer (1946) described fabulized combinations as either having a playful intent or maybe representing a pathological process. Blatt and Ritzler (1974) point to Holt's earlier distinction between two types of fabulized combination, a more pathological type in which there is a threatened loss of boundaries and a less pathological type in which boundaries are relatively intact and well maintained. Blatt and Ritzler found that the more benign type of fabulized combination tended to indicate better prognosis. They did not, however, study the more pathological form of response. For the purposes of our research, we have treated fabulized combinations as a single type of response, recognizing that some blurring of pathological and nonpathological responses may occur. (In reviewing the fabulized combinations on a subset of our protocols, very few of the more benign forms of fabulized combinations described by Blatt and Ritzler were found. In a number of studies in psychiatric populations, distinguishing "benign" fabulized combinations from "malignant," i.e., with and without boundary disturbance implied, has shown the "malignant" form to be the most common and correlated with other boundary disturbance measures. Therefore, we believe that the fabulized combinations, as described, here are in fact a type of response more directly related to boundary disturbance.)

OTHER MEASURES OF BOUNDARY
ON THE RORSCHACH

Confabulations

Another type of Rorschach score that has been described as measuring boundary disturbance is the *confabulation response,* and the weaker forms, *confabulation tendency* and *fabulization* (Blatt and Ritzler, 1974; Blatt and Wild, 1976). In the confabulation response, the subject attributes internal states and concerns to the percept, often elaborating in a personalized or bizarre fashion. Confabulations are believed to represent boundary concerns in that they are a blending of internal and external "reality." The confabulation response is similar to what we describe as "intermingling." In Chapter 15, we examine two types of responses derived from the confabulation: *overspecificity,* or elaboration in ideational, associative terms; and *affective elaboration,* involving either attribution of affect to the response or evidence of the subject's own affective response to the percept.

We do not include confabulatory responses in this exploration of boundaries on the Rorschach for a number of reasons. First, the concept of inner/outer boundary is different from boundaries between percepts and ideas. Second, the confabulation response is not considered to be unique or even strongly identified with schizophrenic psychopathology. Recent writers, for example, have focused on confabulation responses in borderline patients (see Kwawer, Lerner, Lerner, and Sugarman, 1980). We examine the aspects of confabulation responses and intermingling elsewhere (Chapter 15), but in this chapter we will not include confabulations as principal examples of boundary disturbance.

The conceptualization of boundaries as a protective or a vulnerable layer between the person and the outside is an extension of the earlier concept of ego boundaries. Reich (1949) developed the concept of boundaries in terms of a "psychic protection mechanism which evolves into a characterological armor both against inner drives that are unacceptable and from events in the outer world that are threatening."

If we carry Reich's formulation somewhat further, boundaries may also be seen as excessively permeable or easily broken through. In this respect, ego boundaries and body image have been typically treated as related constructs. Fisher and Cleveland (1958, 1968) developed one of the first scoring systems of Rorschach responses to assess this aspect of psychological boundary. Two major facets are scored: *barrier* and *penetration*. Barrier responses are those in which the protective covering aspects of boundaries are emphasized—for example, an armored car, an armadillo (an animal with a thick outer covering), or protective surfaces such as emphasis on clothing, fur on animals, and the like. A number of highly suggestive findings have emerged from the study of the barrier response to indicate that it does correspond in some degree to other psychological characteristics of bodily boundaries, e.g., it appears to be related to the vulnerability to disease of the skeletal and musculature systems (Fisher, 1963). The penetration response represents in some sense the opposite of the barrier response: penetration through a boundary or passage through openings are emphasized; for example, "an arrow piercing through a skin" or "water pouring out of a vase." The penetration response as a measure of an aspect of body image has also received some support; for example, persons high in penetration responses tend to develop psychosomatic diseases of the internal organs (Fisher, 1963). Fisher and Cleveland, however, do not emphasize the relationships between barrier and penetration responses and actual properties of body boundaries, but rather in terms of attitudes and expectancies that are expressed in terms of body peripheral boundaries (1968, p. 367). Landis developed a system for scoring the Rorschach that has a high degree of similarity to the Fisher and Cleveland system but with some important differences (1970). The two aspects of boundaries that Landis develops are labeled permeability and impermeability. Impermeability of psychological boundaries is described as involving a relatively solid or impenetrable wall or barrier between ego and non-ego. A person with a high degree of impermeability might tend to isolate himself from others and from several aspects of experience and emotion. The permeability response involves emphasis on boundaries that are easily passed through or have been penetrated. Landis conceptualizes permeability as "a relative openness of demarcation between ego and non-ego. It expresses the extent to which a person's ego is accessible to the world" (p. 40). Permeable scores are given for responses that involve percepts with soft or insubstantial boundaries, x-rays, disintegrated boundaries, responses showing over-involvement with the stimulus, percepts with fluid contours, and Siamese-twin percepts. Impermeable scores are received for scores that clearly express hardness, solidity, or impenetrability of the object, clothing, silhouettes, vista responses, and statue responses. In Landis's system, the subject's score is based on whether or not permeability responses dominate over impermeability responses, or vice versa. A person is labeled as either "P-dominant" or "I-dominant." Landis reports a number of suggestive findings that indicate the dominance of one or the other type of their boundary response is correlated with other aspects of psychological boundaries and with the tests described earlier.

Thus far, the descriptions of the barrier, penetration, impermeability, and permeability responses have been dimensions within the normal range of personality. Some findings do suggest that these dimensions extend into the areas of psychopathology. Landis (1970) applies his scoring system to the protocols used earlier by Zucker (1958). He found that no permeability scores could be given to either ambulatory or hospitalized schizophrenics. Both of these groups were also marked by a decreased incidence of impermeability responses. Landis concluded that "these rather dramatic changes suggest that schizophrenic fluidity may be structurally a decidedly different personality condition from Permeability-Impermeability" (p. 130).

Barrier and Penetration in Psychopathology

In their original work, Fisher and Cleveland (1968) found that barrier responses were lowered in psychoses and penetration responses were higher. Barrier responses, which were predicted to be higher in paranoid as compared to nonparanoid patients, were not in fact higher, although eleven "classical paranoids" were indeed quite high on the barrier score. Not only were penetration responses considerably higher in psychoses but they appeared to be of a different type, of disintegrated body parts rather than symbolic penetration responses. Similar results were reported by Holtzman, Thorpe, Swartz, and Herron (1961), and by Holtzman, Gorham, and Moran (1964). Cleveland (1960) found that there were changes in the boundary response of schizophrenics over time. As patients improve, in general, the number of penetration responses decreased. In those patients who were rated as "most improved," barrier responses were also higher. However, in a later review, Fisher (1966) concluded, as does Landis (1970), that boundary disorganization as measured by barrier and penetration, or permeability or impermeability, is not a necessary characteristic for schizophrenia. There has been some accumulation of evidence that paranoid patients tend to have more barrier responses in their Rorschach, but this has not been a consistent finding.

In our study, we have focused on the barrier and penetration responses initially described by Fisher and Cleveland as instances of boundary imagery, not necessarily measuring the same construct as boundary disturbance.

METHODS OF ASSESSMENT OF BOUNDARIES

Two principal methods of assessing boundary qualities in hospitalized patients were employed. The first was the assessment of the boundary properties and boundary disturbance scores on the Rorschach. The second, an experimental investigation to scoring human-figure drawings for properties related to barrier and penetration.

Rorschach Scores for Boundary Disturbance

Four basic scores were calculated from the Rorschach protocols of the sample of 171 patients in the acute phase of their illness. The *contamination* response was scored on a 0–2 scale: 0 for no contamination, 1 for contamination tendency, and 2 for full contamination. Here, contamination tendencies were scored for those blots where a response would be initially localized as a contamination but later retracted or for which there was evidence of contaminatory thinking but not sufficient for a full contamination. *Fabulized combination* responses were scored according to the original criteria of Rapaport and others (1946), i.e., *all* fabulized combinations, whether or not they involved an incongruous combination of two distinct percepts or whether one percept involved arbitrarily combined components or parts. *Barrier* responses were scored according to the revised criteria of Fisher and Cleveland (1968). In general, their responses are scored for a percept that involves some emphasis on protective surfaces, such as animals with hard skins, animals with particularly notable textures for their coats, clothing, buildings, containers, and the like. *Penetration* responses were also scored according to the Fisher and Cleveland (1968) criteria. These responses include images that involve penetration disruption or wearing away of outer surfaces, e.g., "bullet, penetrating flesh," "squashed bug." Secondly, openings or channels for getting into the interior of things, e.g., "open mouth," "an entrance," and images that involve surfaces that are easily penetrated or fragile, e.g., "clouds," "cotton candy." In addition, references to the body surface being broken, injured, fractured or damaged are scored.

The results of the scoring of boundary disturbance, and barrier and penetration responses are presented in Table 9.1. Both contamination and fabulized combination responses were highly significantly different in frequency among the four diagnostic groups. Contamination responses were higher in the classical schizophrenics than in the depressives, the character disorders, and the borderline schizophrenics, using *a posteriori* tests. Fabulized combinations were also significantly lower in depressives. By and large there were no significant differences for the barrier response among any of the diagnostic groups, and there was a trend for fewer penetration responses to occur among the depressive patients. Furthermore, this was not accounted for in terms of

TABLE 9.1
Boundary Measures by Diagnostic Group

Diagnostic Group	N	Contaminations (%)[c]	Fabulized Combinations (%)	Barrier (%)	Penetration (%)
Schizophrenics	48	11.00[a]	9.96[a]	17.77	15.21[a]
Latent schizophrenics/ borderline patients	35	2.85[b]	7.69[a]	16.77	16.51[a]
Personality disorders	38	4.45[b]	6.05[a,b]	15.84	15.50[a]
Depressives	38	1.24[b]	2.58[b]	16.63	8.84[b]
ANOVA:					
MSError		111.95	73.89	109.81	100.32
$F; df = 3,155$		6.79**	5.47*	0.24	4.61*

*$P < .01$.
**$P < .001$.
[a,b]Within a variable, groups sharing the same letters are not significantly different. Groups not sharing letters *are* significantly different ($P < .05$) according to the Newman-Keuls test.
[c]"Percentage" scores were obtained by dividing each weighted score by the number of responses then multiplying by 100.

From Quinlan and Harrow. *Journal of Abnormal Psychology, 83,* 533–541, 1974. Copyright 1974 by the American Psychological Association, and reproduced by permission of the publisher.

fewer responses since this trend also holds for the percentage of penetration responses.

Since a very strong hypothesis has been forwarded by a number of workers about the presence of even a single contamination response indicating schizophrenia, a chi-square was performed contrasting schizophrenics with nonschizophrenics (excluding borderlines) on the presence or absence of a single contamination response. The tallies are presented in Table 9.2. As can be seen from the table on the highly significant chi-square test, the presence of contamination responses is strongly associated with the diagnosis of schizophrenia, although a few nonschizophrenic subjects did have a scorable contamination response, but only rarely so. As has been true in a number of other studies, the absence of a contamination response does not rule out schizophrenia, as nearly one-third of the schizophrenic group did not have a single contamination response. Thus, the contamination response, when present, tends to be an indicator of schizophrenia, but the absence of a contamination response does not rule out the diagnosis of schizophrenia.

TABLE 9.2
Presence of Contaminations or Contamination Tendencies by Diagnosis

Diagnosis	Absent	Present
Schizophrenia	16	32
Latent schizophrenia	24	11
Personality disorder	24	14
Depression (neurotic and psychotic)	33	5

$\chi^2 = 27.03$, $df = 3$, $P < .001$
Contingency coefficient, $C = .38$

Schizophrenics versus All Others	Absent	Present
Schizophrenics	16	32
Others	81	30

$\chi_c^2 = 20.49$, $df = 1$, $P < .001$ (Yates' correction for continuity).
$\phi = .37$

From Quinlan and Harrow. *Journal of Abnormal Psychology, 83*; 533–541, 1974. Copyright 1974 by the American Psychological Association, and reproduced by permission of the publisher.

CORRELATIONS OF BOUNDARY SCORES WITH OTHER RORSCHACH SCORES

Contaminations, barrier, and penetration were each moderately correlated with the overall number or responses ($r = .22-.28$). Contaminations occurred in protocols with fabulized combinations at a reasonably frequent level, as suggested by their correlation of .40. Contaminations were correlated moderately with penetration ($r = .24$). There was fairly substantial agreement of the measures of boundary disturbance (contaminations and fabulized combinations) with other aspects of thinking disorder, such as the three variables measuring thought quality, affect elaboration, and overspecificity, and the score for the response showing the greatest disruption of "reality testing" the very poor form score. In addition, both contamination and fabulized combination were correlated to a moderate degree with the total weighted score for drive content in the Rorschach.

TABLE 9.3
Correlations of Boundary Scores with Other Rorschach Indices (Reliabilities in Parentheses, $N = 38$)

	Contaminations[a]	Fabulized Combination	Barrier	Penetration
Number of responses	.22**	.10	.28**	.28**
Contaminations[a]	(.85)**	.40**	.00	.24**
Fabulized combination	.40**	(.74)**	.06	.10
Barrier	.10	.06	(.71)**	.20*
Penetration	.24**	.10	.20*	(.63)**
Thought quality	.51**	.51**	.06	.25**
Affect elaboration	.32**	.28**	−.02	.14
Overspecificity	.42**	.51**	.17*	.39**
Very poor form (*F*−)	.23**	.23**	.07	.06
Sum drive content	.31**	.28**	.26**	.58**

*$P < .05$; $N = 171$.
**$P < .01$; $N = 171$.
[a]Since contaminations presented a skewed distribution, a point-biserial correlation was computed for contaminations present/absent. All other correlations are Pearson product-moment correlations.

From Quinlan and Harrow. *Journal of Abnormal Psychology, 83,* 533–541, 1974. Copyright 1974 by The American Psychological Association, and reproduced by permission of the publisher.

The correlations of barrier and penetration with other Rorschach scores showed a different pattern. They were moderately positively correlated with each other. Barrier showed low, though significant, correlations only with overspecificity and the weighted sum of the drive content. Penetration, on the other hand, correlated significantly with poor thought quality, overspecificity, and to a quite high degree with sum drive content. The results suggest that contaminations and fabulized combinations are similar to each other but do not measure the same construct as barrier and penetration scores.

The interrelationship of contamination scores and fabulized combinations in this sample is in contradiction to the lack of such relationships in the Blatt and Ritzler study (1974). As noted before, Blatt and Ritzler excluded from their fabulized combinations score those responses that involved the "violation of the integrity of the boundary," such as a "bear with a chicken's head." As in the practice of Rapaport and others, such responses *were* scored as fabulized combinations within the present study. Therefore, the fact that fabulized combination does correlate with contaminations and shows similar patterns of correlation with other variables would suggest that the occurrence of this boundary-disrupted type of fabulized combination occurs, and occurs frequently enough in acutely disturbed psychiatric patients to serve as another indicator of boundary disturbance.

The relationship of penetration responses to the sum drive content was also quite striking. Fisher and Cleveland (1968) indicated that, in patients, the penetration scores often had a different quality from the penetration scores found in normals. Specifically, they found that the penetration responses of hospitalized patients tended to involve more deteriorated body parts, x-ray responses, and primitive aggression. A more detailed look at the relationship to the various drive categories within this study suggest that penetration is related to various types of drive content, specifically, aggression and sex. The correlation of penetration responses with defended aggressive responses was $r = .29$ $(P < .01)$, and with primitive aggressive responses was $r = .22$ $(P < .05)$. An even stronger relationship is found with sexual responses. Defended sexual responses correlated with penetration, $r = .38$, and with primitive sexual responses $r = .39$ (both $P < .01$). Thus, the correlation between penetration responses and the weighted sum of the drive content occurs in large part owing to aggressive and sexual responses. This finding is plausible, since aggressive content is frequently related to the breaking of the boundary and many sexual responses involve an emphasis on openings.

Relationship to Other Measures of Psychopathology

The relationship of the boundary measures to other variables suggestive of different types of psychopathology are presented in Table 9.4. Depersonalization and derealization (Brauer, Harrow, and Tucker, 1970), and stimulus overinclusion (Harrow, Tucker, and Shield, 1972) were assessed by questionnaire ratings. In addition, therapist ratings for three psychotic behaviors were examined—delusions, hallucinations, and bizarre behavior. The length of hospitalization was included as another measure potentially related to the severity of psychopathology. It is a rough index of one aspect of outcome (Harrow, Tucker, and Bromet, 1971) and is methodologically independent of the patient's Rorschach responses.

There were modest but significant correlations with a number of the

TABLE 9.4
Relation of Rorschach Boundary Measures with Other "Boundary" and Psychopathology Variables

		Contaminations[a]	Fabulized Combination	Barrier	Penetration
Questionnaire scales;	(N)				
Depersonalization	156	.14	.16*	−.02	.04
Derealization	156	.12	.14	−.06	−.02
Stimulus overinclusion	162	.22**	.18*	−.07	−.01
Therapist ratings:					
Delusions	159	.26**	.14	.02	−.02
Hallucinations	159	.15	.11	.09	−.12
Bizarre behavior	159	.34**	.20*	.06	−.06
Length of hospitalization	133	.13	.25**	.08	.11

*P < .05.
**P < .01.
aPoint-biserial correlation coefficients.

From Quinlan and Harrow. *Journal of Abnormal Psychology, 83,* 533–541, 1974. Copyright 1974 by the American Psychological Association, and reproduced by permission of the publisher.

measures examined. Contaminations were significantly positively correlated with stimulus overinclusion, or the report of experiences in which the patient felt flooded by too much stimulation. Contaminations also correlated with the ratings of delusions and bizarre behavior. Fabulized combinations also tended to predict these other aspects of psychopathology. There was a low but significant relationship with depersonalization and stimulus overinclusion and a moderate correlation with bizarre behavior. Fabulized combinations were the only boundary-related response that showed significant correlation with length of hospitalization. Barrier and penetration showed no correlation with these other measures of psychopathology.

The evidence of contamination responses as the clearest measure of psychopathology among the boundary measures is by and large supported. It shows the clearest differentiation among the diagnostic groups, separating the schizophrenics from all other groups including the borderline schizophrenics, or latent schizophrenics. It also showed consistently high relationships to other aspects of the psychopathology, whether assessed by a patient self-report or by a resident's rating. In addition, when a factor analysis is performed on the Rorschach scores (as reported in Chapter 15), the contamination responses receive the highest loading of any Rorschach response on a bizarre-idiosyncratic ideation. Thus, these findings are consistent with Blatt and Ritzler (1974), Zucker (1958), and Jortner (1966).

What is it about the contamination response that makes it such an effective predictor of psychopathology? Blatt and Ritzler (1974) maintain that the response is indicative of a very primitive boundary disturbance that is the core of schizophrenia. In the present study, only eight of the seventy-six nonschizophrenics had one or more full contamination response, while twenty of forty-eight schizophrenics had one or more full contamination ($\chi^2[1] = 14.59$, $P < .001$, corrected for continuity). The problems of such a formulation include the fact that twenty-eight schizophrenics did not have a full contamination response. Second, contaminations correlated highly with virtually every other aspect of psychopathology, such that it is difficult to assign to it a unique role as an index of schizophrenia. The fact remains, however, that contaminations are one of the few responses that significantly separate schizophrenics from every other diagnostic group, and thus the assertion that it is a measure of true thought disorder has some support. A second way of looking at the contamination response is that it represents the grossest form of bizarre-idiosyncratic thinking, violating, among other things, Newton's first law. It is one of the clearest violations of consensual reality testing suggesting the schizophrenics' loss of shared perspective.

As noted before, fabulized combinations were not only correlated with contamination but also tended to have similar, and at times stronger, pattern of relations with other variables, especially length of hospitalization. The discrepancy between the Blatt and Ritzler (1974) findings and the present findings can be accounted for by the scoring of those types of fabulized combinations that represent more clearly disrupted boundaries. Along with the strong empirical evidence showing relationships to psychopathology, the nature of this type of response suggests that it could indicate the presence of boundary problems; in this case, it may be as a precursor of contaminatory thinking.

The fabulized combinations show a different distribution among the diagnostic groups, and tended to occur most frequently in the latent schizophrenics and personality disorders, and least frequently in the depressives. While some support for the fabulized combinations as a measure of psychopathology is found, it does not have the clear relationship to schizophrenia that was true for contamination. Further work distinguishing the two types of fabulized combination—those with and those without the violation of the boundary of the percepts— would further clarify the pathological import of these kinds of responses.

Barrier and Penetration

By and large, the findings for the barrier response are negative, with only slight correlations with overspecificity and the total drive content.

The penetration response did show some relationship to diagnosis and psychopathology, although the pattern was somewhat different from previously reported patterns. Specifically, among this group of relatively severely disturbed patients, the results with penetration were due primarily to a lowered incidence of this type of response among depressives. Previous findings with the penetration response (Cleveland, 1960; Holtzman et al., 1961) suggested that penetration scores were higher among acutely disturbed schizophrenics, and furthermore, that these responses drop with improvement. The patients in the present study may represent a more disturbed comparison group than the neurotic patients typical of the previous studies. Moreover, the relationship of the penetration response to the presence of drive in the Rorschach suggests that penetration responses may be high in groups such as personality disorders because of the relationship of aggression to sociopathy (see Harrow et al., 1976; Chap. 6). A number of authors

(Fisher and Cleveland, 1968; Landis, 1970) have concluded that the penetration or permeability responses in the record of patients with severe psychopathology represent a qualitatively different type of process than penetration responses in neurotics or normals. While this conclusion cannot be directly supported from the data, the relationship of penetration to the drive categories does suggest that the aggressive penetration of boundaries may occur more frequently in a group that has much higher levels of the expression of otherwise-censored drive material that would not appear in records of normals, or even those of neurotics. Further discussion of barrier and penetration will follow the exploration of these variables on human-figure drawings.

BARRIER AND PENETRATION IN HUMAN-FIGURE DRAWINGS

A subsample of the patients in this study were administered the Draw-A-Person test. The subjects were instructed to draw a person of each sex and then to draw themselves. The sample consisted of sixty-one patients, twenty-five males and thirty-six females. The mean age of the sample was 29.6 years; thirty schizophrenics and thirty-one patients of other diagnoses (thirteen depressives, eleven personality disorders, and seven latent schizophrenics). All patients were tested individually within two weeks after admission.

A scoring system was devised for aspects that were related to Fisher and Cleveland's (1958) barrier and penetrations scores for the Rorschach (see Carlson, Quinlan, Tucker and Harrow, 1973). The barrier dimension involved any emphasis on the substantiality and definitiveness of boundaries. In human-figure drawings, the barrier dimension was assessed by such items as decorative patterns on clothing, heavy outlining of the body, containing the body in a frame or circle, or elaborations of particular details of the body. A scale of nine such items was devised. Eight items were devised that suggested boundary penetration. Scoring was focused on aspects of figure drawings that suggested weakness or permeability of boundaries, including such things as erasures, transparencies, and emphasis on openings. On independent ratings of twenty drawings, the interrater reliability for the barrier scale was $r = .87$, and for penetration was, $r = .51$. While the reliability on the penetration score was lower than desired, this is a conservative estimate of the reliability since the scores reported below included the ratings for all three drawings (corrected reliability

= .70). Barrier and penetration were not significantly related in this sample $r = -.23$). Additional scorings on the figure drawings were made for the frequency of features suggestive of body disturbance (Carlson et al., 1973), and for the scale of Witkin and others (1954, 1962) for sophistication of figure drawings.

Both barrier and penetration scores were significantly related to the degree of body disturbance. Subjects with high barrier scores on the figure drawings have less body disturbance ($r = -.57$, $P < .01$), while subjects with high degrees of penetration have *higher* incidence of features suggestive of body disturbance ($r = .54$, $P < .01$). In addition, subjects with higher barrier scores received higher scores for overall sophistication of body concepts ($r = .34$, $P < .01$). Thus, some further support can be found for the concepts of barrier and penetration being related to a person's representation of the human figure or "body image."

A comparison of these two scores was made with barrier and penetration scores on the Rorschach and depersonalization and locus of control (Rotter, 1966). The barrier score was significantly correlated ($P < .05$) with the Rorschach score for barrier, lending some modest support for the generality of the barrier construct across two projective tests. The penetration on the Rorschach was not correlated with penetration signs in figure drawings. Two other findings approach significance for those two scales: subjects with higher degrees of barrier on their figure drawings tended to report more depersonalization ($P < .10$) and to be more external in locus of control ($P < .05$).

The correlation between figure drawing barrier and depersonalization is an interesting finding. Federn (1952) noted that an extreme sensitivity to inner and outer stimulation is present in some types of severe depersonalization; the inability to tolerate any unexpected stimuli may lead to an extreme attempt to ward off, such as isolation from other people. In addition to this clinical observation, studies of depersonalization in psychiatric patients (Brauer, Harrow, and Tucker, 1970) suggested that the depersonalized patients tended to interpret external stimuli such as the hospital milieu as affecting their bodies rather than their emotions or their intrapsychic states. The drawings of depersonalized patients show a strong emphasis on the boundary properties of the body, but not a greater disturbance of the body image.

Fisher and Cleveland (1958) had suggested that at least within normal individuals, persons with a high barrier score on the Rorschach tended to be more internally controlled. The findings of the figure drawings here are in fact contradictory according to the Rotter (1965) scale for locus of control. Within this sample, patients who see events in their lives as resulting from their own actions (internal control) tended to have lower barrier scores, whereas those who felt their lives were determined by external forces, such as chance or fate (external control), showed a higher barrier score on the figure drawings. Although in contradiction to the hypothesis by Fisher and Cleveland, the finding does lend further credence to the interpretation above that, within this sample, a high barrier score on figure drawings may be related to the perception of the environment as threatening and controlling.

The findings with the figure drawings do suggest some utility for the concepts of barrier and penetration as it relates to body image. This is true not only in terms of internal consistencies of barrier and penetration scores with disruption of the figure drawings, but also in correlations with such things as depersonalization and locus of control. Such measures at best represent a very minimal correlation with other measures of barrier and penetration on the Rorschach, however. When assessed through two different methodologies, Rorschach and figure drawings, barrier and penetration qualities of projective tests do not significantly discriminate among the diagnostic groups, with the exception that penetration tends to be lower in depressed patients.

THE CONSTRUCT OF BOUNDARIES

The answer to the question of whether all of the different types of boundary measures are related to a similar construct is negative. There was not a significant relationship between contaminations and fabulized combinations on the one hand, and Rorschach barrier and penetration on the other, when barrier and penetration are measured on the Rorschach or the Draw-A-Person test. Furthermore, only one of the scores was correlated with two measures theoretically linked to boundary disturbance: depersonalization and derealization. Correlations with these two constructs were not as strong as they were with other measures of psychopathology, however. Other studies reported elsewhere with depersonalization and derealization have indicated that the report of these experiences occurs in several diagnostic categories and is related to dysphoric affect as well as to a thought disorder (Tucker, Harrow, and Quinlan, 1973). Depersonalization and derealization may be related in some way to psychological boundaries, but in general they are not measured by the projective indices of boundary disruption.

The major theoretical difficulty in the evaluation of the boundary hypothesis is that there are no unequivocal measures for assessing this construct (see Zucker, 1958; Landis, 1970). Without such measures, it is difficult to test fully the tenability of the hypothesis that schizophrenia is a disturbance of boundaries rather than some other equally explanatory underlying disturbance. One problem is that there are many different kinds of boundaries, or boundary measures, and there is no clear evidence that they are related. Some further support for the presence of a boundary-related disturbance in schizophrenics is found in a study of boundaries in role playing by schizophrenics and normals (Johnson, 1980; Johnson and Quinlan, 1980). In this study, schizophrenics show a greater use of boundary-related imagery, with nonparanoid schizophrenics showing more fluid boundaries and paranoid schizophrenics more rigid boundaries. Fluid boundaries were significantly correlated with contamination ($r = .28, P < .05$). While the correlation is modest, the large difference in method suggests some common underlying construct of boundary disturbance.

The results from this study suggest that boundaries cannot all be subsumed under a similar construct. At the same time, this is not a final criticism of the boundary constructs and some aspects of boundaries may be important in severe psychopathology while other *unrelated* aspects of boundaries may be important in personality, and yet other aspects are unrelated to psychopathology or personality and may be important for some other aspect of human behavior. It can be concluded, however, that patients with Rorschach responses that contain broken-down boundaries as assessed by contaminations do show greater degrees of manifest severe psychopathology and are much more likely to be schizophrenic.

Other measures of aspects of boundary construct could be utilized in addition to the Rorschach and the Draw-A-Person test. One such measure could be the Object Sorting test for which conceptual overinclusion could possibly represent a breakdown of conceptual boundaries (Cameron, 1947; Harrow, Himmelhoch, Tucker, Hersh, and Quinlan, 1972). Some indications that a boundary disturbance comparable to contaminations is found in the dreams of schizophrenics are studies by Brenneis (1971). In scoring the manifest dreams of schizophrenic and nonschizophrenic patients, Brenneis found that he could apply categories comparable to contaminations and fabulized combinations to the dream. The imagery in such dreams again shows that the measures related to the boundary disturbance, contaminations and fabulized combinations, were indeed more frequent in the dreams of schizophrenics. Another possible method that may assess boundary disturbance is Role-Taking tests (Feffer and Schnell, 1960), in which an inability to differentiate roles would suggest a breakdown of conceptual and/or interpersonal boundaries.

One question that could be raised about boundary disturbance is whether pictorial representation such as that found in the Rorschach and in figure drawing is the principal means by which such boundary disturbances are detected. Some support for the hypothesis that such is in fact the case is found in the fact that thus far it has been only with visual or spatially organized materials that the boundary construct has been reliably assessed or has been used significantly to differentiate schizophrenics with nonschizophrenics. Visual imagery has, since Freud's (1965) interpretation of dreams, been postulated to be a more primitive form of image representation and hence may be the area where the most primitive form of disturbance is likely to emerge.

BARRIER AND PENETRATION

Some further evidence is found for considering barrier and penetration as aspects of the body image. For barrier, this construct was most productive when examined in human-figure drawings. Draw-A-Person barrier, unfortunately, was only moderately related to the Rorschach barrier score. Nonetheless, it did show significant relationships to two constructs that are potentially related to body image: depersonalization and locus of control. In the context of the figure-drawing test, efforts to separate the body from the environment, perhaps to protect it in the psychological sense, may become especially prominent when the body is experienced as being particularly vulnerable to environmental stimuli, or when the subject experiences difficulty in processing the incoming stimuli. Another possibility is that high barrier simply expresses the feelings of being estranged from the world, translating them into visual terms. The further findings that subjects with high barrier on their figure drawings were more externally controlled lends some further credence to the hypothesis that in a pathological sample, Draw-A-Person barrier may be related to the perception of the environment as threatening and controlling. Thus, a further aspect of the concept of body image is suggested by these findings, namely, that it is related to the subject's underlying attitudes toward environment. A question to be investigated in future research is whether or not persons with high degrees of protective barriers tend to seek out environmental stimulation or whether they tend to try to reduce stimulation, i.e., are they augmenters or reducers on the kinaesthetic figural aftereffect (KFA)?

The penetration response on the Rorschach was unrelated to indices of penetration on the Draw-A-Person. This lack of result could well indicate only that the methodology for assessment of penetration needs further work on the DAP. While the Rorschach penetration responses did not show the predicted pattern based on Fisher and Cleveland's (1958, 1968) work, the results are nonetheless interpretable along lines that may, in fact, be quite similar to previous findings. In the present study, the fact that penetration responses were significantly lower in depressives than in the other groups may indicate that penetration responses are generally high in severe, acute psychopathology and that the previous findings with schizophrenics have relied on comparison groups that were much less seriously disturbed. The correlations of penetration with other drive-related aspects of the Rorschach suggest further reasons why penetration would be high in psychopathology. As has been described in Chapter 6, patients with acute symptomatology more frequently present manifestations of normally unacceptable drives, especially sexual and aggressive drives. Such broken barriers as "an arrow piercing a chest" or "bears bleeding" receive scores for both penetration and aggression. Emphasis on female sexual openings similarly receive scores for sex as well as for penetration. Fisher and Cleveland (1968) and Landis (1970) all conclude that the penetration or permeability responses of schizophrenics are qualitatively different from those of normals or neurotics. Our data suggest that the source of this difference is the greater infusion of sexual and aggressive drive themes in the responses that are scored for penetration. The lower penetration score in depression may, in fact, be an assessment of the depletion of energy in such patients.

CONTAMINATION AND FABULIZED COMBINATIONS

The data suggest at least two broad workable groupings for boundary scores, namely boundary disturbance and boundary properties. The two measures of boundary disturbance, contamination and fabulized combination, were most highly predictive of psychopathology. Present data are consistent with previous studies that have placed a great deal of weight on the contamination response and, in a number of systems, on the fabulized combinations as an index of major psychopathology. The contamination score is perhaps unique in that it so reliably and consistently separates schizophrenics from even latent schizophrenics. It should be noted, however, those subjects who did have a contamination response generally had more of other signs of psychopathology.

Furthermore, unlike other measures of psychopathology, full contaminations were not higher in nonschizophrenic hallucinogenic-drug users. The data support the inference that contaminations, a failure to maintain boundaries in the visual representation of objects (Blatt, 1971; Blatt and Wild, 1976), are related to schizophrenia.

Such a cognitive disturbance, were it to occur in a representation of persons, could extend to problems in fusion of the self with another, along with the attendant confusion and anxiety described for such a state. This is not to imply that schizophrenics or persons with boundary disturbance are not able to think in terms that require cognitive boundaries, but rather that spontaneous representations of objects and persons occasionally occur with deteriorated and distorted boundaries, particularly in tasks like the Rorschach that do not have clear, well-defined guidelines and therefore allow such distortions to occur.

The fabulized combination response has a somewhat more indeterminant status. The suggestions of Holt (1963, 1970) and Blatt and Ritzler (1974) that two types of fabulized combinations be distinguished but that one type is more pathological than the other (i.e., violation of integrity of a single figure) has yet to be evaluated. As scored according to the original Rapaport criteria in the present findings, the fabulized combination is a strong index of psychopathology extending across Rorschach, questionnaire, and therapists' rating indices. In fact, it was the only response to show a significant prediction of length of hospitalization. Further work in sharpening the definition of fabulized combination may lead to another index of boundary disturbance. A type of fabulized combination, the playful combination, was in the protocols of a few patients in this study. Yet such responses could occur in imaginative or playful subjects without necessarily indicating a boundary disturbance. Alternately, such responses may in fact represent the capacity to disrupt boundaries, but in a more controlled and less threatening fashion.

Boundaries versus general ego pathology

An alternate way to look at the present results is to view contaminations as representing a severe general pathological disturbance in thinking that is not unique for a specific boundary problems. One such viewpoint—that schizophrenia is marked by a general ego disturbance—was suggested by Bellak (1949) and by Weiner (1966). Other investigators have used a view of schizophrenia as involving other specific types of disturbed thinking and/or reality testing. Looked at in this way, the overall results might be interpreted as suggesting the importance of disordered and distorted thinking (and perception) in general during the acute stage of schizophrenia.

Further research must certainly be more explicit in describing the nature of boundary problems, especially in distinguishing boundary disruption from other properties of boundary, such as measured by barrier and penetration. The former appeared to be strongly related to psychopathology, the latter less clearly to psychopathology than to other aspects of personality. The boundary hypothesis remains a tenable one in view of its unique property of distinguishing schizophrenics from all other groups. Further extension of the construct validity of the boundary-disruption hypothesis must await other equally valid assessments of boundary disturbances before it can be considered a construct that is independent of one specific test, the Rorschach. Recent results with boundaries on a role-playing test (Johnson and Quinlan, 1980), offer such further support.

10
Conceptual Overinclusion

Overinclusion, defined at one point by Norman Cameron as an inability to limit oneself within the boundaries of a problem, and which we have briefly discussed in the introduction, has been one of the more popular constructs in the area of thought pathology (Cameron, 1939, 1944, 1947). An example of overinclusion can be seen when a patient of ours was administered the Object Sorting test and asked to sort with a *ball* the objects that belong with it. The subject's response was "a kindergarten class," and he began to sort a large number of objects he felt could be found in a kindergarten class. These included silverware (since children eat with them) and matches (since children like to play with them). The sorting of a large number of items only remotely related to the ball illustrates the overinclusive tendency of some acute schizophrenics.

Although the concept of overinclusion was formulated by Cameron on the basis of his work on schizophrenic thinking, it has been utilized repeatedly since then, with a variety of instruments used to assess its role in psychotic disorders, and a variety of both positive and negative results (Foulds, Hope, McPherson, and Mayo, 1967a, 1967b; Payne and Hewlett, 1960; Payne, Hochberg, and Hawks, 1970; Watson, 1967). Among the various instruments used to assess overinclusion have been several paper-and pencil tests, constructed by workers such as Epstein (1953) and L. Chapman (1961). Other instruments also have been used to assess overinclusion and to evaluate the construct. But perhaps the most systematic and widely discussed line of research on overinclusion centers on the test battery devised by R. Payne, and the work done by Payne and his colleagues (Payne, 1968; Payne, Ancevich, and Laverty, 1963; Payne and Caird, 1967; Payne and Friedlander, 1962; Payne and Hewlett, 1960; Payne and Sloane, 1968). Payne's definition of the term overinclusion is the *patient's difficulty in maintaining the usual conceptual boundaries,* along with a tendency to include in one's concepts elements that are not essential or are irrelevant.

After a careful series of studies, Payne and colleagues have suggested that the central deficit in schizophrenia is a problem of overinclusion in the schizophrenic's attentional processes. According to this view, an inhibitory "filter" mechanism that normally allows the narrowing of attention to a central focus is impaired, such that irrelevant stimuli intrude into awareness. Several tasks have been successfully used to suggest that schizophrenics seem to pay more attention to distracting and erroneous cues than do other patients. One of the tasks frequently employed is the Object Sorting test. Thus, Payne and others who have followed in this line of research (Payne, 1966; Payne and Friedlander, 1962; Payne, Friedlander, Laverty, and Haden, 1963; Payne and Hewlett, 1960) have attempted to put the concept of "over-inclusion" into operational terms. Their operational measure for the Object Sorting test involves the inclusion of too many items in each category when sorting the objects. While Payne's early research on overinclusion was extremely promising, the results since then have been more mixed, resulting in considerable confusion in the area (Andreasen and Powers, 1975; Broga and Neufeld, 1977; Craig, 1965; Gathercole, 1965; Goldstein and Salzman, 1965; Hasenfus and Magaro, 1976; Hawks, 1964; Lloyd, 1967; Phillips, Jacobsen, and Turner, 1965; Payne, Hawks, Friedlander, and Hart, 1972; Payne, Hochberg, and Hawks, 1970; Sims-Knight and Knight, 1978).

Our own procedure for assessing the relevance of the concept of overinclusion has been to step back and analyze the concept, and then to utilize this analysis as the basis for a series of empirical studies. We believe that some confusion in this area has arisen because the label "overinclusion" has been applied to phenomena that are quite different behaviorally, and that may, or may not, have different origins. We have proposed that the various types of "overinclusion" be studied individually (Harrow, Himmelhoch, Tucker, Hersh, and Quinlan, 1972).

We have identified three types of overinclusion:

1. The first type is *stimulus overinclusion* or a difficulty in attending

selectively to relevant stimuli, and a tendency to be distracted by a wide range of irrelevant stimuli. Our view is that stimulus overinclusion is primarily a disorder of attention, rather than one that is related to conceptual difficulties.

2. The second type of overinclusion is *behavioral overinclusion* based on overresponsive behavior, which can be assessed by *quantitative* aspects of a patient's test performance. This type is closest to Payne's operationalization of the concept, i.e., the number of items sorted into a category on a sorting task, or the number of words used in responses to a proverbs test. In Cameron's later works on overinclusion (Cameron, 1947; Cameron and Margaret, 1951), he often tended to emphasize overresponsive behavior, "a relative inability to exclude contradictory, competing and irrelevant reactions." (Cameron, 1947, p. 59).

3. The third type of overinclusion is *conceptual overinclusion*, which involves the quality of the patient's thinking about the boundaries of concepts (as measured by indices centered about the patient's reasons for, or the concepts he uses in, his sorting of objects into categories in the sorting test).

It is possible that all three of these types of behaviors that have been labeled by others as "overinclusion" may occur together, but this has not yet been examined. At present, the evidence that might suggest that they represent similar or identical phenomena is scant. In light of this, it would seem best to regard them as different, perhaps unrelated, phenomena.

We have endeavored to identify which of these phenomena is most typical of disordered schizophrenic cognition, since each type may have very different implications for the nature and origin of disordered cognition. In addition, more precise evidence on the relationship, or lack of it, between these three phenomena would be of value.

In this book we have described major aspects of our research on two of these types of behaviors that have been labeled by others as "overinclusion." These two are conceptual overinclusion and stimulus overinclusion. Our investigations on conceptual overinclusion are described in this chapter. We have presented aspects of this research on conceptual overinclusion, and other related investigations of ours, in a series of previous reports (Harrow, Bromet, and Quinlan, 1974; Harrow, Harkavy, Bromet, and Tucker, 1973; Harrow, Himmelhoch, Tucker, Hersh, and Quinlan, 1972; Harrow and Quinlan, 1977; Harrow and Silverstein, 1980; Harrow, Tucker, Himmelhoch, and Putnam, 1972; Quinlan, Schultz, Davies, and Harrow, 1978; Tucker, Harrow, and Quinlan, 1973). Our investigations to clarify the role of stimulus overinclusion are described later in Chapter 12.

Our research to determine the role of the third of these three types of "overinclusion," namely behavioral overinclusion, is outlined briefly in this book, since we believe it is less important in schizophrenia. Our research on behavioral overinclusion has produced a series of results that have led us to believe that very high scores on behavioral overinclusion are often a functon of excessive behavioral activity, and that high scores are infrequent in chronic schizophrenia. Since an *absence* of excessive behavioral activity may be a characteristic of most chronic schizophrenics, and of impoverished schizophrenics who are beginning to undergo deterioration, it is possible that behavioral overinclusion may have mild-moderate prognostic implications (i.e., schizophrenics very *high* on this factor may tend to have a more positive outcome). Recent research by Payne and by our own group suggests this (Payne, 1968; Bromet and Harrow, 1973), although further replication of these results is needed. For the interested reader, our results on behavior overinclusion are presented in several previous reports (Bromet and Harrow, 1973; Harrow, Himmelhoch, Tucker, et al., 1972; Harrow and Silverstein, 1980; Harrow, Tucker, Himmelhoch, and Putnam, 1972).

ASSESSMENT OF CONCEPTUAL OVERINCLUSION OVER TIME

Our research on conceptual overinclusion, which would be viewed as one type of positive symptom, is based on the study of several samples of patients at different phases of their disorder, as follows:

1. At first we studied a pilot sample of fifty-one patients during early stages of their disorder, and then assessed a more formal sample of ninety-one patients, investigated at the acute phase of their disorders (first two weeks of hospitalization).
2. These ninety-one patients were then assessed again during the phase of partial recovery (weeks 8–9 of hospitalization).
3. Seventy-four of these patients were assessed a third time, an average of eleven months after the acute phase.
4. A new sample of seventy-five young patients also were assessed an average of three years after hospitalization.
5. To study a different phase of the disorder, we assessed a sample of thirty-one multiyear, chronic schizophrenics (mean length of *current* hospitalization = 9.8 years), and compared them to our earlier samples of acute schizophrenic and nonschizophrenic patients.

The Goldstein-Scheerer Object Sorting Test was used to assess conceptual overinclusion, employing a system with criteria we have outlined previously (Himmelhoch, Harrow, Tucker, and Hersh, 1973), with satisfactory interrater reliability established within each sample. The major types of behavior used to assess conceptual overinclusion included the following: (a) using a vague, distantly related concept as a categorizing principle when there are obviously more closely related and relevant concepts available; (b) using several dimensions of the original "starting object" without seeming to recognize that each dimension is discrete; (c) attempting to force-fit an object into a chosen dimension of the starting point which does not really belong in that dimension; and (d) arbitrarily changing starting points.

The patients also were evaluated on other cognitive indices, and on psychotic symptoms, and behavior, to analyze the relationship between these variables and conceptual overinclusion.

Conceptual Overinclusion at the Acute Phase of Schizophrenia

The first step in our research on conceptual overinclusion was to investigate its presence in a sample of schizophrenic and nonschizophrenic patients admitted to Yale-New Haven Hospital during the acute phase of their disorder. This sample consisted of patients who had not been chronically hospitalized. In our initial pilot work in this area with the first fifty-one patients, we did not control carefully for the phase of the disorder and assessed patients at varying periods during the first seven weeks in the hospital. We found data suggesting that the acuteness of the illness was an important factor, in terms of results indicating that they did not show as much conceptual overinclusion when we assessed patients *after* the first two to four weeks in the hospital, at a less acute period. Thus, in our subsequent work we began to control more carefully for the phase of the patients' disorders.

As a consequence, the next ninety-one patients were assessed carefully for conceptual overinclusion during the first ten days to two weeks of hospitalization, at the more acute phase. These results on conceptual overinclusion for this sample of ninety-one acute patients are presented in Table 10.1. The schizophrenics were compared to nonschizophrenic patients on our Object Sorting measure of conceptual overinclusion, which utilized both qualitative and quantitative aspects of the patients' responses. The differences were significant ($P < .001$): at the acute phase of their disorder, schizophrenics showed significantly more conceptual overinclusion. In addition, eighteen of the twenty-eight schizophrenics (or 64 percent) showed signs of severe degrees of conceptual overinclusion. Another 14 percent of the schizophrenics showed signs of mild levels of conceptual overinclusion. Overall, at the acute phase, twenty-two of the twenty-eight schizophrenics (or almost 80 percent of these patients) showed at least some signs of conceptual overinclusion, and only six of the twenty-eight did not show evidence of conceptual overinclusion.

Other data were collected on the patients' symptom levels. The relationships between therapists' ratings of the patients' potentially pathologic behavior and our indices of conceptual overinclusion were analyzed. The results indicate that at the time of the acute phase, there were significant positive relationships between the presence of conceptual overinclusion and behavioral ratings of the major indices of psychosis. These included the behavioral ratings of delusions, of bizarre speech and behavior, of paranoid thoughts, and the overall ratings of psychopathology. In contrast, behavioral ratings of depressed mood and of neurotic-type behavior were not significantly related to the index of conceptual overinclusion. Thus, conceptual overinclusion seems to be related to psychotic features and to severe overall psychopathology, but does not show a strong relationship to depressive and neurotic types of symptoms.

The overall results at the acute phase of the patients' disorders showing a significant difference between the schizophrenic and nonschizophrenic patients on conceptual overinclusion are in agreement with other reports about the importance of conceptual overinclusion in the acute or active stages of schizophrenia. Perhaps even more important in attempting to understand conceptual overinclusion,

TABLE 10.1
Percentage of Patients at Each Level of
Conceptual Overinclusion at the Acute Phase*

Patient Group		Level of Conceptual Overinclusion		
		None	Mild-Moderate	Severe
Classical schizophrenics	(N = 28)	21%	14%	64%
Latent schizophrenics and borderline patients	(N = 24)	46%	21%	33%
Nonschizophrenic patients	(N = 39)	51%	31%	18%

*Schizophrenics versus nonschizophrenic patients: $t = 4.78$; 65 df; $P < .001$.

From Harrow, Tucker, Himmelhoch, & Putnam. *American Journal of Psychiatry, 128*, 824–829, 1972. Reproduced by permission of the publisher.

the results showed that among young schizophrenics during the most acute or active phase of their disorder, conceptual overinclusion is extremely frequent, with some degree having been present in over three-quarters of these acute schizophrenics.

Our research indicating that conceptual overinclusion was more common during the earlier part of acute hospitalization suggested to us that the high scores may be related to other factors, in addition to schizophrenia and active psychosis. At least at the acute phase, however, conceptual overinclusion seems to be extremely frequent, and probably a very important part of schizophrenic psychopathology.

Conceptual Overinclusion during the Phase of Partial Recovery in Schizophrenia

When the acute schizophrenics were systematically compared to the nonschizophrenics after seven weeks in the hospital, during the phase of partial symptomatic remission (or partial recovery), the picture showed some change. The mean scores on conceptual overinclusion at the phase of partial recovery are reported in Table 10.2, along with the mean scores at the acute phase. As can be seen in Table 10.2, at partial recovery the absolute level of conceptual overinclusion in the schizophrenics had diminished. The schizophrenics were still significantly more pathological than the nonschizophrenics, but the differences between the two types of patient groups on conceptual overinclusion

TABLE 10.2
Mean Scores on Conceptual Overinclusion
at Acute Phase and Phase of Partial Recovery

		Phase of Disorder		
Patient Group	*N*	*Acute Phase: Mean*	*Partial Recovery Mean*	*Acute Phase versus Partial Recovery*
Classical schizophrenics	28	3.18	2.61	$P < .01$
Latent schizophrenics and borderline patients	24	2.33	2.25	NS
Nonschizophrenic patients	39	1.74	1.79	NS
Schizophrenics versus nonschizophrenic patients		$P < .001$	$P < .05$	

From Harrow, Tucker, Himmelhoch, & Putnam. *American Journal of Psychiatry, 128,* 824–829, 1972. Reproduced by permission of the publisher.

were smaller. The decrease in conceptual overinclusion for the schizophrenics was significant. Overall, these data showed a reduction in the level of conceptual overinclusion for these patients, but still indicated a prominent degree of conceptual overinclusion in a number of schizophrenics, and severe levels in some schizophrenics.

We also analyzed the changes over time in conceptual overinclusion for the other diagnostic groups, with some interesting results emerging. While the schizophrenics showed a significant diminishing of conceptual overinclusion during the phase of partial recovery, the nonschizophrenics did not show a significant reduction in conceptual overinclusion as they began to enter into clinical remission. This was partly because of low initial levels. The data also suggest, however, that while conceptual overinclusion may be found in only some nonschizophrenics during the acute stage, for a few of these patients moderate levels of conceptual overinclusion may be a permanent or a semi-permanent feature of their thinking that does not diminish with symptomatic improvement.

Other data on the symptom level of the sample were also assessed to confirm that the period of partial recovery represents a period of reduced symptomatology. These results showed that the patients as a group were indeed in partial symptomatic remission during the stage we have labeled partial recovery. This was seen in the therapists' behavioral ratings of the patients' psychotic symptoms for the two different phases (the acute phase and the phase of partial recovery). As we have noted in earlier chapters, the ratings of delusions, bizarre speech and behavior, and paranoid thoughts showed significant or near-significant declines during the partial recovery phase for the total patient sample and for the schizophrenic sample considered alone. In addition, the therapists' behavioral ratings of overall psychopathology also showed a significant decline during the phase of partial recovery for the total patient sample and for the schizophrenics alone.

During the phase of partial recovery, the acute symptomatology and signs of a thought disorder had diminished. At this period the relationship between the indices of thought pathology and of psychotic behavior were generally not significant. Thus, as the scores declined on overt signs of psychopathology, the relationship that had existed earlier between conceptual overinclusion and psychotic behavior also diminished.

One possible explanation for these results could be that conceptual overinclusion may be influenced by several factors. One of these is acute psychopathology and psychosis. In other sections of this book we have discussed the possibility that a general psychosis factor at the acute or active phases of schizophrenia influences the clinical picture at that stage of psychopathology. We would propose that at the acute phase, conceptual overinclusion is one component of this general psychosis factor for most schizophrenics as well as for some other types of psychotic disorders. Seven weeks later, at partial recovery, the acute psychopathology has diminished and much of the remaining conceptual overinclusion is more a function of other factors (longstanding trait factors) not related to acute disturbance.

Overall, the results in this area indicated that as the acute schizophrenics began to enter into clinical remission, they showed diminished evidence of conceptual overinclusion. These data support our formulation about a general psychosis factor for schizophrenics, most prominent at the acute phase, and suggest that at least some of the disturbed thinking at that stage is related to acute psychopathology and factors associated with it. These findings on conceptual overinclusion for a second sample of patients at two different phases confirmed our initial results on the fifty-one patients assessed during our pilot work, when we had failed to control for the phase of disorder during the early stages of schizophrenia. It provided clear evidence that even during the early stages, the phases of the disorder and the period of hospitalization are important factors in accounting for some of the variance associated with conceptual overinclusion.

Conceptual Overinclusion during the Early Part of the Posthospital Period

A subsample of seventy-four of these patients (twenty-two classical schizophrenics, twenty-two latent schizophrenics and borderline patients, and thirty nonschizophrenic patients) were reassessed about a year after their original acute-phase evaluation. This reassessment allowed further evaluation of formulations about the importance of conceptual overinclusion at a phase of disorder that has not been studied previously. Table 10.3 presents the results at this one-year posthospital phase for the twenty-two schizophrenic and thirty nonschizophrenic patients, evaluating differences in conceptual overinclusion between the acute phase and the posthospital phase.

The following results were found:

1. The schizophrenics had a significant decline in conceptual overinclusion during the postacute period, as compared to their scores during the acute phase. This supports other observations of ours, and our earlier data, indicating that conceptual overinclusion is influenced by acute psychopathology.

2. The results do not show a significant difference between schizophrenic and nonschizophrenic patients on conceptual overinclusion during the follow-up period.
3. Perhaps equally important, the data do not even indicate a trend toward meaningful differences between the two diagnostic groups at the follow-up period.

One view of ours is that very high scores on conceptual overinclusion are partly determined by disorganization and acute psychopathology. Looked at from this viewpoint, these data could suggest that among young patients, most former acute schizophrenics are not more disorganized during the posthospital period than former nonschizophrenic psychiatric patients. The lack of a difference between the diagnostic groups on conceptual overinclusion at follow-up considered in conjunction with the large differences during the initial assessment at the acute phase, also indicates that the pathological scores during the period of acute hospitalization for schizophrenics are partly a function of the acute stage of the disorder. Indeed, as we have noted elsewhere, acute disturbance and acute psychopathology may account for a large amount of the symptomatic picture at the acute stage for schizophrenic patients. Acute disturbance and upset does not seem to have as drastic an effect on nonschizophrenic patients.

TABLE 10.3
Mean Scores on Conceptual Overinclusion at Acute Phase and Posthospital Phase (One-Year Follow-up)

| Patient Group | N | Phase of Disorder | | Acute Phase versus Posthospital Phase |
		Acute Phase: Mean	Posthospital Phase: Mean	
Classical schizophrenics	22	2.73	2.05	P < .05
Nonschizophrenic patients	30	1.70	2.30	P < .05*
Classical schizophrenics versus nonschizophrenic patients		P < .01	NS	

*Contrary to expectations, the nonschizophrenic patients showed an increase in conceptual overinclusion at follow-up.

From Harrow, Harkavy, Bromet, & Tucker. *Archives of General Psychiatry, 28*, 179–182, 1973. Copyright 1973, by the American Medical Association, and reproduced by permission of the publisher.

4. The nonschizophrenic patients scored significantly higher on conceptual overinclusion at follow-up than at the acute phase of hospitalization. This result was not expected and we found it rather puzzling. Since the initial levels of conceptual overinclusion during the acute stage may influence subsequent increases or decreases, this factor was analyzed separately. Using several types of analyses, we found that these results were not just a function of initial low scores during the acute stage followed by regression toward the mean. Thus, for instance, almost all nonschizophrenic patients with some conceptual overinclusion during the acute stage also exhibited some at follow-up, and a number of them who had shown no signs during the acute stage showed some increases at follow-up. When the data were analyzed still further, it appeared that a number of patients with considerable personality pathology or character pathology who had previously not shown high scores on conceptual overinclusion at the acute period later showed at least moderate levels of conceptual overinclusion during the postacute period. The significant increase in conceptual overinclusion for the nonschizophrenics during the follow-up period was due mainly to the increases for this subgroup of patients with character pathology, although the reason for it is still not clear.

5. Despite the decline in conceptual overinclusion found for the schizophrenics, a mild to moderate level of conceptual overinclusion was still present in some of the schizophrenic patients at the follow-up period. The lack of differences between the schizophrenic and nonschizophrenic patients was mainly due to both groups showing at least a mild degree of conceptual overinclusion during the follow-up period.

What the data seem to reflect is that conceptual overinclusion declines in schizophrenics with the decline in acute psychopathology. However, it is of key importance in understanding the phenomenon of conceptual overinclusion itself that after the decline in conceptual overinclusion, and after the acute phase, some patients were still left with a mild degree of conceptual overinclusion. These patients included both schizophrenics and nonschizophenics. The schizophrenics showed a large absolute decline in conceptual overinclusion, but this seemed to be partly a function of their earlier very high scores at the acute phase.

We have described conceptual overinclusion in terms of the

influence of acute psychopathology and acute disturbance, and have suggested that for many schizophrenics, very high levels of conceptual overinclusion form some component of a general psychosis factor. A question that arises is what specific factors associated with the acute episode seem to be related to conceptual overinclusion. We have hypothesized that disorganization is such a factor, with our observations at the time of the cognitive assessments having suggested to us that conceptual overinclusion was influenced by disorganization. Cameron also seemed to believe that there was some link between conceptual overinclusion and disorganization. In terms of the definition of disorganization, some of the phenomena usually rated under the label "conceptual overinclusion" would seem to fit in with the concept of disorganization. As the results from our research indicate, conceptual overinclusion may be influenced by several factors, with disorganization being one important influence on *severe* levels of conceptual overinclusion. Thus, during acute periods, disorganization could be a prominent influence in leading to very high scores on conceptual overinclusion.

As we have noted, a look at the types of behavior assessed in the test situation shows that the actual sorting behavior rated under conceptual overinclusion can easily fit under the category of disorganized behavior. One of these types of behavior, which occurred in a moderate percentage of the ratings of overinclusion, involved using several dimensions of the original "starting object" without seeming to recognize that each dimension is discrete. This type of behavior, and several other types that were assessed under the category of conceptual overinclusion, could easily be influenced by confusion and disorganization.

It appears that in addition to disorganization, other traitlike features may be related to the phenomenon of conceptual overinclusion and these may be important influences in *milder* forms of conceptual overinclusion. Our data would suggest that for at least some nonschizophrenics, conceptual overinclusion is a permanent or semipermanent feature. The follow-up data revealed that some nonschizophrenics, who have a relatively good clinical picture and who are not disorganized, show mild or moderate levels of conceptual overinclusion. Thus, older hypotheses about conceptual overinclusion's prominence as a schizophrenic feature were not supported by our data, except during select phases of the disorder. Mild levels of conceptual overinclusion would seem to be a more long-lasting characteristic of some people, including nonschizophrenics as well as schizophrenics.

Conceptual Overinclusion during the Posthospital Period: Three-year Follow-up

Our results indicating that conceptual overinclusion was not more severe in schizophrenic than in nonschizophrenic patients a year after the acute phase do not fit theoretical views on this phenomenon. To confirm this finding we collected data on an additional, separate sample of seventy-five young patients from a different hospital setting whom we assessed on conceptual overinclusion at an even later follow-up phase. These patients were assessed at a mean follow-up period of three years after hospitalization.

Table 10.4 reports the distribution of scores for the schizophrenic and nonschizophrenic patients on conceptual overinclusion three years after discharge from acute hospitalization. The data are presented using a revised scoring system that is more sensitive for detecting mild and moderate levels of conceptual overinclusion (e.g., some patients with mild levels of conceptual overinclusion who did not show sufficient signs of it, and thus who formerly had been placed in the "none" category, would now be placed in the "mild" category using this more sensitive system).

These data indicate the following:

1. There were no significant differences between the schizophrenics and nonschizophrenics on conceptual overinclusion three years after hospitalization. The mean scores of the two major groups were almost identical, indicating the lack of any trends toward diagnostic differences.
2. A large number of both schizophrenics and nonschizophrenics showed at least mild levels of conceptual overinclusion, suggesting that at least some degree of this type of overinclusion is common in a variety of different types of former inpatients.

TABLE 10.4
Percentage of Patients at Each Level of Conceptual Overinclusion Three Years after Index Hospitalization*

Patient Group		None	Mild	Moderate-Severe	Very Severe
				Level of Conceptual Overinclusion	
Schizophrenics	(N = 46)	37%	28%	33%	2%
Nonschizophrenic patients	(N = 29)	24%	45%	24%	7%

*Schizophrenics versus nonschizophrenics : t = 0.00, nonsignificant.

The overall results on this separate sample of young patients assessed three years after hospitalization support the conclusions from our earlier study, with no differences between schizophrenic and nonschizophrenic patients on conceptual overinclusion when in non-acute phases. During the acute or active stages of the schizophrenic disorder, a severe level of conceptual overinclusion can be a prominent factor. After the most acute phase, however, during the recovery period, conceptual overinclusion is not a distinguishing characteristic.

While the focus of this chapter is on conceptual overinclusion, we should note that the inpatient and follow-up samples we tested for conceptual overinclusion were also assessed simultaneously for bizarre-idiosyncratic thinking. When we take an overview of the data on both of these concepts, we can observe that our results showed consistent differences at the acute phase between schizophrenic and nonschizo-phrenic patients on both conceptual overinclusion and bizarre-idio-syncratic thinking. However, as we have noted, by the time of assessment at the various follow-up periods, the pathological scores on conceptual overinclusion of the schizophrenic patients had diminished. By this phase of their disorder, there were not even near-significant differences between the major diagnostic groups on conceptual over-inclusion. In contrast to these results, at follow-up, the schizophrenics consistently showed either significantly or near-significantly more pathological scores than the parallel samples of nonschizophrenics on the indices of bizarre-idiosyncratic thinking. Similar results of this type have been obtained with several follow-up samples. They support our analysis suggesting that conceptual overinclusion is more closely related to acute and active phases of psychopathology, and to factors such as the disorganization present at that time. In contrast, some degree of bizarre-idiosyncratic thinking persists in a number of schizophrenic patients. As such, severe conceptual overinclusion would seem to be related to variables associated with the acute phases of schizophrenia or psychosis and is less important as a permanent or sustained schizophrenic feature.

Conceptual Overinclusion during the Chronic Phase of Schizophrenia

Table 10.5 reports data on a sample of chronic, multiyear, hos-pitalized schizophrenics, and a comparison with a sample of acute schizophrenics. These results help to answer questions concerning the extent of conceptual overinclusion present in the chronic schizophrenic patient.

In regard to the quality of the chronic schizophrenic's thinking, the results on conceptual overinclusion indicated that chronic schizophrenics had moderate-high scores. The scores of the chronic schizophrenics were higher than those of the sample of nonschizophrenic patients. However, the chronic schizophrenics showed *less* conceptual overinclusion than a sample of acute schizophrenics.

Thus, in looking at the overall results, chronic schizophrenics showed some degree of conceptual overinclusion. Our other evidence indicated a relative impoverishment of thinking in these chronic patients. We have discussed this general trend toward impoverishment among multiyear, chronic schizophrenics in Chapter 7 in conjunction with similar impoverished thinking in a *different* sample of chronic, multiyear schizophrenics whom we assessed for concrete thinking. Despite the impoverishment of thinking in these mulityear schizophrenics, traces of various types of positive thought disorder appeared in these patients, including conceptual overinclusion. As we have noted, there was less conceptual overinclusion in these chronic patients than in our sample of acute schizophrenics, although some evidence of overinclusion still appeared.

These results would suggest that, for many schizophrenics, the chronic phase of their disorder, like the acute phase, is also a stage of active disorder. In our research with this type of multiyear, chronic schizophrenic, we have found considerable variability in the level of overt thought pathology (i.e., some were extremely thought disordered and a few showed little overt evidence of it). However, conceptual overinclusion was still one factor present in the clinical picture of a number of these chronic schizophrenics. We would assume that while the chronic phase of schizophrenia is an active stage of psychopathology with some degree of disordered thinking, there is a relative

TABLE 10.5
Mean Scores on Conceptual Overinclusion of Chronic, Multiyear Schizophrenics Compared to Acute Schizophrenics and Nonschizophrenic Patients

Patient Group	N	Means	Comparison with Chronic Schizophrenics
Chronic schizophrenics	31	2.45	—
Acute schizophrenics	28	3.18	$P < .05$
Nonschizophrenic patients (acute)	39	1.74	$P < .05$

From Harrow, Tucker, Himmelhock, & Putnam. *American Journal of Psychiatry, 128,* 824–829, 1972. Reproduced by permission of the publisher.

impoverishment of thinking at this chronic phase, and some "burnt-out" quality in these patients These latter factors can reduce the *overt* manifestation of positive symptoms. Nevertheless, multiyear hospitalized patients in the chronic phase of schizophrenia still show an active level of idiosyncratic thinking and other positive symptoms. At this chronic phase, conceptual overinclusion is still a factor, but apparently is not as prominent as it is at more flagrant phases of the schizophrenic disorder.

SUMMARY OF RESULTS ON CONCEPTUAL OVERINCLUSION

In summarizing our results and conclusions about conceptual overinclusion, using several different samples, we have found the following results:

1. Severe conceptual overinclusion is prominent during early, active, acute phases of the schizophrenic disorder.
2. Conceptual overinclusion diminishes as acute psychopathology begins to remit.
3. Severe conceptual overinclusion is not present to any important degree during nonactive stages of the schizophrenic disorder or during periods of remission.
4. Conceptual overinclusion is present in some chronic schizophrenic patients, and is still a factor at that stage, but it is less important than other pathological features at that phase.
5. Severe levels of conceptual overinclusion are related to active psychosis, and to confusion and general disturbance.

There are a number of implications from these data concerning conceptual overinclusion.

1. The phase of the schizophrenic disorder is an extremely important factor in this area, since it influences patients' immediate overall clinical conditions, and this is one determinant of whether or not patients will have conceptual overinclusion.

2. Very severe degrees of conceptual overinclusion are related to psychotic symptoms and to severe overall psychopathology, and constitute part of a general psychosis factor for many schizophrenics.

3. Conceptual overinclusion is a prominent factor in schizophrenia during acute phases of the disorder. Apparently, while conceptual

overinclusion is influenced by acute psychopathology in general, this seems to interact with other tendencies of schizophrenics (perhaps the tendency to become disorganized under pressure or upset). Hence, conceptual overinclusion is especially prominent in schizophrenia during the acute stage. At that phase, it is a very important part of their psychopathology, with this apparently being a function of the above-noted *interaction* between increased upset or disturbance and other characteristic tendencies of schizophrenics. This interaction between (a) acute upset and disturbance, and (b) characteristic tendencies of the schizophrenic to respond more flagrantly and severely to disturbance, is an important factor since nonschizophrenics do not show this tendency to the same extent. Thus, acute disturbance and upset may increase conceptual overinclusion in nonschizophrenics, but if it does, it increases conceptual overinclusion to a much less severe degree in these patients.

4. Conceptual overinclusion is also found in schizophrenics during other active stages of the disorder, although it is not as prominent as it is during the height of the acute phase.

5. Disorganization, often present during active stages of psychopathology, increases the patient's level of conceptual overinclusion. In this respect, severe levels of conceptual overinclusion are one workable index of disorganization. Severe conceptual overinclusion, however, is only an approximation of disorganization, since conceptual overinclusion is influenced by other factors as well, and some disorganized patients may not show conceptual overinclusion.

6. Mild to moderate levels of conceptual overinclusion show a limited degree of consistency over time in many types of patients, suggesting that at the milder levels, conceptual overinclusion is influenced by longstanding traitlike characteristics in select schizophrenics and nonschizophrenics.

Overall, severe conceptual overinclusion is influenced by disorganization and confusion, and by active psychosis. Mild levels of conceptual overinclusion may be found as longstanding traitlike features in some schizophrenics and nonschizophrenics. While severe conceptual overinclusion is prominent and important during the acute stages of schizophrenia and can also be found in active chronic phases, it is not a permanent, sustained, or fundamental characteristic of schizophrenia.

11

Depersonalization*

"**I** feel I am unreal; I am a stranger to myself." Such complaints frequently occur in psychiatric patients of all diagnoses experiencing acute stress. The depersonalization state comes and goes; it may last for a few minutes or hours, or it may persist for days. Depersonalization experiences, along with a related but distinct experience (namely derealization), have been noted in a wide range of disorders and in normal persons. Theories have been proposed to account for depersonalization as a neurological symptom, as a defense, a distortion of body image, or ego state (in analytic writing), an outcome of a specific syndrome, or as a precursor of the schizophrenic process.

Depersonalization is an experiential state, particularly distinct in character. The person feels *the self*, and in particular the body, detached and distant from the world, with the result that he or she feels strange and unreal. Depersonalization is a symptom frequently attributed to schizophrenia. In one sense, it could be considered to be a form of disordered thinking since it involves a distortion of fundamental aspects of thinking—the reality of one's own body and bodily experiences. Depersonalization is also reported in nonschizophrenic and in border-

---

*Dr. Gary Tucker joined the authors in their research on depersonalization, directed major phases of these studies, and thus the research in this area evolved from joint collaboration with him.

line states. The phenomenon can be described further by some of the items we used to assess depersonalization:

1. Have you ever had the feeling you were two people, one going through the motions, while another you is observing?
2. Have you ever had the feeling as if there were a wall or veil between you and other people?
3. Have you at any time experienced the feeling as if you were unreal?
4. Do you ever feel like a stranger to yourself?

Persons who have had such a feeling state recognize the state immediately from such questions; it is a distinct state in the awareness and memory of those experiencing it.

Two other experiential states have been associated with depersonalization: *derealization* and *déjà vu.* In derealization, it is the surrounding world that is unreal or "uncanny." This has been found frequently in persons experiencing depersonalization but does not occur as often, and depersonalization can occur alone. A third state, déjà vu, is the sense that one has been in a situation before. It is described by some writers as a distortion of the time sense (e.g., Lewis, 1934).

The possibility that depersonalization is a result of organic factors was suggested by Mayer-Gross (1935). Impressed by the similarity of the condition from person to person, he postulated a "pre-formed cerebral mechanism" analogous to an epileptic fit, as the neurological basis of depersonalization. A variety of neurological conditions have been described as causing depersonalization; temporal-lobe epilepsy in particular has been cited as a disorder accompanied by depersonalization (Sedman, 1970). Roth and Harper (1962) found depersonalization and related states to be frequent in patients with temporal-lobe epilepsy. Sedman and Kenna (1965) studied organic "psycho-syndromes" in thirty-two epileptic patients and found depersonalization only in patients with psychomotor attacks or more than one type of attack. Depersonalization, however, was not related to other forms of epilepsy or organic psychosis. Levitan (1969, 1970) described depersonalization as a universal process in the sleep cycle, related to activity of the Reticular Activating System.

PSYCHOANALYTIC THEORIES

Psychoanalytic theorists have interpreted depersonalization in a variety of ways. Nunberg (1932) treated the phenomenon of "estrangement" as a sudden transposition of libido from objects back onto the libido. Bergler and Eidelberg (1935) viewed the state as a defense against exhibitionism transformed into voyeurism and accepted by the ego in the form of self-observation. Several writers, in particular Jacobsen (1964), emphasize a narcissistic predisposition in persons who develop neurotic experiences of depersonalization.

One line of analytic thought has characterized depersonalization as an ego state, especially involving the body image. Schilder (1928) emphasized the role of bodily precursors of depersonalization such as dizziness. Federn (1952) described depersonalization as an "ego disease" in which libido is withdrawn from the ego boundaries (estrangement) and from the core of the ego (depersonalization). Jacobsen (1964) described depersonalization occurring in female political prisoners who become overinvested in thought processes at the expense of bodily ego. Shorvon (1945–46) found that the nonpsychotic patients with depersonalization had a strong obsessional quality, with a high emphasis on intellectual defenses.

As an ego state, depersonalization has been described as a splitting within the ego, a "detachment and disowning" of a regressed, diseased part of the ego (Jacobsen, 1964). At the same time, the bodily part of the ego is subject to close observation (Schilder, 1914). While such an ego state could occur in a well-functioning person under stress, such as in the political prisoners described by Jacobsen, most analytic theorists place depersonalization and estrangement or derealization in the pathological spectrum. Before considering the question of normal versus pathological states of depersonalization, however, another view of depersonalization is relevant.

DEPERSONALIZATION AND DYSPHORIC AFFECT

Several writers have suggested that depersonalization is closely linked to dysphoric affects, whether anxiety, or depression, or both. Roth and Harper (1962) examined thirty cases of "phobic anxiety depersonalization syndrome." They found that the subjects were similar to temporal-lobe epileptics on a number of symptoms, but that as a group they were more neurotic in their personality structure. Roth (1960) suggested that the basic personality syndrome of people experiencing depersonalization included obsessional traits and anxiety proneness. Kelly and Walter (1968) studied the physiological correlates of anxiety in depersonalized subjects. They reported an extremely high "basal" anxiety (without experimental stress) in patients with prolonged and chronic depersonalization. On a broader sample of subjects with depersonalization, Sedman's (1968) findings challenged the thesis that anxiety is an important etiological factor, and instead found greater similarity with depression.

Depression, particularly as a clinical syndrome, has been linked with changes in bodily functions such as sleeping, eating, and sexual interest (Beck, 1967). Sedman (1968) found that the depersonalized subjects scored equally high on the Beck Depression Inventory (Beck, Ward, Mendelson, Moch, and Erbaugh, 1961) as clinically depressed subjects. Sedman (1970) attributed depressed *mood* as an important but not necessary correlate of depersonalization. Ackner (1954) included "depressive depersonalization" as a syndrome in his categories of depersonalization. Within analytic writings, there are similarities between the "withdrawal of libido" described in depersonalization and the analytic description of depression. There appears to be strong support for an association between depersonalization and depression as an affect, although not necessarily between depersonalization and the clinical syndrome of depression.

NORMAL VERSUS PATHOLOGICAL STATES

Depersonalization has been reported in persons judged to be normal, neurotic, manic-depressive, and schizophrenic. Roberts (1960) found depersonalization experiences reported by 39 percent of college students. Dixon (1963) used a questionnaire technique to determine that 46 percent of 112 college students had experienced deper- sonalization within the previous year. Sedman (1970) found that twenty-seven of fifty normal subjects had at one time or another experienced the state. Further inquiry revealed that the depersonalized state was often experienced with some contributing context such as fatigue, anxiety, or alcohol use. Moreover, the experiences were brief, usually lasting a few seconds to a few minutes. Subjects reporting depersonalization tend to be young, and females report it more often than males (Sedman, 1970).

Several writers treat depersonalization as a neurotic symptom. Oberndorf (1950) and Roth (1960a, and 1960b) both linked deperson- alization to anxiety; depersonalization was viewed as a defense against the anxiety. Fenichel (1945) treated the state as a special type of defense mechanism.

Depersonalization is frequently described as a symptom of schizophrenia or a prodromal state that may be an early sign of ego weakness. Weiner (1966), for example, includes depersonalization under indicators of "loss of reality sense," which in turn are suggestive of schizophrenia. Ego-analytic writers such as Federn (1952) and Jacobsen (1964) view depersonalization as an "ego disease" that may indicate the weakening of the ego prior to schizophrenia. Levitan (1970) suggests that when depersonalization persists in the wakened state, "often psychosis is not far behind or already present." Galdston (1947) explicitly wrote of depersonalization as a prodromal state of schizophrenia. In a review of theories of depersonalization, however, Sedman (1970) concludes that while depersonalization is frequent in schizophrenics, its occurrence in other states cannot allow the assumption that depersonalization is a "form frusté" of schizophrenia.

PERSPECTIVE AND DEPERSONALIZATION

Depersonalization and derealization can be analyzed in terms of whether or not impaired perspective is involved. In one sense, in depersonalization the patient seems to have problems in taking an accurate perspective on him or herself, particularly concerning his body. Similarly, in derealization, one's perspective on the world might appear to be distorted. These symptoms, however, do not involve the type of impaired perspective about what is socially appropriate that we have discussed earlier in this book. Thus, the patient experiencing depersonalization is able to use, effectively, his long-term stored knowledge about himself, is *simultaneously* aware of what is appropriate and real, and aware of the state of affairs concerning himself as it "should be." Finally, since depersonalization and derealization are by definition subjective symptoms, unobservable by others, potential faulty monitoring of one's thinking and verbal behavior is not at issue. While depersonalization and derealization involve a type of psychopathology, they do *not* relate to those aspects of disordered thinking that involve a faulty perspective of the general other, nor do they involve faulty monitoring.

This brief and selective review of depersonalization and related states raises a number of questions about the nature and role of depersonalization in schizophrenia and other disorders:

1. To what degree is the severity and frequency of depersonalization different among different diagnostic groups? In particular, to what extent is depersonalization a symptom of schizophrenia?

2. To what degree is depersonalization associated with disordered thinking, especially "ego-boundary disturbances"?
3. What happens to the experience of depersonalization over the course of inpatient hospital treatment? In particular, do medications affect the experience of depersonalization?
4. Does depersonalization reflect changes in aspects of bodily awareness in either quality or degree of awareness?
5. To what degree do depersonalization, derealization, and déjà vu occur together? In other words, are they manifestations of the same process or do they occur independently?
6. To what degree do depersonalization experiences occur with dysphoric affects, such as anxiety and depression, or with other symptoms, such as delusions?

These questions, which we have outlined above, were studied by Dr. Gary Tucker and the current authors in a series of systematic investigations. Aspects of our research in this area are described in greater detail in several reports by Dr. Tucker and ourselves (Brauer, Harrow, and Tucker, 1970; Tucker, Harrow, and Quinlan, 1973).

A problem of studying depersonalization

Depersonalization is a phenomenological or *experiential* state. Unlike the experiential states of depression or psychosis, however, there is no known observable correlate of depersonalization. The depersonalized subject may go about his daily activity without manifesting any distinctive change of behavior. It is, however, a distinct state, with a high degree of agreement among persons reporting it.

As with other distinctly subjective experiences (such as pain), the investigation of depersonalization and related phenomena must rely on the individuals' self-report. To study depersonalization, questionnaire items were written to describe the depersonalized state; they were presented earlier in the chapter. To study derealization, a similar procedure was used to produce these items:

1. Have people well known to you seemed changed or unfamiliar?
2. Have you ever experienced the feelings that your surroundings were unreal?
3. Do things with which you have been comfortable ever appear strange?

To assess déjà vu, the patients were asked: "Everyone has had feelings of familiarity when visiting new places. How often have you had them?"

A random sample of forty patients who had responded to our items about depersonalization, derealization, and déjà vu were interviewed about those experiences. Pilot work involving clinical interviews and observations of a sample of patients indicated that their verbal descriptions agreed with their questionnaire responses. As feeling states, depersonalization and derealization have an especially distinct quality that patients report in a consistent way. The self-report items were therefore utilized in a detailed questionnaire interspersed with items from other scales. Each item was responded to on a five-point scale (1 = never, 5 = all the time).

Patient samples

Three separate samples of patients were assessed for depersonalization, derealization, and accompanying traits and symptoms. Each sample was collected within a separate time period. The first, Sample A, consisted of 84 consecutively admitted patients; the second, Sample B, 155 patients; and the third, Sample C, 111 patients. Samples A and B were administered the questionnaire in the first week of hospitalization; sample C took the questionnaire at the first week and again at the fifth week of hospitalization. Each of the samples consisted of approximately 40 percent males and 60 percent females. In each sample, the median age was between 23 and 25 years, with a few patients (5–10 percent) under 15, and a few over 60 years (5–15 percent), and approximately equal numbers in the 16–20, 20–25, and 26–45 age ranges (see Brauer, Harrow, and Tucker, 1970). The diagnostic distribution for Sample B in Table 11.1 is representative of the other groups; there are no differences in mean values as proportions for age, sex, or distribution of diagnoses across the three samples.

Frequency of depersonalization

The frequency of degrees of depersonalization are presented by diagnostic groups in Table 11-1. Fifty-nine percent of all patients report at least more than minimal experiences of depersonalizatoin, 46 percent experiencing "considerable" depersonalization. The highest proportion of patients reporting considerable depersonalization is the borderline or latent schizophrenic group, followed by the schizophrenics. The overall variations among diagnostic groups (combining "minimal" with "some" versus "considerable") is highly significant ($P < .01$). The latent schizophrenics are higher in depersonalization than the nonschizo-phrenic groups ($P < .01$), while the "classical" schizophrenics also tend to be higher than nonschizophrenics ($P < .05$), and are not significantly lower than latent schizophrenics. Only the personality disorder group considered alone has a tendency to approach the frequency of "considerable" depersonalization of the borderline or latent schizo-phrenics. Thus, there is some support for the assertion that deper-sonalization is associated to a limited degree with schizophrenic psychopathology, although it is more often found in latent schizo-phrenics. It is possible that the tendency to occur in *latent* schizo-phrenics has resulted in some writers viewing depersonalization as a *prodromal symptom*. Evidence in the field, however, does not suggest that a huge percentage of borderline patients and latent schizophrenics later have schizophrenic breaks.

Relationship among experiential states

The association or co-occurrence of depersonalization, dereali-zation, and déjà vu was explored in the first sample. Depersonalization was highly correlated with derealization (r [82] $= .64$; $P < .01$) and not significantly correlated with déjà vu experiences ($r = .18$, ns). As will be seen in the correlations of each of the states with other variables, depersonalization and derealization show a similar pattern, while déjà vu shows a different pattern of correlations with other variables.

TABLE 11.1
Severity of Depersonalization by Diagnostic Group

Diagnosis	Degree of Depersonalization*			N
	Minimal	*Some*	*Considerable*	
Depression : neurotic	10	3	6	19
psychotic	9	4	9	22
Personality disorder	12	4	13	29
Latent schizphrenia	8	2	21	31
Schizophrenia	13	6	21	40
Others (including manic-depressive)	11	2	1	14
				155

*For statistical comparisons reported in the text, "Minimal" and "Some" depersonalization are combined to contrast with "Considerable" depersonalization.

From Tucker, Harrow & Quinlan. *American Journal of Psychiatry, 6*, 130, 1973. Repro-duced by permission of the publisher.

Therefore, for the most part, we will narrow the examination of results to depersonalization.

Perceptual experience and psychomotor functions

For the first sample, the depersonalization questionnaire included questions assessing specific perceptual and psychomotor experiences previously attributed to patients with depersonalization, as well as information on age, sex, marital status, and the use of LSD. (See Table 11.2) The data indicated that younger patients experienced more depersonalization and derealization. There was no difference between the sexes, or between married and unmarried patients. Use of LSD was assessed because depersonalization is reported to occur frequently during drug use. No relations to frequency of depersonalization phenomena were found between either frequency or type of LSD experience and the states studied. (The patients were not using hallucinogens during hospitalization.)

A number of relationships between depersonalization phenomena and other variables were found. There was little relationship to other perceptual changes in color or time. Depersonalization and derealization were related to problems in attention, especially the questions related to the need for extra effort in attention. In addition, when depersonalization was related to an impairment in selective attention (Table 11.3), subjects high in depersonalization reported themselves to be readily distracted, i.e., high on stimulus overinclusion. The feelings of depersonalization and derealization were strongly related to questions assessing patients' *awareness* of their bodies, increased restless activity (but not a sense of drivenness to maniclike activity) and to patients' feelings of their bodies being dead. One aspect is of special interest: namely, that patients high on depersonalization experience their bodies as affected by the hospital milieu. The changes experienced in depersonalization suggest, as several writers have reported, that depersonalization is accompanied by a heightened attention to the body. Moreover, patients with high depersonalization and derealization tend to experience psychological changes in bodily terms.

This last point is further elaborated by the experience of medication effects. Not only do patients high in depersonalization experience more personality change due to medications, they also report more physical side-effects. They experience an *increase* in depersonalization (rather than relief) and report more behavior change due to medications than comparable patients low on depersonalization or derealization. Thus, depersonalized patients react more to medications, and experience medication-induced changes as bodily changes. In the sense that depersonalized patients attend more to their body, feel "dead," and experience the hospital and medications as affecting their bodies more, these patients have an altered body image.

The relationship to psychotic and depressive symptoms was also explored. Forty of the patients in Sample A were selected randomly for

TABLE 11.2
Correlations of Depersonalization Phenomena with Demographic Variables, Perceptual Functions, "Body Image," and Medications Effects

| Variable | Sample A (N = 84) | | |
| | Correlation Coefficients | | |
	Depersonalization	Derealization	Déjà Vu
A. Identifying information:			
Age	−.22*	−.24*	.02
Sex (M = 1, F = 2)	.09	.11	.08
Married (1 = No, 2 = Yes)	.04	.04	.04
B. Perceptual alterations:			
LSD frequency	.16	.14	.05
LSD type of experience	.10	.10	.15
Changes in color	.16	.17	.19
Changes in time	.11	.25*	.20
Effortful attention	.47**	.54**	.15
C. "Body image" changes:			
Increased body awareness	.45**	.45**	.47**
Increased restless movement	.42**	.40**	.10
Amount of organized physical activity	.23*	.14	.01
Increased drive to motor activity	−.37**	−.35**	.10
Bodily feelings affected by milieu	.27*	.26*	.05
Feelings of deadness	.51**	.60**	.24*
Depressed mood	.43**	.35**	.14
D. Medications effects:			
Personality affected	.54**	.35**	.07
Behavior affected	.21*	.15	.05
Increased depersonalization by meds	.35**	.21*	.32**
Body tenseness or tiredness affected	.41**	.41**	.29**

*P < .05
**P < .01

From Brauer, Harrow, and Tucker. *British Journal of Psychiatry*, 117, 509–515. 1970. Reproduced by permission of the publisher.

TABLE 11.3
Depersonalization and Personality Scales
Samples A and B

Scale	Sample A N = 49	Sample B N	Sample B r	Correlation with Social Desirability Partialled out (Sample B)
Maudsley Personality				
Inventory: Neuroticism	.19	115	.43**	.38**
Extraversion	−.32*	115	−.24**	−.22*
Lie scale	−.08	115	−.14	
Stimulus overinclusion	.35*			
Taylor Manifest Anxiety	.32*	152	.50**	.46**
Semantic differential:				
Self-evaluation	−.42*	115	−.43**	−.38**
Self-potency	−.17	115	−.16	
Self-activity	−.28	115	−.16	
Srole and Brimm scales:				
Anomie	.35*	133	.31**	.32**
Autism	.54*	133	.44**	.38**
Cycloid thinking	.32*	133	.32**	.26**
Emotionality	.56**			
Frustration	.42**	133	.39**	.34**
Withdrawal	.53**			
Authoritarianism		132	−.12	
Dominance		133	−.14	
Fatalism		133	.02	
Optimism		133	−.26**	−.22*
Originality		133	−.01	
Pessimism		133	−.09	
Reflectiveness		133	.04	
Rigidity		133	.00	
Self-confidence		133	−.33**	−.28**
Guilt (Buss-Durkee)	.41**	140	.35**	.35**
Cyclothymia	.48**			
Symptom ratings:				
Sadness		140	.12	
Thought retardation		140	.30**	.24**
Motor retardation	.13	140	.25**	.19**
Diurnal variation		126	.06	
Confusion	.21	141	.38**	.32**
Concentration	−.20	145	−.30**	−.24**
Zung Depression Scale		135	.46**	.41**
Zuckerman MAACL:				
Depression		136	.32**	.29**
Anxiety		136	.32**	.28**
Modified Q-sort (self-esteem)		136	−.53**	−.49**

*P < .05

**P < .01

From Brauer, Harrow, and Tucker. *British Journal of Psychiatry, 117,* 509–515, 1970. Reproduced by permission of the publisher.
and
From Tucker, Harrow and Quinlan. *American Journal of Psychiatry, 6,* 139, 1973. Reproduced by permission of the publisher.

further analysis in an interview with a psychiatrist who was unaware of their depersonalization and derealization experiences. Separate ratings were obtained from the therapist treating the patient. Patients high on depersonalization had significantly more hallucinations (both visual and auditory), but were not higher in delusional thinking. There were no other major symptoms significantly related to depersonalization, but the psychiatrist rated the patients who were high on depersonalization as more dysfunctional ($P < .01$) and rated their prognosis less favorably ($P < .05$). Patients high in depersonalization, nonetheless, stayed in the hospital no longer than other patients. Other indices of progress through the hospital, however, such as time to reach privilege status in the milieu "ladder," were related to depersonalization; patients with depersonalization took longer to reach higher positions of responsibility for themselves and others. It may be that depersonalization is overweighted by interviewers and observers in the staff as a sign of poor prognosis; in fact, it does not predict any better or poorer course in the hospital. To assess whether depersonalization may disappear after the acute period, a separate Sample C of 111 patients was given the depersonalization questionnaire in the first week and again in the fourth week of hospitalization. Unlike other symptoms such as delusion, hallucinations, and suicidal thinking, which decline after the initial weeks, depersonalization did not show a significant decrease after the acute phase.

Personality and Affect Scales

At the same time that patients completed the depersonalization questionnaire, most of the patients completed a battery of other tests and questionnaires which are summarized in Table 11.3. The battery was somewhat different for Sample B, since the earlier work with Sample A had suggested further inquiry into dysphoric affect and its relation to depersonalization.

In addition, scales were examined in Sample B to rule out the possibility that depersonalized patients are simply reporting themselves in a bad light, whether through malingering, exaggeration of their symptoms, or whether subjects low on depersonalization are concealing symptoms in an attempt to present themselves in an especially favorable and socially desirable light. Two scales were used—the lie scale incorporated in the Maudsley Personality Inventory and the

Marlowe-Crowne Social Desirability Scale (Crowne and Marlowe, 1964). The Maudsley lie scale was not significantly related to the depersonalization scores, but the Marlowe-Crowne was related ($r = -.25, P < .05$). Subjects low on depersonalization appear to present themselves in a favorable light, but do not appear to have the exaggerated desire to deceive themselves and others about minor flaws. Even here, however, the correlation is low. Nevertheless, where significant relationships were obtained between depersonalization and other scales, a partial correlation was computed correcting for the Marlowe-Crowne score. As can be seen in Table 11.3, such a correction makes very little difference in the correlations.

Depersonalization tends to be related to neuroticism, although this is significant only in Sample B. In both samples, depersonalized patients tend to be introverted, cyclothymic, and to have more stimulus overinclusion, thought retardation, confusion, and impaired concentration. Thus, the personality structure is an introverted one, with mood swings and problems in attention and concentration. These findings are consistent with previous descriptions of depersonalization. More striking, however, was the relationship to dysphoric affect. Depersonalized patients had a general lowering of self-esteem both on the Semantic Differential Evaluation Scale and the modified Q-sort self-rating. They report more manifest anxiety, anomie, autism, cycloid thinking, emotionality, frustration, withdrawal, and guilt. Their symptoms more often include those ususally related to clinical depression (Colbert and Harrow, 1967). They are significantly higher and report more depressive symptoms on the Zung Depression Scale and more depressive and anxious affect on an adjective checklist. These findings are relative to dysphoric affect and symptoms, but not to primary depression as a diagnostic grouping.

The co-occurence of depersonalization and depressive symptoms and affect would appear to be a reliable and stable finding. The findings are internally consistent and reasonably high for personality and psychopathology scales that are taken during periods of acute stress early in hospitalization, conditions that usually work against reliable findings. Even stronger evidence for stability is the replication of almost all findings over two samples taken at two distinct time periods. The correlations are always in the same direction and of approximately the same size. Thus, the relationship of depersonalization to dysphoric affect appears to be a stable and reliable finding. The findings for aspects of disordered thinking are not as clear and were studied further.

DISORDERED THINKING AND DEPERSONALIZATION

The previous reports of the frequency of depersonalization in schizophrenic or pre-schizophrenic patients and its description as an ego disease suggested further measures of disordered thinking be studied for their relation to depersonalization. Subsamples of Sample B were given the Rorschach ($N = 60$) and the Object Sorting test ($N = 150$). Federn's (1952) description of depersonalization as a boundary disturbance suggested the specific evaluation of boundary disturbance scores on the Rorschach (see Chapter 9) as well as the study of nondisturbed measures of boundary properties, barrier, and penetration. In addition, general indices of disordered thinking were calculated from the Rorschach and Object Sorting tests.

A composite index of boundary disturbance composed of a weighted combination of fabulized combinations, contamination tendencies, and full contaminations yielded a low but significant correlation (r [58] $= .28; P < .05$). Contaminations, the type of response most strongly indicating boundary disturbance, had a significant correlation with depersonalization when examined by itself (r [59] $= .25; P < .05$). This is a low to moderate level of correlation. While patients with manifestations of boundary disturbance on the Rorschach do have more depersonalization than other patients, the relationship is not sufficiently large to rule out other contributions to depersonalization phenomena.

Barrier responses did not correlate with depersonalization ($r = .04$), while penetration showed a nonsignificant tendency to be correlated ($r = .22; P < .10$). While depersonalized patients show a greater awareness of their body and report experiencing milieu influences and medication effects as bodily changes, these findings are corroborated only to a weak degree by the indirect measures of body image (penetration). The multiple meanings of "body image" and the lack of direct measures of body image make the concept a particularly difficult one to study.

An index of general thinking disturbance utilizing the extreme levels of disrupted verbalization (thought quality, affect elaboration, overspecificity, but excluding contaminations) showed a significant degree of correlation with depersonalization. (r [58] $= .35; P < .01$). Other measures of disordered thinking from the Object Sorting test did not yield significant correlations with depersonalization: behavioral overinclusion (r [148] $= .07$), idiosyncratic thinking (r [148] $= .05$), or conceptual overinclusion (r [148] $= .00$). While the Object Sorting test may assess a different aspect of disordered thinking, depersonalization does not show a uniform relationship to thinking disruptions. As is the case in its relationship with schizophrenia, depersonalization is related (to a moderate degree) with some measures of disordered thinking. However, depersonalization is *not* related to all measures of disordered thinking. The relationship of depersonalization to dysphoric affect is more clear-cut and not attributable solely to diagnosis or disordered thinking.

Implications

What is surprising about the findings for depersonalization phenomena is not that so many of the hypotheses about depersonalization are disproven but rather that so many receive support. Very clearly, depersonalization phenomena are not specific to a single disorder but range in severity across several disorders. Thus, several seemingly contradictory theories each describe one or more aspect of these states. Several of the questions posed earlier in this chapter can be answered.

First, depersonalization and derealization do tend to occur together, while déjà vu appears to be predominantly an independent phenomenon. The degree of intercorrelation of depersonalization and derealization ($r = .65$ to $r = .72$) accounts for over 40 percent of the variance, but each experience clearly has some measures of independent occurrence as well.

Body image, at least in some aspects, is related to experiences of depersonalization and derealization. Depersonalization appears to involve; (a) an increase of attention and awareness of the body, (b) an experiencing of the body as "dead," and (c) an interpretation of psychological and medication effects as changes in body sensation. Schilder's (1928) emphasis on bodily awareness is supported, as are other theorists who emphasize the ego's observation of part of itself as though diseased and disowned (e.g., Jacobsen, 1964). In particular, Federn's (1952) description of depersonalization as an ego-boundary phenomenon receives some support from the boundary disturbance found in patients who score high on depersonalization.

Those investigators who stress that depersonalization is a precursor or prodromal symptom of schizophrenia (e.g., Galdston, 1947) do not receive strong support. The fact that latent or "borderline" schizophrenic patients are highest in depersonalization sheds some light on why previous clinical observers felt that this state occurs before, rather than as a part of, the "classical" schizophrenic picture. In addition, depersonalization is related to some but not all measures of attention disturbance and disordered thinking. These findings, considered together, are not sufficient to support the view of depersonalization as a chronic symptom.

The experiences of depersonalization very clearly *do* correlate with the dysphoric affects. The relationship with anxiety is sufficient to explain the appearance of depersonalization in the phobic anxiety-depersonalization syndrome (Roth and Harper, 1962). More striking are the relationships with a broad variety of phenomena associated with clinical depression: dysphoric affect, guilt, feelings of deadness, restless activity, and feelings of bodily changes. Depersonalization, however, is not related to primary depressive *disorder*. Depersonalization is a characteristic of patients with chronic depressive trends or with chronic depressive characters. Hospitalized depressed patients, however, represent only a subsample of clinically depressed persons. Further study of less disturbed depressed patients is in order.

The data obtained from well over 300 patients suggest that depersonalization and derealization are "core symptoms" that, like anxiety and depressed affect, occur to a greater or lesser degree in most or all psychopathological states. This view is in agreement with Lewis (1934), who suggested that in depressive states there is possibly little more than a verbal difference between the loss of interest and enjoyment and feelings of unreality. Lewis, however, rejected equating depersonalization with depression (Sedman, 1970). The findings here are sufficient to support viewing depersonalization as a distinct and separate experience, but one that is related to other affective states. After a review of the literature and of his own work, Sedman (1970) concluded that the strongest relationship of depersonalization was with affective states.

The present findings have clinical implications. As was true with the rated prognosis given by the psychiatric interviewer, clinicians may tend to overrate tha pathological meaning of depersonalization, possibly because of its previous association as a schizophrenic symptom. The occurrence of this experience in all forms of disorder, and its lack of relationship to prognosis, should modify the view of depersonalization. When this experience occurs in a context of relatively mild symptoms, depersonalization may be best treated as a nonspecific symptom and may often be a nonspecific depressive symptom. Further clinical studies would be helpful in investigating the *treatment* of depersonalization.

The categorization of such "signposts" as depersonalization into separate disorders may cloud the many similarities that exist across diagnostic groups. In general, we seem to be dealing with a chronic sense of discomfort of the self in the world. The strong association of depersonalization with dysphoric affects suggests a core symptom-atology in mental illness in general, which finds different degrees of expression in different disorders. The existence of a primary distur-bance denoted by depersonalization experiences (Shorvon, 1946; Roth, 1960; Roth and Harper, 1962) does not seem to be supported. Rather, the continued experience of depersonalization may occur in a char-acterological picture that is best described as a chronic depressive char-acter.

12
Disorders of Attention and Stimulus Overinclusion

As we have noted in Chapter 10, one type of potential disorder in schizophrenia is what we have labeled "stimulus overinclusion," which involves difficulties in selective attention. We have defined stimulus overinclusion as *perceptual experiences characterized by the individual's difficulty in attending selectively to relevant stimuli or by the person's tendency to be distracted by or to focus unnecessarily on a wide range of irrelevant stimuli.*

Members of our research group have come across a number of examples of stimulus overinclusion in patients' autobiographical accounts of their experiences (Bowers, 1974; Freedman, 1974; Kaplan, 1964; Sommer and Osmond, 1960), as well as in other aspects of the literature on psychosis based on clinicians' reports about their patients (Chapman, 1966; McGhie and Chapman, 1961). We also have observed them in our own clinical experience with both schizophrenic and nonschizophrenic patients. These types of aberrant perceptual experiences involving a disorder in selective attention can best be exemplified by the self-reports of schizophrenic patients studied by J. Chapman. One schizophrenic patient reported that he was attending to everything at once and as a result could not really attend to anything. Another schizophrenic patient reported that it was hard for her to focus selectively on one thing because she found herself distracted by every possible object, line, and color within sight (MacDonald, 1960). In our own research in this area (Harrow, Silverstein, Quinlan, and Lazar, 1978; Harrow, Tucker, and Shield, 1972; Shield, Harrow, and Tucker, 1974; Tucker Harrow, Detre, and Hoffman, 1969), presented in this chapter, we have studied the issues raised by both of these reports of schizophrenic patients, as well as other reports such as: "I have found that background noises seem louder than the main noises I am trying to pay attention to," and "I have found myself paying attention to the silliest little things going on around me and wasted a lot of energy that way."

As can be seen by both the definition listed above and the examples cited, stimulus overinclusion could be viewed as a disorder in one aspect of the perceptual process, and could most precisely be categorized as a disorder in attention. A number of new formulations about schizophrenic psychopathology being related to disturbed attention, or to other aspects of information processing, have appeared in the literature (Asarnow, Steffy, MacCrimmon, and Cleghorn 1978; Broen, 1968; Callaway 1970; Callaway and Naghdi, 1982; Garmezy, 1978; Maher, 1972; Neuchterlein, 1977; Reed, 1970; Spring, Neuchterlein, Sugarman, and Matthysse, 1977; Venables, 1964; Witkin, Dyk, Faterson, Goodenough and Karp, 1962; Yates, 1966). There have been a large number of carefully designed research studies related to theories in this area (Braff and Saccuzzo, 1981; Erlenmeyer-Kimling and Cornblatt, 1978; Keith, Gunderson, Reifman, Buchsbaum, and Mosher, 1976; Knight, Sherer, Putchat, and Carter, 1978; Koh, 1978; Kornetsky and Orzack, 1978; Neale and Cromwell, 1968; Oltmanns, Ohayan, and Neale, 1978; Pogue-Geile and Oltmanns, 1980; Rochester, 1978; Rochester and Martin, 1979; Saccuzzo and Braff, 1981; Salzinger, Portnoy, Pisoni, and Feldman, 1970). Theories about impairments in information processing and/or disordered attention might be considered among the most popular types of modern pathological theories of schizophrenia.

Several investigators, including Shakow (1979), Payne (1966), Maher (1972), and Silverman (1964, 1968), have hypothesized that disordered schizophrenic thinking and abnormal perceptual experiences in schizophrenia may be due to a general impairment in focusing attention, or in stimulus processing. As we have noted in Chapter 10, investigators such as Payne have hypothesized that this is due to a defect of a hypothetical "central filter mechanism" that normally functions to exclude irrelevant stimuli (both internal and external) so as to allow efficient processing of incoming information. Silverman has considered the disturbance we call "stimulus overinclusion" as one dimension of attention that plays a role in the altered states of consciousness found in various types of people, prominent among which are schizophrenics.

In an attempt to focus on this phenomenon with more precision, McGhie and J. Chapman have hypothesized that the basis of these perceptual abnormalities arises from an "ego defect" peculiar to schizophrenics. This "ego defect" appears to be similar in some respects to the defective "filter system" that Payne postulates. McGhie and Chapman, in a series of reports based on detailed study of a population of what they regarded as early schizophrenics, attempted to focus in on stimulus overinclusion (J. Chapman, 1966; McGhie and Chapman, 1961). Their research involved a series of interviews with schizophrenic patients. They reported positive results on the presence and importance of stimulus overinclusion in schizophrenics.

In some respects McGhie and Chapman's work represents a pioneering effort. However, there also is reason to question aspects of their method. It is unclear from their reports whether their patients with stimulus overinclusion and other disorders of attention were selected from a larger unspecified sample of patients, some of whom did not have these problems, or whether the sample they reported was exhaustive. There is a hint that some patients from their original sample were excluded if the diagnosis was not "confirmed" at follow-up, although it is unclear what specific criteria were used for such confirmation. Most important, it is unclear how frequently these perceptual phenomena would be found in a parallel sample of disturbed nonschizophrenic patients given the same intensive scrutiny. In addition, when we examined the information reported about McGhie and Chapman's "early" schizophrenic population, we found that this sample included patients who had been ill for two years or longer, and possibly hospitalized some or all of that time. This leaves open the suspicion that some of these patients were not early schizophrenics, but rather may have been more chronic schizophrenics.

Our research team felt that while the vivid clinical reports on schizophrenic patients' subjective experiences have contributed to the literature, it was important for these reports to be supplemented by a more rigorous, systematic investigation of the extent to which the phenomena described occur in both schizophrenic and *nonschizophrenic* patients. As a result, we have undertaken a program of research to study stimulus overinclusion, and disorders of selective attention. We should note in describing the efforts of our research team, that almost all of our work in this area, as in several other areas concerning disordered thinking, were facilitated by our joint collaboration with Dr. Gary Tucker, at first while he was a colleague of ours on the faculty at Yale

University School of Medicine, and later after he moved to assume a senior faculty position at Dartmouth Medical School. Detailed accounts of our previous research with Dr. Tucker on stimulus overinclusion and of our more recent research in this area can be found in a series of reports of ours (Harrow, Silverstein, Quinlan, and Lazar, 1978; Harrow, Tucker, and Shield, 1972; Shield, Harrow, and Tucker, 1974; Tucker, Harrow, Detre, and Hoffman, 1969). The major trends of this research on stimulus overinclusion are described in the current chapter, along with some of our later thinking in this area.

There were several background factors that stimulated the research of Dr. Tucker and ourselves on stimulus overinclusion during the early course of our thinking in this area. These factors highlighted for us the importance of documenting attentional and perceptual experiences such as stimulus overinclusion more precisely in schizophrenia and of providing data on how unique they are to schizophrenia (and even whether these experiences are more frequent in schizophrenia than in other disorders). In the first case, we noted when lecturing to undergraduate classes on theories about disordered attention that a number of "normal" students seemed to turn pale when we mentioned views that it is a phenomenon important or unique to schizophrenic patients, and when we provided specific examples of what stimulus overinclusion was like. These students later reported to us, at times in alarmed tones, that the phenomenon we have labeled stimulus overinclusion was not uncommon to them. The second reason for documenting the frequency of this phenomenon in schizophrenia was, as we have noted earlier, because of the increasing number of theories of schizophrenia that have hypothesized that this difficulty in attention and in stimulus processing is a key factor which may contribute to, or even cause, much of the schizophrenic disorder.

In this phase of our research we attempted to quantify the subjective perceptual experiences noted above which have most frequently been reported to be characteristic of schizophrenia, and to relate them to various subjective and objective phenomena in order to answer the following questions:

1. Is stimulus overinclusion found in all schizophrenics or only a portion of them?
2. Is stimulus overinclusion and disordered attention peculiar to schizophrenics alone or is it also found in many nonschizophrenic patients, and even in normals?
3. What factors influence stimulus overinclusion, and what is stimulus overinclusion related to?

4. What degree of importance does stimulus overinclusion play for both disturbed patients, and possibly for normal people as well?

PERCEPTUAL EXPERIENCE INVENTORY

Our method of studying stimulus overinclusion and disordered attention was to compile a list of representative statements selected from the detailed anecdotes of McGhie and Chapman (J. Chapman, 1966; McGhie and Chapman, 1961), and from the descriptive literature on the subjective experiences of schizophrenic patients. The statements selected, which in general assessed what we call stimulus overinclusion, were chosen on the basis of how pervasive and characteristic they were of the subjective experiences that have frequently been attributed to schizophrenic patients. In some phases of our research we administered this series of statements in the form of a structured interview conducted by a clinician, and in other phases of the research we administered the statements in the form of a questionnaire.

In the final questionnaire and structured interview, which we call the *Perceptual Experience Inventory* (PEI), these statements were interspersed with other filler items to get at test-taking attitudes and to detect possible biases in responses by the patients. The final questionnaire and structured interview consisted of a series of statements, all asked in terms of how frequently the patient had experienced them. Several of the questions that assess stimulus overinclusion have already been cited as examples earlier in this chapter. Several other questions on stimulus overinclusion that we used in various forms of our inventory are: "Lately, when you try to pay attention to something have you found a very great many different stimuli or events distracting you?"; "Recently, have you found that if people talk in simple sentences you can understand it, but when they use long sentences you lose the meanings?"; "Lately, when you are doing something, do you find that you have to pay attention to every little movement, even those you once did automatically?"; and "Recently, does it seem like everything is brighter, or louder and noisier?"

A list of six of the statements on stimulus overinclusion that we used as the central core in our research on stimulus overinclusion is presented in the box on page 275. The responses were scored on a five-point scale, depending on the frequency with which the subject has experienced stimulus overinclusion (e.g., 1 = not all, to 5 = almost all the time). We have utilized the Perceptual Experience Inventory in a series of three studies on stimulus overinclusion, using a number of samples of different types of patients and of normals.

INITIAL STUDY OF STIMULUS OVERINCLUSION AND DISORDERED ATTENTION

In the first investigation we used a fourteen-item form of our Perceptual Experience Inventory as the basis for a study involving detailed, individual, structured interviews with a first sample of seventy-three acute inpatients from our psychiatric services at Yale New Haven Hospital. This first sample included twenty-three schizophrenics. In this initial research effort in this area, we attempted to explore the relationship between schizophrenia and stimulus overinclusion, and also analyzed other aspects of personality, symptoms, and behavior to explore whether stimulus overinclusion might be related to personality or other factors. Hence, we used our Perceptual Experience Inventory as the basis for a study involving personal interviews (based on our structured interview format) with seventy-

---

SIX KEY STATEMENTS ON DISORDERED ATTENTION COMPRISING SCALE ON STIMULUS OVERINCLUSION

1. Recently have you found yourself paying attention to everything at once and as a result found that you were not really attending to anything?
2. Lately has it been hard to focus on one thing because you found yourself distracted by every possible object, line, and color within sight?
3. Lately when doing things that were once automatic have you had to think of your movements every second and found that it took a lot of extra energy?
4. Recently have you found that background noises seem louder than the main noises you are trying to pay attention to?
5. Lately when you try to pay attention to something, have you found a very great many different stimuli or events distracting you?
6. Recently have you found yourself paying attention to the silliest little things going on around you and wasted a lot of energy that way?

From Harrow, Tucker, & Shield. *Archives of General Psychiatry, 27,* 40–45, 1972. Copyright 1972, by the American Medical Association, and reproduced by permission of the publisher.

three acute inpatients. In this research we related the interview material to diagnosis, and the results from other indices of psychopathology, to a number of attitude scales, and a series of personality measures, to get some estimate of the role played by stimulus overinclusion in acute patients.

The results from our first sample of seventy-three acute inpatients began to provide some systematic data in support of our earlier observations that stimulus overinclusion is not limited to schizophrenics, and can be found in many nonschizophrenics. Those frightened reports by some of our students that they too had experienced stimulus overinclusion were beginning to be vindicated! Thus, we found no significant differences between diagnostic groups, although there was a nonsignificant trend for a larger amount of stimulus overinclusion in schizophrenic patients. In addition, there was a slight trend toward more stimulus overinclusion in severe borderline patients, and in our latent schizophrenics (patients who had not had clear psychotic breaks, but who had a combination of many severe personality difficulties, along with anxiety and depressive features, chronic difficulties in adjusting to life problems, and some odd or peculiar features). Thus, a slightly larger percentage of both the classical schizophrenic, and also the latent schizophrenic, patients tended to report stimulus overinclusion, but the differences among diagnostic groups were not significant.

Some of the reports by the schizophrenic patients about stimulus overinclusion and difficulties in attention were quite dramatic, but these types of dramatic reports could almost be matched by other dramatic accounts by nonschizophrenic patients about difficulties they experienced in this area. The results from this first study left us with some lingering questions about the possibility that when schizophrenics experience stimulus overinclusion, the consequences may be different and more severe than when nonschizophrenics experience it. But this possibility—and it is a real possibility—was not studied in our sample, and still remains unconfirmed.

In addition to our comparison of diagnostic groups, we also assessed the relationship between the scores on stimulus overinclusion and a variety of clinical behaviors that were rated by the patient's therapists, and the nursing staff. The correlations that emerged are reported in Table 12.1. As can be seen in the table, the behavior and symptom data included ratings of delusions, of paranoid ideas, of hallucinations, and of bizarre speech and behavior. Again, we did not find strong relationships between the presence of stimulus overinclusion and these types of psychotic behaviors.

The results we obtained from this first sample clearly suggested that stimulus overinclusion is not unique to schizophrenia. If stimulus overinclusion is more frequent in schizophrenia, the differences are relatively small, and on the basis of this sample of seventy-three patients the differences between diagnostic groups were not significant.

When we analysed our results on stimulus overinclusion, in conjunction with the data from our personality tests, a number of other features emerged that we had not completely expected. These results on the relationship betwen stimulus overinclusion and the series of personality tests are presented in Table 12.2. The most surprising of the results was a moderately high relationship between stimulus over-inclusion and our indices of trait anxiety. A correlation of $r = 0.38$ was found between stimulus overinclusion and scores on the Taylor Anxiety Scale (Bendig, 1956). Similar correlations of about $r = 0.40$ were found between the patients' scores on stimulus overinclusion and their scores on a scale of "nervousness," and also on the "neuroticism" scale of the Maudsley Personality Inventory (Eysenck, 1956). Thus, a picture emerged of patients who were high on stimulus overinclusion also being high on trait anxiety. This would suggest that patients high on stimulus overinclusion also tend to become anxious more easily, and to respond more quickly and more poorly to stress. Looked at in another way, patients who frequently experience stimulus overinclusion are probably patients who tend to respond to disturbing events or stress by becoming anxious. They are more susceptible to outside pressures,

TABLE 12.1
Relationship of Stimulus Overinclusion
to Symptom and Behavioral Data

Variables	Correlation
1. Stimulus overinclusion r Isolation	.05
2. Stimulus overinclusion r Withdrawal	.04
3. Stimulus overinclusion r Regression	−.11
4. Stimulus overinclusion r Paranoia	−.15
5. Stimulus overinclusion r Delusions	.00
6. Stimulus overinclusion r Hallucinations	.04
7. Stimulus overinclusion r Bizarre speech or behavior	.11
8. Stimulus overinclusion r Disorientation	.08
9. Stimulus overinclusion r Depressed mood	.06
10. Stimulus overinclusion r Hypochondriasis	−.12
11. Stimulus overinclusion r Hospitalized before	−.09

more easily disrupted and aroused by environmental stimuli, and also by internal pressures or stimuli. Probably as a result of these factors, they tend to be anxious a larger percentage of the time.

On the face of it, these trends would seem to be in contradiction to the Estabrook hypothesis that, in anxiety, attention is narrowed. This paradox is resolvable, however. It is quite possible that the anxious subject is able to use stimuli from a narrower central range, but may be more *distractable* as well. The two phenomena, narrowing and stimulus overinclusion, may operate in complementary fashion (i.e., the narrowing may result from the increased distractability). Another important possibility is that there may be basic differences in the effect on attention and perceptual processes between the presence of mild versus severe anxiety. Thus, it is possible that severe anxiety may lead to difficulty in focusing and an impairment in selective attention.

In addition, with this first sample we also assessed the relationship between stimulus overinclusion and locus of control (the internal-external scale). Locus of control, a concept elaborated by Rotter, has been widely used as a measure of the extent that people believe events occurring to them are determined by their own behavior (internal locus of control), as opposed to being determined by fate, luck, or chance (external locus of control) (Rotter, 1966). Locus of control or internal-

TABLE 12.2
Relationship of Stimulus Overinclusion
to Personality Variables

Variables	Correlation
1. Stimulus overinclusion *r* Taylor Anxiety Scale	.38**
2. Stimulus overinclusion *r* Neuroticism scale	.36**
3. Stimulus overinclusion *r* Nervousness	.41**
4. Stimulus overinclusion *r* Anomie	.22
5. Stimulus overinclusion *r* Lie scale	−.04
6. Stimulus overinclusion *r* Marlow-Crowne Scale	−.26*
7. Stimulus overinclusion *r* Locus of control	.31**
8. Stimulus overinclusion *r* Introversion	−.03
9. Stimulus overinclusion *r* Authoritarianism	.10
10. Stimulus overinclusion *r* Depersonalization	.16
11. Stimulus overinclusion *r* Derealization	.33**
12. Stimulus overinclusion *r* Concentration difficulty	.18
13. Stimulus overinclusion *r* Confusion	.32**

*$P < .05$.

**$P < .01$.

From Tucker, Harrow, Detre, & Hoffman. *Archives of General Psychiatry, 20,* 159–166, 1969. Copyright 1969, by the American Medical Association, and reproduced by permission of the publisher.

external control, is an important concept that has been used widely in social-psychological research and in personality research. Our own research group has studied this concept in the past, in relation to psychiatric patients (Harrow and Ferrante, 1969). When we did analyze locus of control in relation to stimulus overinclusion (see variable 7 in Table 12.2), we found that the correlation ($r = 0.31$) suggested that patients high on stimulus overinclusion generally tended to feel that they do not have much control over the events in their lives.

In terms of our initial data indicating that stimulus overinclusion is related to a tendency to be upset more easily by stress or anxiety, it should not be surprising that patients high on stimulus overinclusion, who have problems with selective attention, would tend to have external locus of control. One might almost expect patients with such difficulties to tend to see events in their lives as being out of their control and in the hands of destiny. Thus, it would be easy to view one's fate as not being under one's control, and not a consequence of one's own actions, if during one's life one's equilibrium is frequently disrupted by minor (or major) events and upsets, and shifts in outside pressures as well as internal pressures. In a sense, the lives of these patients really are determined by the vicissitudes of external forces, and their view of external locus of control may be partly accurate for themselves.

On the basis of the results with our first sample of seventy-three inpatients we now had formal data that suggested that: (a) the link between schizophrenia and stimulus overinclusion is an unclear one, and not the simple unidimensional relationship many seem to have formulated; (b) there was some more solid basis for believing that stimulus overinclusion, or a disorder in selective attention, may be found in many nonpathological conditions, although this would have to be verified with a larger nonschizophrenic sample and with a normal sample; (c) there was a possibility that conditions of anxiety, general upset, and disturbance might contribute to stimulus overinclusion; and (d) more general features of personality may be related to stimulus overinclusion.

SECOND STUDY OF STIMULUS OVERINCLUSION, USING PATIENTS AT TWO PHASES OF THEIR DISORDER AND USING A SAMPLE OF NORMALS

Having devised a method of investigation, applied it to a first sample of patients, and used the data to formulate a series of hypotheses about the role of stimulus overinclusion in schizophrenia and about what factors stimulus overinclusion might be related to, we felt we had completed the first phase of our research in this area. In our second phase we set out to utilize our methodology and evaluate our formulations with a new, larger sample of patients (sample 2) and with a sample of normals. We also set out to evaluate more directly our formulations about the importance of acute upset and disturbance as a contributor to stimulus overinclusion by studying patients at two phases of their disorder, the acute stage, and then seven weeks later, reassessing the same patients when the influence of acute disturbance had diminished.

In this second investigation we used the material we had collected from the personal interview in the first study as a basis for a paper-and-pencil questionnaire consisting of our six core questions assessing stimulus overinclusion, with these being embedded with other questions that tap other perceptual experiences and symptom material. We administered the questionnaire to a new sample of 199 consecutive psychiatric inpatients.

This second sample, composed of consecutive admissions to our psychiatric inpatients services at Yale New Haven Hospital, included 42 classical schizophrenics, 38 latent schizophrenics, and 119 other psychiatric inpatients. The nonschizophrenics were primarily depressives and severe personality disorders. In addition, to compare the schizophrenic sample with both a comparable disturbed patient population and a normal sample, we obtained and studied a sample of fifty-three "normals" from a small college. These normals were also administered the Perceptual Experience Inventory and a series of personality tests.

In this second stage of our research we studied the patients systematically at two phases of their disorders. These included the acute phase (first ten days of acute hospitalization) and the phase of partial recovery (six to eight weeks later). This allowed us to explore more directly the role of acute upset and acute psychopathology on stimulus overinclusion, and disordered attention, and to investigate patient changes on stimulus overinclusion as they began to emerge from the period of extreme upset.

Stimulus Overinclusion at the Acute Stage of Hospitalization

Table 12.3 presents the mean scores of each diagnostic group on stimulus overinclusion at the acute stage, in this second phase of our research. Analysis of these results indicated that when a very large sample was used, the small to moderate differences between classical schizophrenics and nonschizophrenic patients on stimulus overinclusion and problems in selective attention became significant $(P < .01)$. The use of large sample sizes creates a more sensitive experimental design in which true, but small, differences between groups will emerge as statistically significant. Interpretation of this type of significant difference must be conducted with caution. It sometimes indicates that there is a genuine difference between the groups (in this case the classical schizophrenics at the acute phase show more stimulus overinclusion than the acutely disturbed nonschizophrenic patients), but the differences may be relatively small.

There also was a trend for the most disturbed and most psychotic patients to have higher scores on stimulus overinclusion regardless of diagnosis. This was most apparent in the scores on stimulus overinclusion for the psychotic depressive group, with this severely disturbed group having relatively high scores on stimulus overinclusion. When the scores of the group of psychotic patients (classical schizophrenics and psychotic depressives) were combined and compared to those of the nonschizophrenic, nonpsychotic patients, the results also were statistically significant ($t = 3.26$, 159 *df*, $P < .01$). These data and other subsequent data we collected at a later point in our research in this area could suggest that severely disturbed depressive patients are high in general on stimulus overinclusion. This possible relationship to severe depression deserves further investigation.

TABLE 12.3
Mean Scores on Stimulus Overinclusion at the Acute Phase for Sample 2

	Mean	N
Classical schizophrenics	16.76	42
Latent schizophrenics	14.34	38
Psychotic depressives	15.39	23
Neurotic depressives	13.60	25
Personality disorders	13.66	44
Other nonschizophrenics	12.00	27
Normals	12.91	53

From Harrow, Tucker, & Shield. *Archives of General Psychiatry, 27*, 40–45, 1972. Copyright 1972, by the American Medical Association, and reproduced by permission of the publisher.

Stimulus Overinclusion in Normals

The data from our sample of "normals" are also presented in Table 12.3. The "normal" sample included fifty-three students from two undergraduate psychology classes at a small local college. Our earlier hypothesis, based on observations of normals and based on the trend beginning to emerge with our first sample of patients, had been that we would also find some normals who experience stimulus overinclusion. The data on the normals confirmed these earlier indications that stimulus overinclusion is not a phenomenon that is limited only to patients. Select normals reported high levels of stimulus overinclusion. In addition, a number of other normals showed some degree of stimulus overinclusion, although as a group they were significantly lower than the schizophrenic samples.

Overview of Results on Acute Patients and Normals

Overall, these data collected on a second sample of patients at the acute phase of their disorders (and on normals) should be looked at in conjunction with the results on stimulus overinclusion, a type of impaired attention, from our first sample of seventy-three patients. In both samples the schizophrenics showed the highest scores on stimulus overinclusion. In the previous, smaller sample the schizophrenics were not significantly higher than the nonschizophrenic patients, and in the current larger sample a significant difference emerged. Thus, in the current sample the schizophrenics showed the most stimulus overinclusion, the other acute patients were the second highest, and the normals were the lowest on stimulus overinclusion, although a number of normals showed at least a moderate level of stimulus overinclusion. Perhaps of most importance for hypotheses about the unique role of stimulus overinclusion, a number of disturbed patients of all types, and some normals experienced stimulus overinclusion. Many of the formulations in this area about schizophrenia are based on ideas that stimulus overinclusion and disorders of attention play a key etiological role in leading to other psychopathological features, especially thought pathology and other aspects of psychosis.

In view of the high scores on stimulus overinclusion by many acute nonschizophrenics, the question could be asked, if stimulus overinclusion is a major etiologic factor in schiozophrenia, why are there so many nonschizophrenic patients and normals who are high on stimulus overinclusion? And also, why is there a certain percentage of schizo-phrenics who are not high on stimulus overinclusion? These results would seem to indicate that while stimulus overinclusion may (or may not) play some role in schizophrenia, in itself it is unlikely to be the major etiologic factor. It is still quite possible that when schizophrenics do have stimulus overinclusion, they experience it as more upsetting and it interferes with their functioning to a great extent. If this were the case, then stimulus overinclusion would play some role in the schizophrenic picture but would not be a major etiologic factor. However, even this role for stimulus overinclusion is currently undocumented.

Stimulus Overinclusion during the Phase of Partial Recovery

The data on stimulus overinclusion or impaired attention, during the phase of partial recovery (seven to eight weeks after the acute assessment) are presented in Table 12.4. These results, in particular, bear on our formulation that stimulus overinclusion is influenced by acute upset and acute disturbance. Thus, they alowed us to make a comparison of schizophrenic patients (and nonschizophrenic patients) at the acute phase with the same sample of patients at the phase of partial recovery seven to eight weeks later (75 percent of the acute patient sample presented in Table 12.3 were still available in the hospital and reassessed seven to eight weeks later). The mean scores on stimulus overinclusion for each of the diagnostic groups had dimin-ished after the acute phase. The overall sample of patients had declined

TABLE 12.4
Mean Scores on Stimulus Overinclusion
at the Phase of Partial Recovery for Sample 2

	Mean	N
Classical schizophrenics	14.31	32
Latent schizophrenics	13.26	31
Psychotic depressives	11.94	18
Neurotic depressives	11.61	18
Personality disorders	11.21	29
Other nonschizophrenics	11.27	22

From Harrow, Tucker, & Shield. *Archives of General Psychiatry, 27*, 40–45, 1972. Copyright 1972, by the American Medical Association, and reproduced by permission of the publisher.

significantly on stimulus overinclusion, and on disorders of attention, and this was true for each of the major diagnostic groups (the classical schizophrenics and the nonschizophrenic patients). These data, as well as several other aspects of the overall results, can be interpreted as providing evidence that acute disturbance, stress, and turmoil play some role in stimulus overinclusion. These factors lead to a higher level of stimulus overinclusion and an increase in attentional disorders in all diagnostic groups during the most acute phase. Fitting in with this, seven weeks later at the phase usually associated with partial recovery, when patients' symptoms and other psychological features had been reduced considerably, there was very little difference on stimulus overinclusion between the nonschizophrenic patients and the sample of normals.

The data on diagnostic differences during the phase of partial recovery again showed the classical schizophrenics as having significantly higher scores than the nonschizophrenic patients ($P < .01$). These results, at the phase of partial recovery, would suggest that either schizophenia and/or severe psychopathology (both are factors that characterize the schizophrenic sample) lead to a somewhat more severe level of stimulus overinclusion, when the differences are assessed with large samples.

One caution concerning the interpretation of these results relates to the significant differences between the schizophrenic and nonschizophrenic sample at the phase of partial recovery. At the period of seven to eight weeks later, acute schizophenic disorders (although diminished in intensity) are often in a more flagrant form than can be found in other disorders. Thus, schizophrenia takes longer to remit than most other psychiatric disorders. As a result, some of the schizophrenics were still more acutely disturbed than patients from the comparable sample of nonschizophrenics. Other independent ratings of various aspects of psychopathology showed the schizophrenic group as more pathological at the acute phase and at the phase of partial recovery. Because of this, a slightly larger percentage of schizophrenics were still in the hospital available for assessment eight weeks after the acute phase. The poorer adjustment of the schizophrenics, their lower level of functioning, and their higher degree of psychopathology, may have been an influence contributing to their higher scores on stimulus overinclusion during the phase of partial recovery.

STIMULUS OVERINCLUSION IN OUR THIRD SAMPLE OF PSYCHIATRIC PATIENTS

Having obtained the above clues indicating that stimulus over-inclusion, or impaired attention, occurs in nonschizophrenics as well as in schizophrenics, and having obtained evidence that stimulus over-inclusion seems to be influenced by acute disturbance and periods of upset, we attempted to focus on these findings in a further study. We therefore designed subsequent research entailing a third investigation assessing 109 new patients. These 109 patients were acute psychiatric admissions to the inpatient services at Yale New Haven Hospital. The 109 psychiatric patients included 27 classical schizophrenics and 25 latent schizophrenic patients.

In this phase of our research we used the hypotheses derived from the first two studies to serve as a basis for another series of personal structured interviews. In these interviews we examined formulations derived from the first two studies, especially those about the role of anxiety and acute upset as having an influence on stimulus over-inclusion. Hence, we evaluated the frequency of stimulus overinclusion in this third sample and attempted to assess under what kinds of conditions stimulus overinclusion occurs. We also looked at whether it is influenced by other enviromental and external events, such as drug use, whether it disrupts patients' daily activities, and a series of other similar issues to help determine the role of stimulus overinclusion and its importance in patients' lives.

Since there has been a great deal of discussion about stimulus overinclusion and psychotomimetic drugs, we also explored the frequency of this type of impaired attention in a subsample of patients who had LSD experiences. LSD and psychotomimetic drugs in general have been of interest to people in the mental-health field for a number of reasons, one of which is a belief by some that LSD experiences simulate schizophrenia. In the past our own observations have not been in complete accord with this belief about typical LSD expeiences, although we have noted many striking similarities between reactions to a different type of drug, namely amphetamine psychosis, and certain types of schizophrenic reactions. In Chapter 13 we present some of our research with patients who could be classified as chronic hallucinogen-drug users, and the relationship between this phenomenon and thought pathology.

In this third major sample of 109 patients, 69 of these patients (constituting 63 percent of the sample) reported a moderate or high level of stimulus overinclusion. As with our previous sample, we investigated this population for possible diagnostic differences in the level of stimulus overinclusion. The results on the sample indicated slightly higher scores for our sample of schizophrenics, but the schizophrenics were not significantly higher on stimulus overinclusion than nonschizophrenics. There was again a trend for psychotic depressive patients and other severe depressives to have experienced considerable stimulus overinclusion. Overall, the results in our analysis involving all the diagnostic groups again indicated somewhat higher scores for the schizophrenics, but failed to show significant diagnostic differences. These data are in accord with the results from our previous samples suggesting a consistent trend for more stimulus overinclusion among schizophrenics, but the trend was small enough that it sometimes just achieves statistical significance, and sometimes fails to achieve it.

The sixty-nine patients from this sample who did have stimulus overinclusion were examined more closely concerning anxiety, with a focus on the relationship between the occurrence of stress and stimulus overinclusion. Extensive structured interviews were conducted with the patients about the details of their experiences of stimulus overinclusion. In our investigation of stress and its relation to stimulus overinclusion, we have used the term "stress" to refer to periods of increased upset. The upset could be related to external environmental events or to internal or subjective stress.

The data from our interviews on the possible occurrence of stimulus overinclusion under conditions of stress are presented in Table 12.5. The data on stress indicated that 75 percent of the sixty-nine patients with stimulus overinclusion reported some relationship between stress and stimulus overinclusion. Our results in this area indicated that for the great bulk of these patients, stress and stimulus overinclusion were related, either in terms of these patients reporting that stimulus overinclusion, or impaired attention, was directly "caused" by stress for them, or else by stimulus overinclusion, or impaired attention, being exacerbated by stress. The majority of this subsample (60 percent) reported that stimulus overinclusion was exacerbated by stress, and the other 40 percent felt it was directly caused by it. These results, obtained using a different technique than we had used in our previous studies and suggesting a strong relationship between increased stress and stimulus overinclusion, fit in with our earlier data on the relationship between stimulus overinclusion and trait anxiety. The relationship between stress and stimulus overinclusion was not a perfect one, but it was a relatively high one.

Our investigation with this sample of 109 patients also explored whether or not stimulus overinclusion disrupts ongoing activity and interferes with current adjustment. The results were positive in this area, indicating that over 80 percent of the patients who had stimulus overinclusion found that it disrupted their immediate ability to function.

We explored whether stimulus overinclusion is more common during specific affective states, such as periods of anger, anxiety, or depression. The results in this area did not show much association between stimulus overinclusion and anger, but they did suggest a relationship with other types of affective states. Thus, the results showed that in the subsample of patients with stimulus overinclusion, slightly over 60 percent reported an increase in this phenomenon during general periods of anxiety, and slightly over 40 percent reported an increase in stimulus overinclusion during more depressed periods. Using different techniques than with our previous samples of patients we obtained results that fit in with the evidence from the earlier samples, which suggested a link between stimulus overinclusion and trait anxiety in many cases. It should be noted that whereas stimulus overinclusion occurred more frequently for many during these types of

TABLE 12.5
The Occurrence of Stimulus Overinclusion
under Conditions of Stress

	Number of patients in each category	% of total patient sample in each category	% of patients from among 69 patients who experience stimulus overinclusion
Has stimulus overinclusion, it is persistent, and exacerbated by stress.	31	28%	45%
Has stimulus overinclusion, but only during stress.	21	19%	30%
Has stimulus overinclusion, it is persistent, but it is not related to stress.	12	11%	17%
Has stimulus overinclusion, but it is not stress related or persistent.	5	5%	7%
Does not experience stimulus overinclusion.	40	37%	—
TOTAL PATIENT SAMPLE	109	100%	99%

From Shield, Harrow, & Tucker. *Psychiatric Quarterly, 48*, 109–116, 1974. Copyright 1974 by Human Sciences Press, Inc., New York, NY, and reproduced by permission of the publisher.

emotional states, it also occurred at times in the absence of any enviromental occurrences or obvious internal events.

STIMULUS OVERINCLUSION AND THE USE OF PSYCHOTOMIMETICS

Our research on the relationship between stimulus overinclusion and psychomimetic drugs produced somewhat unexpected results. At times clinical observation has suggested a strong relationship between LSD use and stimulus overinclusion. Our results did not support these observations. A large number of our hallucinogen users reported little or no stimulus overinclusion, although some of the other users of psychomimetics did report stimulus overinclusion. In contrast, many of our patients who did not use LSD regularly reported experiencing some stimulus overinclusion on those rare occasions when they did use hallucinogens. Thus, in this area there was a tendency toward a negative relationship between the use of LSD and stimulus overinclusion. The results of marijuana use and its relationship to LSD were less clear-cut.

A possible explanation for these results is that some or many of the patients who use LSD and tend to experience both stimulus over-inclusion and other upsetting and disruptive perceptual experiences learn to avoid psychotomimetics after a while. This would leave us with a situation in which patients (and other people) who tend to use LSD are those who find that its use brings less upsetting perceptual difficulties.

It is still possible that there is a relationship between stimulus overinclusion and the use of psychotomimetics, and that the lack of a strong relationship is due to sampling errors. Thus, our results occurred with the use of patient populations, and it is possible that with the investigation of a "normal" sample, the results would show a stronger relationship. It also is possible that a strong relationship exists between stimulus overinclusion and hallucinogen use but that other unique characteristics of the sample obscured this relationship. In our sample, however, where patients chose whether or not they would use LSD, rather than being randomly assigned to it, no relationship was found between stimulus overinclusion and hallucinogen use. In the absence of clear evidence to the contrary, it remains for those who believe in such a relationship to produce overt evidence in support of their hypothesis.

CONCLUSIONS ON STIMULUS OVERINCLUSION

Summary of Our Main Results on Stimulus Overinclusion and Disorders of Attention

On the basis of our assessment of three large samples of patients, and a sample of normals, a number of results emerged concerning disorders of attention and stimulus overinclusion. These include the following:

1. Stimulus overinclusion is not found in all schizophrenics, or in all delusional patients.
2. Stimulus overinclusion is not unique to schizophrenia and can be found in many nonschizophrenic patients and nonpsychotic patients.
3. Stimulus overinclusion can also be found in some normals.
4. Stimulus overinclusion cuts across the usual diagnostic lines. If there are diagnostic differences concerning stimulus overinclusion, they are relatively small and not the major factor in accounting for stimulus overinclusion.
5. The results from our three large samples suggest that stimulus overinclusion is more frequent in patients who are high on trait anxiety and who are more susceptible to, and more easily disrupted by, environmental pressures or stimuli, or by internal pressures or stimuli. Perhaps stimulus overinclusion is more likely to occur in people with autonomic nervous systems that are more easily disrupted and tend to be less stable.
6. Acute upset and general disturbance are key factors that influence stimulus overinclusion, and during periods of partial recovery, when severe disturbances diminish, patients experience less stimulus overinclusion.

A Negative View of Stimulus Overinclusion as the Etiologic Factor in Schizophrenia

Perhaps of most importance, our overall results on the formulation of stimulus overinclusion and an impairment in selective attention as a major etiological factor in schizophrenia were negative. Recently, in a separate study in a different setting, Freedman and Chapman (1973) reported results from a study of stimulus overinclusion and a variety of other types of disorders, of attention and perception, in a psycho-pathological sample. These investigators found some trend toward more pathological levels of stimulus overinclusion and disorders of attention in schizophrenics, but when phenomena such as stimulus overinclusion were considered alone, the schizophrenic-nonschizo-phrenic differences were not as large as might have been expected. In some respects these results are in accord with our findings.

We should comment on the point that a number of seemingly positive results on stimulus overinclusion and related factors have been reported by other investigators. However, these results are usually based on experiments in which a performance deficit is found in schizophrenics, with the deficit then being ascribed to stimulus overinclusion or some other aspect of attention. In this type of research, poor performance by schizophrenics, or a deficit shown by schizo-phrenics, is interpreted as being due to stimulus overinclusion. It is quite possible that stimulus overinclusion is a major factor in these deficits, but it is also possible than any one of a number of other factors, or a combination of other factors, is the critical feature in the poorer performance by schizophrenics in this type of research by others.

A View of Stimulus Overinclusion and an Impairment in Selective Attention as Arising from Several Sources and its Role in Schizophrenia

In relation to the data we have collected on stimulus overinclusion and impaired selective attention, we have noted the indications from our series of investigations that it occurs in both schizophrenics and disturbed nonschizophrenic patients, but perhaps somewhat more frequently in schizophrenic and borderline patients. Thus, a relation-ship with schizophrenia seems to exist, although the relationship is not a very strong one. We must explain why, (1) on the positive side, there is some positive relationship between stimulus overinclusion and schizophrenia; and yet, on the negative side (2) the relationship is not strong; (3) stimulus overinclusion is not a necessary condition for schizophrenia (i.e., some schizophrenics do not have stimulus over-inclusion); and (4) stimulus overinclusion is not a sufficient condition for schizophrenia (i.e., many nonschizophrenic patients and normals experience stimulus overinclusion, and this is not sufficient to make them schizophrenic).

Part of the dilemma in thinking about stimulus overinclusion and an impairment in selective attention is that it is sometimes viewed as being related to only one factor, such as schizophrenia. It seems likely that the perceptual and the attentional systems can be disrupted by more than one means, as well as by a number of different interacting factors.

Hence, one outlook would consider that several factors can influence stimulus overinclusion, and that stimulus overinclusion or an impairment in selective attention can occur through several means. One means would be by anxiety or extreme disturbance. This may upset a number of different aspects of attention and perception, with ability to attend selectively to relevant stimuli being one such aspect of attention that is disrupted. Our data suggest that this is one of the most common means by which stimulus overinclusion occurs, and that this is experienced by many schizophrenics, disturbed nonschizophrenics, and some "normals."

A second way that stimulus overinclusion could occur is as a concomitant of disorders that involve or are centered in a disruption of higher-level executive processes. Thus, stimulus overinclusion could occur as a concomitant of schizophrenia, which we believe involves disruption of specific aspects of executive processes, and of aspects of functioning regulated by central mechanisms. Schizophrenia could be viewed as a centrally based disorder involving a disturbance in executive processes, one in which there is a malfunctioning of a variety of specific aspects of functioning, with some aspects of executive functioning characteristically being disrupted and others rarely showing dysfunctioning. These higher-level functions characteristically showing malfunctioning in schizophrenia would involve the internal regulation of thought processes and judgment, and perspective about reality (or reality testing) and about the appropriateness of one's own behavior. These have been discussed in earlier chapters, and will be treated in the last chapter of this book.

While the above central distrubance may play a major role in many of the features involved in active psychosis, other perceptual functions could also be affected. As a concomitant of this type of central disorder involving disruption of central control mechanisms, the regulation of a number of aspects of external stimuli, such as that involved in attention and perception, might be disrupted, with the possibility that these perceptual functions are less uniformly influenced. Indeed, with such a central disorder, the regulation of internal stimuli might be impaired more frequently and this may be a more important feature, although our research has not focused on this aspect of functioning.

The formulation here concerning stimulus overinclusion would be that perceptual and attentional dysfunctioning also occur in many schizophrenics, but that no one aspect of perceptual functioning is uniformly disrupted by such a disturbance in the central control mechanisms. As a result, any of a number of routine aspects of perceptual functions of schizophrenics could be interfered with, and probably other functions as well. For some of these schizophrenic patients, disorders of attention, such as stimulus overinclusion, would appear, and for other schizophrenics different aspects of perceptual functioning would show disorder. In some other schizophrenic patients, both stimulus overinclusion and a variety of other types of perceptual disorders would appear, and in some schizophrenic patients there would be no gross impairment in perceptual functioning. Since we believe that no one aspect of perceptual functioning is uniformly disrupted in schizophrenia, we would propose that if one used a composite score combining a variety of different types of perceptual dsyfunctioning, one would find a bigger difference between schizophrenics and nonschizophrenics than would be found studying stimulus overinclusion or an impairment in selective attention alone.

Viewed in the manner we have discussed above, stimulus overinclusion would not be an etiologic factor in schizophrenia, but rather would be a condition that could be influenced, increased, or made manifest by several factors. One of these would be the underlying disorder associated with schizophrenia. This underlying factor sometimes may lead to stimulus overinclusion in schizophrenia, along with its leading to other pschopathological conditions. However, in this model other factors can contribute as well to stimulus overinclusion in schizophrenics, and would be important in nonschizophrenic patients and normals as contributors to more pathological levels of stimulus overinclusion, and to an impairment in selective attention.

## PART V

OTHER IMPORTANT
ASPECTS OF DISORDERED
THINKING AND
OVERVIEW

13

The Use of Hallucinogenic Drugs and Their Effect on Disordered Thinking

Soon after I was placed in my room at home, all of my senses became perverted. . . . The tricks played upon me by my perverted sense of taste, touch, smell, and sight were the source of mental anguish. . . . Familiar materials had acquired a different "feel." In the dark, the bed sheets at times seemed like silk.

My sense of sight was subjected to many weird and uncanny effects. Phantasmagoric visions made their visitations throughout the night. . . . Moving pictures, often brilliantly colored, were thrown on the ceiling of my room and sometimes on the sheets of my bed. . . . I remember one vision of vivid beauty. Swarms of butterflies and large and gorgeous moths appeared on the sheets. That sight I really enjoyed, knowing that the pretty creatures were not alive; and I wished that the usually unkind operator would continue to minister to my aesthetic taste by feeding it colors so rich and faultlessly combined. [Beers, 1908, pp. 30–33]

This description by Clifford Beers could easily be mistaken for the account of a "trip" on psychedelic drugs. Voluntarily, many thousands of people have sought out what were expected to be temporary experiences through self-administration of a whole host of mind-altering drugs and combinations, some with what appear to be lasting changes in their thoughts, feelings, and relationships with others. In this chapter, we ask the question: Do the long-term effects of hallucinogenic drugs mimic the changes in schizophrenia?

One of the problems of studying disordered thinking in any population that includes a large number of young patients is how to assess the contribution of past or current hallucinogenic drugs to the disordered thinking that one sees in a clinical test protocol? The early research with such chemicals and the later uncontrolled casual use both suggested that the mental states produced by these chemicals were similar in many ways to the kind of changes in speech and thinking found in schizophrenia. Over and above the immediate effect of such drugs, the "youth culture" in which they were taken transformed those signs of mental disorders that we commonly associate with psychosis into parts of a popular, if limited, subculture. Some forms of the changes in speech and thinking became a more lasting aspect of the presentation of some of the drug users, even when they were not under the immediate influence of such drugs. Some biochemical theories of schizophrenia have raised the question of whether the effects of such chemicals on the neurotransmitters may not be, in fact, similar to a process that some suspect to be underlying schizophrenia.

There are some tantalizing similarities between the immediate effects of the hallucinogenic drugs and the symptoms found in acute schizophrenic reaction. Bowers and Freedman (1966) presented data suggesting that the experiential states during lysergic acid, diethylamide (LSD) in fact have some clear parallel with the symptoms of the acute psychotic state of schizophrenia. An earlier study by Rinkel in 1952 showed that normal subjects during the height of reaction to LSD showed changes such as autistic thinking, poor mental organization, contaminatory reponses, and illogical thinking on the Rorschach; each of these has been associated with schizophrenia. It is perhaps because of the manifest pathology found during the acute drug use that there have been few planned experimental studies of the continued use and long-term effect of these drugs. Prospective studies such as those of McGlothlin, Arnold, and Freedman (1967) and Shagass and Bittle (1967) looked at the effects of single doses of LSD.

The ethical limitations of studying a drug that may have deleterious long-terms consequences requires investigators to look at populations that have voluntarily participated in "recreational" use of such drugs. An example of such a study can be found in research by Welpton (1968) who used psychological testing to investigate ten long-term LSD users. He concluded that the users manifested problems of sexual identity and dependency as well as regressing easily into the production of idiosyncratic responses. Glass and Bowers (1970) presented three cases in which the psychotic patient appeared to have a clear contribution from the history of heavy use of hallucinogenic drugs. Smart and Jones (1970), using the MMPI, compared the profiles of 100 LSD users and 46 nonusers. There was a higher incidence of psychopathology among the users. Naditch (1974, 1975), using self-administered questionnaires, concluded that the use of LSD and mescaline was related to regression and negatively related to adjustment. Heaton and Victor (1976) studied the characteristics associated with psychedelic flashbacks in natural and experimental settings and they found that the test profiles associated with previous flashbacks tended to show less reality-oriented thinking. They concluded that flashbacks are possibly exacerbations of underlying psychopathology, rather than a specific reaction to the current drug use.

While these previous studies are of interest, they usually have two major drawbacks: (1) the actual drugs used and their exact chemical composition are unknown; and (2) whether or not there was preexisting psychopathology is also unknown. In a number of the studies, comparable samples of nondrug users are not used when clinical patients have been studied, or only those people that have remained relatively well functioning have been studied.

Aware of these shortcomings and paying some specific attention to the variety and length of drug use, we attempted to examine the possible differences in thinking in a group of drug-using patients and comparable group of non-drug-using psychiatric patients. A detailed account of this research, which was conducted in collaboration with Dr. Gary Tucker, can be found in a separate report of ours (Tucker, Quinlan, and Harrow, 1972).

Four different groups of patients were identified for this study: (1) sixteen schizophrenic patients with a reliable history of heavy drug use; (2) twenty-eight schizophrenic patients without drug use and a reliable history; (3) fourteen nonschizophrenic patients with reliably reported heavy drug use (most diagnosed as having personality disorders); and (4) twenty-one nonschizophrenic patients without drug use (most diagnosed as having personality disorders). For this sample of patients, we obtained Rorschach protocols and used the system of analysis of thought pathology reported elsewhere in this book, which is outlined in greater detail in a comprehensive manual (Quinlan, Harrow, and Carlson, 1973). A number of questions could be addressed using these four groups:

1. Is there a similarity in thinking of nonschizophrenic patients with heavy drug use and schizophrenic patients with and without drug use?

2. Does the thinking of schizophrenic patients with heavy drug use show any similarity or difference from schizophrenic patients without drug use?
3. Are there any specific signs of disordered thinking that might be attributable to drug use alone, independent of diagnosis?
4. What could be the relationship between the length and variety of drug use and signs of changes in thinking as measured by the Rorschach. While these groups of patients show some of the same kinds of difficulties as found in any self-selected group of individuals, they nonetheless represent those groups of patients practitioners must deal with on a day-to-day basis in psychiatric practice.

PLAN OF STUDY

The four groups of patients described above were drawn from the consecutive admissions to the Yale-New Haven Hospital used as part of the overall study described in Chapter 2. The ages and sex composition of the groups are presented in Table 13.1. There tended to be more male drug users and female nondrug users, although generally, there are no significant within-group sex differences on the variables we describe below. The samples tend to be relatively young, ranging in mean age from eighteen to twenty-four. There were no significant correlations of measures with age.

We devised scales for this particular study to describe the relative frequency of drug use for both the length and quantity as follows: (1) for the length of use, one equals zero to six months, 2 equals six months to a year, 3 equals one to two years, 4 equals more than two years; (2) intensity of the drug use (hallucinogens: LSD, DMT, STP and so on) was scored as follows: 1 equals no hallucinogenic drug use, 2 equals one to four trips, 3 equals five to ten trips, 4 equals ten to twenty, and 5 equals more than twenty trips; (3) frequency of marijuana use: 1 equals rare; 2 equals monthly; 3 equals weekly; 4 equals daily use for one to two week periods; (4) frequency of amphetamine use—same scale as for marijuana, (5) use of other mind-altering drugs (glue sniffing, heroin, etc.). The length-of-use scale described first was applied separately to the hallucinogens, marijuana use, amphetamine use, and other drug use. The total score for the use of combined hallucinogens, marijuana, and amphetamines was derived as well. Table 13.1 also

TABLE 13.1
Drug Use

	Drug Users		Nondrug Users	
	Schizophrenic patients (N = 16)	Nonschizophrenic patients (N = 14)	Schizophrenic patients (N = 28)	Nonschizophrenic patients (N = 21)
Age (median year)	20	18	20	24
Men	13	10	8	4
Women	3	4	20	17
Hallucinogens[1] (mean use)	3.8	4.2	0	0
Length of hallucinogen use[2]	2.6	2.3	0	0
Marijuana[3] (mean use)	3.5	3.1	0	0
Length of marijuana use[2]	2.5	2.6	0	0
Amphetamines[3] (mean use)	2.3	2.3	0	0
Length of amphetamine use[2]	2.5	2.6	0	0

[1] 1 = no use; 2 = one to four trips; 3 = five to ten trips; 4 = ten to twenty trips; 5 = more than twenty trips

[2] 1 = zero to six months; 2 = six months to one year; 3 = one to two years; 4 = more than two years

[3] 1 = rare or none; 2 = monthly; 3 = weekly; 4 = daily use for one -to two week periods

From Tucker, Quinlan, & Harrow. Archives of General Psychiatry, 27, 443–447, 1972. Copyright 1972, by The American Medical Association, and reproduced by permission of the publisher.

reports the extent of drug use in the sample. Within the group of drug users there were no significant differences between the schizophrenics and the nonschizophrenics as to frequency or length of drug use.

While the drug users were able to be fairly clear about the amount of LSD-type drugs used (except those reporting very heavy use), the extent of amphetamine and marijuana use was less accurately and consistently reported. In all cases, the drug users at one time or another had used all of the substances, although in different amounts and frequencies. LSD-type drugs were the most frequently used (none of the drug-use sample used either amphetamines or marijuana exclusively). Thus, the data reported represent young people who have used primarily LSD-type drugs, although many have also used amphetamines and/or marijuana occasionally to frequently. The data on amphetamine use are somewhat less clear than for other drugs. The primary route was oral ingestion; intravenous administration was occasional except for three of the patients who had used intravenous amphetamines on a regular basis for intermittent periods. Consequently, the dosage, route of administration, and drug-combination effects may influence the findings in an unknown way and will be considered further later on.

As with the other samples using the Rorschach, the test was given during the first week and a half after admission. As we have noted, protocols were scored using the scales reported elsewhere for signs of disordered thinking on the Rorschach. We chose for a specific examination the ratings of verbalization, thought quality, affective elaboration, and overspecificity, along with boundary responses including contaminations, barrier, and penetration, and ratings of primitive- and socialized-drive content.

Patients were selected for this portion of the study on the basis of a clear schizophrenic diagnosis or a clear nonpsychotic diagnosis (i.e., patients with borderline schizophrenia, psychotic depressions, or organic disorders were excluded). In addition, only those patients were selected for whom a reliable history of drug use or abstention with some substantiating information, usually from the family, was available. This was determined by the chief psychiatrist of the ward who was not aware of the test productions of the patients. Two approaches to analyzing the data were used. First, an analysis of variance of diagnosis by drug use/nonuse and, second, relationship of individual types of Rorschach reponses to type and extent of drug use.

FINDINGS—DRUG USE BY DIAGNOSIS

Number of responses

The number of Rorschach responses obtained in the drug-user groups, regardless of diagnosis, was significantly higher than in the non-drug-using groups. Although the variation in the number of responses was restricted to a degree by the procedure used in the administration, there was still a significantly greater productivity within the drug-user group. As a group, drug users, regardless of diagnosis, may (a) be more prone to use visual imagery, or (b) have greater access to visual imagery as a result of the visual imagery produced by the hallucinogenic-type drugs. In either event, the clinical picture of the presenting drug user is of greater visual imagination. When the number of responses was used as a covariate to control for productivity, only a few of the findings were affected; these will be reported.

Disturbances of formal properties and verbalizations

The mean scores for the various categories of Rorschach responses are presented in Table 13.2. On measures of quality of verbalization, two types, the Thought Quality scale and the Overspecificity scale, showed that drug users had higher scores than nonusers. However, there was a much larger difference between the schizophrenic groups' mean and that of the nonschizophrenic groups. The effects of drug use and schizophrenic diagnosis were both in the same direction. For both drug use and the diagnosis of schizophrenia, patients produced more occurrences of bizarre idiosyncratic responses or reponses representing overly personalized elaborations. Affective Elaboration, describing the response in affective terms, was not different for the groups. The exact nature of the cause of these differences is somewhat unclear; the particular language of the drug-using subculture may be a possible result of the frequency of drug use or a culture artifact of the drug subculture. If the level of productivity is covaried, the differences between drug-using and non-drug-using patients fall below the level of significance. The differences between diagnostic groups, however, remain statistically significant.

TABLE 13.2

Mean Scores for Rorschach Variables by Diagnosis and Hallucinogen Use Analysis of Variance (df = 1,75) and Covariance (df = 1,74)

	Means				Correlation with Responses (R)	Analysis of Variance (Analyses of Covariance in Parentheses)		
	Drug Users		Nonusers			Drug Use	Diagnosis	Interaction
	Schizophrenic	Nonschizophrenic	Schizophrenic	Non-schizophrenic				
A. Responses (R)	27.86	24.50	21.21	21.24		13.23**	1.51	1.55
B. Verbalization								
Thought Quality	31.94	16.79	25.71	7.71	.41**	4.77** (0.65)	22.40** (20.55**)	0.17 (0.86)
Affect Elaboration	2.88	5.00	3.00	3.19	.12	0.54	1.01	0.71
Overspecificity	25.12	17.50	20.21	9.04	.43**	6.71** (1.40)	13.27** (11.40**)	0.47 (1.54)
C. Boundary Diffusion								
Fabulized Combinations	2.75	1.43	2.18	0.67	.13	2.12	9.58**	0.04
Contamination Tendencies	2.00	0.79	0.96	0.28	.30*	4.64* (1.74)	7.09** (5.83**)	0.56 (0.25)
Full Contamination	0.81	0.14	0.50	0.05	.10	1.59	12.04**	0.45
Penetration	5.25	3.14	2.71	2.52	.31**	9.00** (4.96*)	4.77* (3.91)	3.32 (2.60)
D. Drive								
Socialized Drive (Level 2)								
Sum Level 2	6.31	4.86	5.82	4.52	.25*	0.27	2.98	0.01
Aggression 2	3.62	3.14	3.79	2.29	.27*	0.35	2.81	0.74
Sex 2	1.12	0.50	0.68	0.62	.02	0.74	1.49	1.02
Oral 2	1.50	0.71	1.36	1.38	.11	0.75	1.59	0.11
Primitive Drive (Level 1)								
Sum Level 1	2.69	1.14	1.25	0.43	.24*	8.90** (5.95*)	10.76** (9.79**)	1.05 (0.77)
Aggression 1	1.31	1.00	0.86	0.33	.16	4.46*	2.48	0.16
Sex 1	1.06	0.00	0.39	0.05	.36**	1.74	8.98**	2.32
Oral 1	0.38	0.07	0.00	0.05	.02	4.72*	1.94	3.66

*p < .05.
**p < .01.

From Tucker, Quinlan, & Harrow. *Archives of General Psychiatry*, 27, 443–447, 1972. Copyright 1972, by The American Medical Association, and reproduced by permission of the publisher.

Drive content

Drive-dominated content refers to those responses with references to agressive, sexual, oral, or other types of drive-related material. In Chapter 6, our research on drive-dominated content was described. In this research, reported in Chapter 6, we had found a nonsignificant tendency toward higher levels of drive content in schizophrenics, with more agressive drive-dominated thinking being found in patients with behavior that violated social rules. Within the current samples, when drive content was divided into "socialized" and "primitive" types, drug users were not significantly higher on socialized-drive content, but the appearance of "primitive" or more blatant drive content was significantly more frequent in drug users. Within types of drive content, the drug-using groups showed a greater frequency of primitive aggressive and oral responses, but not sexual responses. Schizophrenics showed a greater overall incidence of primitive drive, but the only significant difference in type of drive content was for primitive sexual reponses. Thus, there was an increase in the level of primitive-drive content for both drug use and schizophrenia, but the differences occurred on different types of drive-dominated content. Partialling out the effects of productivity did not change the significance of the findings.

Boundary measures

The measures of boundary properties and boundary disturbances produced a number of significant findings. All of the measures suggestive of boundary problems, including penetration, fabulized combinations, contamination tendencies and full contamination, were significantly higher in the schizophrenic groups. Within the drug users, there was a tendency for contamination tendencies to be significantly higher, although this disappeared when the number of responses was covaried. Penetration responses, not necessarily a sign of pathology, were significantly higher in the drug-use groups even after adjusting for number of responses. Drug users tended to have a somewhat higher level of responses suggestive of boundary permeability, but these responses came from the less pathological end of the boundary-diffusion measures (see Chapter 9).

Correlations within drug users

Reliable information on the frequency of hallucinogenic LSD use was available for twenty-nine of thirty drug-using patients. In Table

13.3, we present the correlations of the amount and length of use in these patients with the Rorschach scores. There were no significant relationships between the Rorschach variables and the amount of use (i.e., the intensity and frequency over a fixed period). When the length of drug use was examined, however, a number of significant correlations were found. Length of use correlated positively with the verbalization scores, i.e., patients using drugs for longer periods of time tended to produce more bizarre, peculiar, and idiosyncratic verbalizations and tended to elaborate to a greater extent in overly specific terms. However, the patients using drugs for a longer period of time tended to elaborate in affective terms less than the shorter-term drug-using patients. The variable showing the strongest correlation with the length of drug use was the presence of contamination responses (a weighted sum), which yielded a highly significant correlation. In general, patients with a longer history of drug use showed higher degrees of thought disturbance.

Overall, the major element appears to be the length of drug use. Thus, if one looks at the relative frequency of use over a fixed period of time, or if one looks at the frequency times the length of drug use, no significant results are obtained. Examination of the trends within marijuana and amphetamine use shows similar relationships, but there were too few patients that reported significantly heavy use of these

TABLE 13.3
Correlations of Hallucinogenic Drug Use (LSD) with Rorschach Variables

Variable	Amount of Use		Length of Use		Total Drug Use	
	r	(N)	r	(N)	r	(N)
Responses	.13	(29)	.02	(29)	−.08	(29)
Thought quality	.21	(29)	.38**	(29)	.09	(29)
Affect elaboration	−.09	(29)	−.32*	(29)	−.08	(29)
Overspecificity	.22	(29)	.35*	(29)	.12	(29)
Primitive drive	.10	(29)	.22	(29)	.01	(29)
Primitive Aggression	−.03	(29)	.16	(29)	−.02	(29)
Penetration	.19	(29)	.10	(29)	.06	(29)
Contaminations	.21	(29)	.58***	(29)	.16	(20)

*$P < .10$.
**$P < .05$.
***$P < .01$.

From Tucker, Quinlan and Harrow. *Archives of General Psychiatry, 27,* 443–447, 1972. Copyright 1972, by The American Medical Association, and reproduced by permission of the publisher.

drugs to provide reliable information. In addition, the reduced accuracy of the reports of these substances made interpretation of such data more doubtful.

Relations with demographic variables

We reexamined those variables producing significant main effects or significant correlations, to see whether age, sex, or amount of education could explain the differences obtained. While younger subjects were found to have used drugs for a shorter period of time ($r = .46$; $P < .05$), age had no relationship to the amount of drug use, either of hallucinogens or of all drugs combined. Patients with longer education tended to have used drugs for a shorter period of time ($P < .10$). An analysis of variance, including the sex of the patient as a third factor, yielded no significant interactions between sex of patient and drug use. None of the variables for which significant correlations were found could be accounted for solely in terms of age, sex, or amount of education. Thus, the findings reported in the tables do not appear to be due to differences in the demographic characteristics of these patients.

IMPLICATIONS AND LIMITATIONS

The data appear to indicate that drug-using patients, independent of a schizophrenic or nonschizophrenic diagnosis, show clear differences from nondrug users. They tend to respond more freely when presented with a visual associative task such as the Rorschach. Their verbalizations responding to that task show more evidence of unusual and peculiar thinking, and of overly specific or overly personalized elaborations, although, to some degree, those differences can be accounted for in terms of the overall productivity. Drug users also tended to present reponses with more primitve-drive content and their responses more frequently contain primitive aggression or primitive oral content. They tended to have responses that had indications of boundary diffusion (i.e., penetration), but these were responses at a lower level of boundary disruption and pathology. When one accounts for the increased level of productivity in drug users, one does not find a strikingly greater incidence of areas of disturbed thinking but one does find more primitive content and some greater diffusion of boundaries.

In comparison to variable results for drug use, the differences between schizophrenic and nonschizophrenic patients, when stratified for drug use, appear to be clear and consistent. These schizophrenics are higher than nonschizophrenics on most of those variables associated with increased pathology and these differences are not reduced by accounting for differences in productivity. The differences between schizophrenics and others appear to be strongest on the most pathological indicators. Perhaps the strongest finding from this analysis is that the differences between schizophrenics and nonschizophrenics cannot be accounted for by differential rates of drug use.

An interesting feature of the data is that it is the length of drug use and not the intensity that correlates most with signs of changed thinking. This fact raises the possibility that it may be the length of time of exposure to either the forms of thinking induced by the hallucinogenic drug or the subcultural milieu associated with drug taking that produces the changes in the patterns of thinking, rather than the pharmacological intensity and extent of the drug use itself. The results from this and other data must be interpreted with care. The current research, as in most studies on this topic, presents data from people who have used hallucinogenic drugs on a self-selected basis. Many of the differences found in this study may be characteristic of the group of people who become attracted to, or tend to seek out, the use of drugs rather than the effect of the drugs themselves. The data might also reflect a selection factor operating in the opposite direction: people who are more constricted and are less likely to be able to tolerate unrealistic experiences may be less likely to use hallucinogenic drugs, even though they may otherwise become disorganized and require hospitalization. In a study of hallucinogen use among adult members of labor unions, Khavari, Mabry and Humes (1977) found that the use of psychedelics was associated with a person's need to seek out new and often unconventional experiences. The findings with current data, that drug users are most responsive to visual associative stimuli and they tend to produce more responses with primitive-drive content, are consistent with the hypothesis that drug users are more likely to seek out novel forms of stimulation and to be more responsive to the stimulation. Thus, even within a population with a considerable level of psychopathology, there may be preexisting differences in terms of the tendency to seek out unusual experiences that account for the differences in final presentation of pathology. It should be noted, however, that the differences found between those areas are not those that most significantly differentiated schizophrenics from nonschizophrenics.

The presence of a greater amount of primitive oral and aggressive drive in the protocols of drug users is interesting. It is not simply that drug users are more open to unconventional expression of normally taboo drive-related topics. First of all, these differences are not found in the more conventional socialized expressions of drive that are normally unusual, if not unacceptable. Second, in the area of sexual drive content, schizophrenics were higher than nonschizophrenics but there was no difference between the drug users and nondrug users. Blacker and others (1968) and Glass and Bowers (1970) described a sense of passivity in their drug-using patients. In the current study, drug use was negatively related to the appearance of affectively elaborated response in the Rorschach and was also accompanied by more primitive oral responses which have been interpreted by some as an indication of passive wishes. Yet, in another sense, the drug users were more active; they were more responsive and they showed more primitive aggressive content, although these latter do not necessarily imply activity. It may be that the passivity at times described in drug users is an openness to a broader variety of stimuli, including those that are not necessarily reality oriented.

Any discussion of the use of hallucinogenic drugs must deal with the complex set of interactions of predisposing factors and the complexity and multiple varieties of drugs, purities, dosages, and means of administration, as well as the complex subculture patterns associated with drug use. Drug use alone may produce some of the changes that we have noted in our patients. It is also possible that drug users who become more familiar with unrealistic forms of thinking while under the influence of the drug persist in using this type of thinking during drug-free periods.

Drug users also may be susceptible to the suggestions and social expectations of a deviant subculture. It is conceivable that such subcultures could give rise to unrealistic patterns of thinking, not as an expression of the direct consequeces of the drugs, but rather in relation to the underlying patterns of the subculture.

Perspective and the use of hallucinogenic drugs

The above discussion on the possible influences of the youth subculture, which in some cases is involved in drug-taking, suggests the possible influence of subcultures on perspective taking. It is possible that the changes in observed thinking were influenced by a change in the perspective of the general other in the direction of a deviant subculture. Frequent and prolonged exposure to a milieu that does not respond to aspects of disordered thinking as if they were signs of pathology may significantly alter the perspective of the general other toward a looser, more lenient audience. As different as this subcultural standard is, however, it does not come close to matching the extreme loss of perspective we often see in schizophrenia, although it may exacerbate the effects.

POSITIVE THOUGHT DISORDER: IMPORTANCE OF SCHIZOPRENIA VERSUS DRUG USE

The data from our research have addressed the issue from the viewpoint of the clinician who must deal with presenting symptoms of patients' arriving for hospitalization. It is difficult to come to any firm conclusions about the origins of differences in thought disorder between drug users and nonusers, concerning whether these differences have been produced by drug use alone, or whether patients with a tendency toward thought disorder tend to use drugs such as LSD, and thus self-select themselves. It is perhaps helpful to note that the changes found to be associated with prolonged drug use are not completely identical with the differences found between schizophrenics and nonschizophrenics. There were no interactions between diagnosis and drug-use status. Thus, the schizophrenics who used drugs showed the same difference from schizophrenics who did not use drugs as the nonschizophrenic counterparts showed. Moreover, the more significant indicators of thought pathology associated most strongly with schizophrenics are not those that tend to differentiate drug users from nonusers within the diagnosis.

Patients who have used psychedelic drugs, particularly LSD, do show differences in terms of changes in their patterns of thinking. While these patterns do have some similarities to changes found in the differences between schizophrenics and nonschizophrenics, they are by no means identical to them. The data suggest that the *lasting* effects of hallucinogenic-drug use, such as LSD use, are only similar in a very few ways to the changes found in schizophrenia. As we have noted elsewhere, in relation to acute psychotic states, our own clinical observations have suggested that psychotic states associated with amphetamine use are much closer in appearance to schizophrenia, and at times are perhaps indistinguishable from schizophrenia.

Studies in both patients and nonpatients, preferably with some kind of pre-drug measure of patterns of thinking and personality, may serve to shed some light on the degree to which self-selection, subcultural influences, and direct influences of the drugs may change the thinking patterns of people using psychedelic drugs. It would also be of interest to follow whether or not other types of experiences associated with other forms of "altered states of consciousness" (e.g., medication) have similar or different effects on the prevailing thought patterns of people subsequent to such experiences.

Some tentative suggestions are made by these data that the prolonged use of LSD and other hallucinogens by nonschizophrenics could serve to heighten changes of thinking that are suggestive of pathological disturbances, but these are similar only to a limited extent to the changes found in schizophrenics.

14

Disordered Thinking in the Families of Schizophrenic Patients*

A meeting took place between a patient, her mother and father, the patient's therapist, and the family's social worker. The patient had recently been in a catatonic state, and was being evaluated for continuing epilepsy. Her tested intelligence was in the Dull-Normal range.

> *Mother*: Can [*the patient*] get out of here by August [*in one month*]?
>
> *Social Worker*: Why do you ask?
>
> *Mother*: We'll need time to find a college for her.
>
> *Patient*: I don't want to go to college.
>
> *Father*: You need something to keep you busy.
>
> *Mother*: Your sister would like you with her.

The patient lapsed momentarily into a blank stare and replied, "I feel my wires are being plugged in."

*We were joined in the studies of families by K. David Schultz and Robert Davies, and select aspects of our research in this area are described in greater detail in a recent report of ours (Quinlan, Schultz, Davies, and Harrow, 1978).

Clinicians working with families of seriously disturbed psychiatric patients report repeated incidents such as the above. Defending against the recognition of their children's pathology, parents try to emphasize restoration to health. After initial protests by the patients, and then recognition that their own problems are being discounted, patients sometimes affirm their need for help with the reoccurrence of symptoms. Many clinicians and research workers have focused on the communication value of the symptoms. In this chapter we will look at a different aspect of such exchanges; do children with severely disturbed thinking come from families with severely distorted patterns of thinking?

Clinical experience and family-oriented research are generally consistent in reporting a higher level of disordered thinking in the families of schizophrenic patients, but the nature of the connection is in doubt: first, there may be a hereditary component of vulnerability to disordered thinking that is passed on to children; second, there may be an influence in the early rearing of the child that reflects the psychopathology of the parents that is transmitted through early experiences to the child; third, the family of the patient may have developed defective and pathogenic means of communication that produce distorted thinking in their offspring over the course of the child's development (not only in early infancy); and fourth, the disruption in the thinking processes of the patient, and disturbed behavior by the patient, may produce stress, conflict, and ambiguity for the immediate family. This latter situation may result in distorted thinking in family members in response to the disrupted and disruptive communication and behavior by the patient.

EARLY CHILDHOOD EXPERIENCE

A longstanding hypothesis about the etiology of schizophrenia has been that early parent-child experiences, especially mother-child interactions, lay the groundwork for subsequent health or pathology. Mahler (1968), for example, focuses on the earliest infantile experiences around individuation, the sense of being a separate individual, and its subsequent effects on development. In order for a satisfactory sense of the self as a separate individual, it is felt that sufficient satisfaction of needs must occur in the earliest stages of fusion and symbiosis, i.e. stage before the infant can experience separation. Blatt and Wild (1976) form a more specific hypothesis, that the infant destined to become schizophrenic fails to establish, firmly and securely, the sense of boundary between the self and the mother, with subsequent disturbances in self-other boundaries appearing in different forms at later stages of life. In Chapter 9 we reported in greater detail data that bear on some of these boundary hypotheses.

Over the years, studies of the possible role of the family in transmitting communication disorders to their offspring have encountered difficult conceptual and methodological problems (Garmezy, 1974; Keith, Gunderson, Reifman, Buchsbaum, and Mosher, 1976). Despite the potential problems, substantive research on the possible role of the family in transmitting communication or thinking disorders has been conducted by Wynne and Singer, by Lidz and Fleck, by M. Goldstein and colleagues, and by a number of other investigators (Goldstein, Rodnick, Jones, McPherson, and West, 1978; Lidz, 1973; Wynne, Singer, Bartko and Toohey, 1977). Lidz, Cornelison, Fleck, and Terry (1958) called attention to the quality of thinking and communication within the families of schizophrenics. Thinking was frequently distorted; communication proceeded along irrational but mutually understood avenues. Distorted thinking and communication were also observed in the marital relationships of the parents (Lidz, Fleck, Alanen, and Cornelison, 1963). In view of the hypothesis of a "schizophrenogenic mother," the finding of distorted and irrational thinking in the fathers of schizophrenic patients points to a more general hypothesis, that disordered styles of thinking and communication are transmitted via the family environment from parents to children. Lidz and others (1958) suggest that the patient becomes prone to withdrawal by means of altering internal representations of reality because the within-family communications have distorted or denied valid interpretations of the enviroment (p. 314).

Operational measures of distorted communications within individual family members have been developed, using projective techniques such as the Rorschach, by Wynne and Singer (1963a, 1963b; Singer and Wyne, 1965a, 1965b). Disturbed modes of thinking in family members, parents and siblings, parallel the thought disturbances found in the patient offspring/siblings. Two hypotheses follow from such studies: (1) that family transactional styles are related to cognitive development in the offspring; distortion, invalidation, and denial of affect impair the establishment of a stable and validatable view of the world; and (2) the disturbed interpersonal relationships are also reflected in disordered thinking in the patients and family members at the time of acute psychological illness; families with a disturbed pattern of functioning will also show disturbances in the thinking of individual members outside of immediate family interactions. In this approach, the communication patterns come from and persist beyond the immediate parent-child interactions.

An alternate set of hypotheses have been proposed by Mishler, Waxler, and others; the degree of disturbance found in the family members is a reaction to, rather than a cause of, the disturbance in the offspring-patient (Mishler and Waxler, 1968a, 1968b; Waxler, 1974). Waxler (1974) constructed "artificial families" of normal and schizophrenic parents with normal and schizophrenic patient offspring. Liem (1974) pointed out a limitation of such designs: that disordered communication may be highly specific and idiosyncratic to particular family constellations. Using families with schizophrenic sons with poor premorbid histories in a VA hospital, and normal families with nonpatient sons of comparable demographic background matched on relevant demographic variables, Liem found consistent differences between patients and nonpatients on communication variables in children, but not in their parents. Sons were no different in response to patient-parent and normal-parent communications, but normal and patient parents both made significantly better identifications through communications of normal sons versus patient sons. Parents of schizophrenic sons made more errors in responding to their children's responses, and fewest in response to normal children's responses. Normal and schizophrenic sons were not differentially affected by communications of parents of normal children versus parents of schizophrenics. Liem's conclusion was that parents learn peculiar communication in response to their offspring

A different hypothesis is offered by Rosenthal, Wender, Kety, Schulsinger, Welnar, and Rieder (1975), that there is genetic transmission of psychopathology. Their study examined subjects who were (a) adoptees with a maternal parent, with or without mental illness, (b) adoptees with normal parents but with abnormal adopting parents, and (c) nonadopted children with natural parents with schizophrenic or manic-depressive illness. Extensive ratings were obtained from retrospective-interview descriptions of parent-child relationships, and separate independent ratings were made of psychological disorder in the offspring. There was a stronger association between natural parents and offspring psychopathology than between the quality of rearing-parent relationship and offspring pathology. The rearing-parent-child relationship was associated to a small but significant degree with pathology, but accounted for a median of 6 percent of the covariance. Greater incidence of pathology in genetic offspring of pathological parents than of nonpathological parents was found. Children of pathological parents, whether or not they were raised by those parents, had a higher incidence of psychopathology. Thus, genetic factors were clearly implicated in the pathology of the offspring. It should be noted, however, that neither parental environment nor genetic contribution accounted for more than a small portion of the total variance of psychopathology.

FAMILY COMMUNICATION AND IMPAIRED PERSPECTIVE

It is possible that the role of families may be of particular importance in understanding the children's development of adequate perspective about what types of thinking and behaviors are socially appropriate. Usually, the individual initially learns about societal expectations of appropriate behavior and speech from his parents and other family members. The child learns not only what is "right" and expected, but also what is odd, peculiar, and unexpected. A child growing up in an environment with unusual, vague, or distorted communication faces a larger task in learning what is generally socially appropriate. Other influences, to be sure, are found in school, peers, and other outside contacts. Adolescents and young adults potentially have additional socialization about what is expected and unexpected, at times in a peer culture that is consciously different from adult culture, often involving specific types of speech, dress, and behavior. In any given instance, one or another set of influences may predominate in the shaping of the set of general expectations for speech and behavior but few influences are as universal, as early in influence, or as pervasive in potential effect as the influence of one's family. It is logical to look at the occurrence of bizarre-idiosyncratic thinking in the immediate family of patients who experience difficulty in monitoring their speech and behavior from the perspective of a general "other."

ISSUES IN ASSESSING DISORDERED THINKING IN PATIENTS AND FAMILIES

One issue in the assessment of familial similarity of disordered thinking is: What sample of thinking does one obtain? Singer and Wynne's research successfully demonstrated familial similarities using the Rorschach, an open-ended unstructured technique. Wild and her colleagues (Wild, Singer, Rosman, Ricci, and Lidz, 1965) carried over the concept of "transactional thinking," or the disturbance of attention and blurring of meaning, to the Object Sorting test. The Object Sorting test is suggested for study not only for scoring transactional thinking, but also for scores on overinclusion, discussed in Chapters 3 through 5, and 10. Another technique we had previously used with success in discriminating schizophrenic patients from others was the score for bizarre-idiosyncratic thinking derived from a subject's responses to the WAIS Social Comprehension subtest. Inclusion of the WAIS Comprehension items allowed evaluation of whether "generalized decrement" could account for group differences, and allowed for a comparison of two different measures of positive thought disorder.

Comparison of schizophrenic patients and their parents with nonschizophrenic patients and their parents allowed us to ask a number of questions:

1. Are transactional thinking, overinclusion, and other aspects of distorted communication unique to schizophrenics or schizophrenics and their families, or does some degree of these indices occur around acute disturbances in other disorders?
2. Is there a similarity between the distortions of thinking of the offspring and those of one or both of the parents?
3. Are schizophrenic patients and their parents higher on indices of transactional thinking, overinclusion, and other aspects of disordered thinking in comparison to disturbed nonschizophrenic patients and their parents?
4. Do one or the other measures of disordered thinking present clearer evidence of discriminating schizophrenics from nonschizophrenics and/or reveal greater similarity of offspring and one or both parents?

METHOD

Patient Sample

The patients studied were twenty acute schizophrenic patients and their parents, and twenty acute nonschizophrenic patients and their parents admitted to the psychiatric inpatient services of two New

Haven–area hospitals. In three instances in the nonschizophrenic group and in one instance in the schizophrenic group the father was deceased or was divorced from the wife prior to the patient's hospitalization. Only one family approached refused to participate. Major characteristics of the schizophrenic and nonschizophrenic patients and their families are outlined in Table 14.1

Demographic characteristics

The schizophrenic patients and families and the nonschizophrenic patients and families were matched with regard to age and education. There were ten males and ten female schizophrenic patients and eleven male and nine female nonschizophernic patients. All schizophrenic patients met or exceeded the NHSI criterion score for a diagnosis of schizophrenia and none of the nonschizophrenic patients exceeded this criterion.

Measures of Transactional Thinking and of Cognition

Each patient and his or her parents were tested separately and asked not to discuss the test until all family members were tested. Each family member was given a six-item set of items from the WAIS Comprehension test to induce a test-taking context for the Object Sorting test and to provide an independent assessment of bizarre-idiosyncratic thinking or positive thought disorder on a different measure. The Object Sorting test was then presented according to standard instruc-

TABLE 14.1
Characteristics of Sample Studied

Category	Schizophrenic Patients			Nonschizophrenic Patients		
	Patient	Father	Mother	Patient	Father	Mother
No. of Ss	20	20	20	20	17	20
Sex: Females	10			9		
Males	10			11		
Mean age (yrs.)	18.3	47.5	45.4	17.3	49 8	45.9
Mean education level (yrs.)	12.1	13.9	13.1	11.3	14.3	13.6

From Quinlan, Schultz, Davies, and Harrow. *Journal of Personality Assessment, 42,* 401–408, 1978. Reproduced by permission of the publisher.

tions. Verbal responses were recorded on tape and later transcribed. Object Sorting responses were scored for:

a. *transactional thinking disorder,* including scores for fragmentation of attention, inability to maintain the role of a subject, blurring of meaning, and pathological thought or language; scoring was according to a manual developed by Wild (1972);
b. *behavioral overinclusion,* or total number of objects sorted
c. *conceptual overinclusion,* or the tendency to include conceptual elements not essential or irrelevant (see Chapter 10);
d. *bizarre-idiosyncratic thinking* (scored on both the OST and the Comprehension subtest);
e. *richness of associations* (a positive aspect of OST responses);
f. *concreteness;* and
g. *underinclusion,* including failure to sort objects, incomplete sortings, and repeated use of the same categorizing principle.

As we have noted earlier, the scoring of the OST measures is described in a separate manual by Himmelhoch, Harrow, Tucker, and Hersh (1973). Responses to the Comprehension items were scored for accuracy according to the WAIS manual, and for bizarre-idiosyncratic thinking, using a manual developed by our research group (Adler and Harrow, 1973). A revised and expanded version of this manual can be found in the appendix. Two raters scored the protocols blind to diagnosis, sex, and family position; they achieved interrater reliabilities ranging from $r = .81$ (concreteness) to $r = .99$ (transactional thinking), with a median reliability of .93. To assure comparability of these ratings with the Wild scoring system, one of the raters scored twelve cases from Wild and colleagues' (1968) data; a reliability of $r = .87$ with Wild's scoring was found.

Sex differences on Measures of Transactional Thinking and Cognition

Before combining across sexes, male and female patient offspring were compared on the various measures in a sex-by-diagnosis design. Only one difference was found: females showed more bizarre responses, and no significant interactions occurred. This number of significant findings could have been expected by chance. Since females were slightly higher than males on some measures of disturbed thinking and lower on others, the two sexes were combined for further analyses.

Diagnostic Differences

The means scores for offspring, mother, and father are presented in Table 14.2, and the analyses of variance for family groups are presented in Table 14.3. Analyses of covariance in Table 14.2 partialled out effects of age and education (the analyses without the covariation procedure are quite similar).

Overall diagnostic differences between diagnostic groups (averaging over all three family members) are found for four variables: transactional thinking, conceptual overinclusion, and bizarre-idiosyncratic thinking on the OST and the Comprehension test. In each case, the schizophrenic patient family scores were higher than those for the nonschizophrenic patients.

A comparison sample of ten college volunteers, four females and six males, and their parents was gathered for comparison. On all measures significantly differentiating nonschizophrenic patients and families, the nonhospitalized control sample produced scores in the same direction as the nonschizophrenic group. No significant differences between the nonschizophrenic and nonpatient groups were found. Thus, the schizophrenic scores are significantly more pathological than nonschizophrenic scores, and these are in the direction of being more disordered than nonpatient scores.

Family member differences

A surprising result occurred in the comparison of family members for degrees of disturbed thinking, namely, that only one significant difference occurred: parents tended to be *more* underinclusive in their sorts than their offspring. On one measure, transactional thinking, parents tend to score higher than offspring, while on bizarre thinking, patient offspring score at a more pathological level than that of their parents. Over an assortment of different measures of disordered thinking, parents are at the same level as their children, even though only the children are currently defined as patients.

The comparisons of patient children, mothers, and fathers separately across diagnostic groups support the overall picture: on three of the four measures that are significantly different across diagnostic group, the comparisons for patient children only are also significant—conceptual overinclusion is the exception is *not* differentiating between patient groups. On two of the four measures showing overall differences, the schizophrenics' mothers and fathers *also* show significantly more pathological scores, although on different measures. Thus, the

TABLE 14.2
Comparison of Samples on the Thinking Disorder Variables
Analysis of Covariance, Age and Education Partialled Out

Variable	1 Schiz. Mean	2 Nonschiz. Mean	Analysis of Variance Comparisons Schiz. versus Nonschiz. $F^1(1, 36)$
Transactional thinking			
Child	4.25	1.90	5.28[2]
Father	5.55	3.71	2.74
Mother	5.50	2.75	4.59[2]
Behavioral overinclusion			
Child	47.60	40.10	0.21
Father	39.35	32.24	2.64
Mother	47.60	33.15	3.85[3]
Conceptual overinclusion			
Child	3.05	2.25	2.46
Father	3.65	2.65	5.97[2]
Mother	3.45	2.65	5.06[2]
Richness of association			
Child	1.65	1.75	0.02
Father	1.60	1.59	0.02
Mother	1.40	1.20	1.03
Bizarre thinking (OST)			
Child	2.30	1.60	4.20[2]
Father	2.90	2.24	2.86
Mother	2.95	2.00	5.82[2]
Concreteness			
Child	2.85	2.50	1.07
Father	2.95	2.71	0.22
Mother	3.40	2.75	3.82[3]
Conceptual Underinclusion			
Child	1.50	1.35	0.30
Father	1.65	1.94	1.90
Mother	1.70	1.65	0.02
Bizarre thinking (Comprehension test)			
Child	5.45	2.90	11.63[4]
Father	4.30	2.88	4.91[2]
Mother	3.75	2.80	1.45

[1]*df* = 1,33 for fathers' comparison
[2]$P < .05$.
[3]$P < .10$.
[4]$P < .01$.

TABLE 14.3
Analysis of Variance of Thinking Disorder Variables
Diagnosis by Family Member

Variable		MS	F[1]
Transactional thinking	Diagnosis (D)	137.98	6.19[2]
	Family member (F)	24.40	3.00
	D × F	1.10	0.14
	MS error	22.29	
	MS error, F, D × F	8.13	
Behavioral overinclusion	Diagnosis (D)	2334.81	2.46
	Family member (F)	761.15	0.96
	D × F	243.85	0.31
	MS error	950.87	
	MS error, F, D × F	796.70	
Conceptual overinclusion	Diagnosis (D)	16.58	9.11[3]
	Family member (F)	2.39	1.56
	D × F	0.37	0.24
	MS error	1.82	
	MS error, F, D × F	1.53	
Richness of association	Diagnosis (D)	0.17	0.22
	Family member (F)	1.81	2.11
	D × F	0.29	0.34
	MS error	0.79	
	MS error, F, D × F	0.86	
Bizarre thinking	Diagnosis (D)	14.94	9.48[3]
	Family member (F)	3.91	2.64
	D × F	0.17	0.11
	MS error	1.58	
	MS error, F, D × F	1.48	
Concreteness	Diagnosis (D)	3.21	1.59
	Family member (F)	1.34	1.24
	D × F	0.38	0.35
	MS error	2.02	
	MS error, F, D × F	1.08	
Underinclusion	Diagnosis (D)	0.00	0.00
	Family member (F)	1.53	3.83[2]
	D × F	0.60	1.49
	MS error	0.92	
	MS error, F, D × F	0.40	
Bizarre thinking	Diagnosis (D)	86.81	13.30[4]
(Comprehension test)	Family member (F)	7.60	1.46
	D × F	6.63	1.28
	MS error	6.53	
	MS error, F, D × F	5.20	

[1]For diagnosis $df = 1,35$, and for Family Member and Diagnosis by Family Member, $df = 2,70$. Families with father absent were deleted from this analysis.
[2]$P < .05$.
[3]$P < .01$.
[4]$P < .001$.

parents of schizophrenic offspring show higher levels of disordered thinking than parents of nonschizophrenic offspring.

Several measures fail to show significant differences between groups: behavioral overinclusion, richness of association, underinclusion, and concreteness. The last three can be viewed as measuring variables related to richness or impoverishment of thinking, and all four of these measures can be viewed as assessing features related to the presence or absence of negative symptoms. The negative results for behavioral overinclusion replicate similar negative findings of ours with three different samples of acute patients.

Family similarities

Up to this point we have examined the overall levels of disordered thinking among patient offspring and their parents. In Table 14.4 we present the correlations between the offsprings, the mothers, and the fathers on the Object Sorting measures, also including their scores for bizarre-idiosyncratic responses. The results for the whole sample and for schizophrenics and their families alone are both presented. Transactional thinking reveals the highest degree of association among the family members. In the overall sample, all three possible correlations among the three family members are significant for transactional thinking. Of the seven remaining variables, significant correlations are found between one parent and the child; for three variables, the correlation of the child with the mother is significant while the child-father correlation is not. For one variable, bizarre-idiosyncratic responses, the child-father correlation is significant, while the child-mother correlation falls just short of significance ($r = .29$; $P < .05$, versus $r = .24$, $P < .10$). While in each case the *difference* between correlations is not significant, the overall pattern tends to point to a higher degree of association between mother and offspring as compared to father and offspring.

The correlations in the right half of Table 14.4 are for the schizophrenic patients and their parents alone. Fewer correlations reach statistical significance, but the overall pattern is generally the same as for the group as a whole. While greater differences could possibly have been obtained if the groups were larger, the similarity of correlations within the data do not lend themselves to interpretations of differences in patterns of association. One possible exception is the significant negative correlation between mothers and fathers of schizophrenics on bizarre thinking. While this is an isolated finding that needs to be interpreted cautiously, trends in this direction would be consistent for

TABLE 14.4
Correlations among Family Members, Overall and Within the Schizophrenic Group Only[1]

	Patients and Controls			Schizophrenics Only		
	Child-Father (df = 44)	Child-Mother (df = 48)	Father-Mother (df = 44)	Child-Father (df = 18)	Child-Mother (df = 18)	Father-Mother (df = 18)
Transactional thinking	.39[3]	.53[4]	.38[3]	.26	.51[2]	.37
Behavioral overinclusion			.37[3]			.29
Conceptual overinclusion		.34[2]				
Richness of association				.42		
Bizarre thinking (OST)		.44[3]			.33	-.54[2]
Concreteness		.39[3]			.61[3]	.26
Underinclusion						
Bizarre thinking (Comprehension test)	.29[2]	.24	.27	.61[3]	.41	-.27

[1] Correlations below r = .24 are deleted.
[2] p < .05.
[3] p < .01.
[4] p < .001.

the hypothesis of *skewed* family pathology, in which one parent is more pathologically disturbed while the other is more nearly normal. The absence of negative correlations between mothers and fathers of schizophrenic patients on other variables requires that we view this finding cautiously.

Implications

From a sample of acutely disturbed patients and their families, several findings stand out with our current data. First, the *level* of disturbed thinking is higher for schizophrenic families as compared to acutely disturbed nonschizophrenic patients and families. Comparisons of mothers and fathers support the general findings that: (a) disturbed thinking is higher in parents of schizophrenics than in parents of nonschizophrenic patients; and (b) parents are not significantly lower or higher than their offspring on major aspects of disordered thinking. The findings do not offer differential support for the reactive versus the transmission theories of disordered thinking. Whatever the mechanism of transmission of disordered thinking between parents and children, it is clear that the parents, who generally do not share the other positive symptoms of the acute episode, do share in the higher levels of disordered thinking.

The finding of nearly *equal* levels of disordered thinking in mothers and fathers suggests that disturbed thinking may be a pattern of the family as a whole. This finding has implications for the treatment of schizophrenic patients, namely that their families are also symptomatic, and restoring such patients to their families could be aided by treatment directed at the parents and family unit as a whole.

Differences among measures of disordered thinking

At first glance, the measures of transactional thinking and of bizarre-idiosyncratic responses would appear to be better indices of disordered thinking as a whole (i.e., they show the clearest differences between diagnostic groups of patients and their families), and as measures of similarity of thinking disorders among family members. Such a conclusion is premature, since the other measures (e.g., conceptual overinclusion) are relatively specific indices, while measures such as transactional thinking represent more global indices that include within them many varieties of disordered thinking. A more general finding suggested by the data is that the vulnerability to disordered thinking is common to members of the same family; the specific manifestations that disordered thinking take may reflect the influences of one or the other (e.g., mother) and the unique pattern of the child.

Overinclusion

The present data allow further analysis of the measures of conceptual and behavioral overinclusion examined in Chapter 10. Within patients alone, behavioral overinclusion was not significantly different for schizophrenics and nonschizophrenics (mean for schizophrenics = 47.60, for nonschizophrenics = 40.10; $F = 0.38$, ns), while for conceptual overinclusion, there was a near-significant trend (schizophrenics $\bar{x} = 3.05$; nonschizophrenics $\bar{x} = 2.25$; $F = 3.25$; $P < .10$). When family members were combined with patient offspring, conceptual overinclusion (Table 14.2) did yield significant difference between families of schizophrenics and families of nonschizophrenics, but not behavioral overinclusion. By comparison, transactional thinking and idiosyncratic response measures yielded significant differences for both patients alone and their families as a whole. In general, the results tend to support the conclusion in Chapter 10 that aspects of disordered thinking other than overinclusion are more important when studying differences between schizophrenia and other psychiatric disorders.

Perspective and monitoring and disordered thinking in families

The findings of high levels of disordered thinking in parents of schizophrenics offer several possibilities for the generation of faulty perspective and monitoring. One avenue is that of providing models of faulty perspective. If the child grows up in an environment in which faulty perspective about bizarre and idiosyncratic responses occurs, the child might model his or her thinking after the most immediate example. A second potential route for transmission of disturbance is the failure by the parents to provide feedback. If the child's initial attempts to test appropriateness of his thinking do *not* receive corrective feedback, or worse, if the child receives distorted feedback, opportunities for developing adequate perspective and monitoring may be impaired. Both mechanisms—modeling and the absence of feedback— could operate simultaneously. The modeling mechanism, however, would require that one or both parents provide faulty models (i.e., have high levels of pathology), while the absence of a feedback mechanism would require only that parents fail to respond to the child's inappropriate responses, without requiring that the parents themselves have disordered thinking.

Overview

Parents of schizophrenics show levels of disordered thinking similar to their patient offspring. The findings do not specifically differentiate among hypotheses about family/genetic transmission versus family reaction, but do indicate that the mothers and fathers of schizophrenics, as compared to the parents of other acute inpatients, show higher levels of disordered thinking. Further understanding of disordered thinking must take the potential role of familial transmission/reaction into account. Whatever the etiology of disordered thinking, treatment of patients with disordered thinking must take into account the fact that patients live in environments that often show similar patterns of distorted and disturbed thinking.

15

Disordered Thinking and Rorschach Assessment: A Factor-Analytic Approach

A patient responded to a Rorschach card with the response "my boss," "a shark." On inquiry, the examiner asked why the card looked that way; the patient replied, "It just looked that way." When locating his percepts, however, he said, "Actually, it's only my boss's sunglasses. Here is a mark the shark has made on the beach, and the shark has eaten away the rest of my boss." His responses to the Rorschach card were constructed out of two large dark circles and two long black lines, that do not remotely resemble either a face or a shark.

The Rorschach is one of the more frequently used vehicles for assessing disordered thinking. In this chapter we will bring together several techniques brought to bear on Rorschach responses. Because of this, and since we have employed it as one of several key instruments to assess thought disorder, with several earlier chapters having focused on aspects of our research with the Rorschach, a few words are in order here about various properties and characteristics of this instrument.

In the process of responding to the inkblots, which are ambiguous visual forms, the patient must locate possible visual images, assess whether the match is close enough, and then describe the image to the examiner. As such, the Rorschach lends itself as a tool for assessing bizarre thinking as well as impaired perspective about how inappropriate one's responses are in terms of the standards of the general other.

The study of the Rorschach or other inkblot techniques suffers from an inherent ambiguity: an inkblot technique is not a test in and of itself. Rather, the Rorschach and similar "projective" techniques are complex sets of behaviors elicited in a more or less standard manner. It utilizes a specific set of stimuli, a subject who is instructed implicitly or explicitly to see forms in the inkblots, and an examiner who records the verbalizations of the subject and inquires about details of the subject's responses. The Rorschach becomes a "test" when aspects of the behavior are scored and analyzed against criteria of personality or pathology. It is the scoring method that is the "test," not the technique itself. The Rorschach is regarded as an "unstructured" test. The subject's answers are not restricted to a limited list of possible answers; there are no strictly correct or incorrect answers. Nonetheless, there is a good deal of structure to the Rorschach setting. A few aspects are:

a. The subject is expected to see forms and images, and these forms are judged for their "goodness or fit" to the areas of the inkblot chosen; subjects who attribute auditory, olfactory, or gustatory characteristics engage in atypical behavior.
b. The subject must communicate his images to the examiner in understandable language.
c. The subject anticipates that some unspecified quality of his answers will be used to infer something about his personality or pathology.

The contribution of the setting and of the relationship between examiner and subject is often insufficiently appreciated. As we have noted earlier with other tests, there are some problems in comparing the responses of patients who anticipate treatment consequences to follow from their answers with the responses of nonpatient "controls" who have no reason to anticipate any serious consequences. In fact, nonpatient subjects may often interpret the Rorschach technique as an invitation to appear "creative" and deliberately embellish responses in unusual ways. For purposes of assessing the clinical utility of the Rorschach to serve as an indicator of perception, thinking, and communication, we have looked at schizophrenic and nonschizophrenic patients' responses in a clinical setting.

In considering the relationship of the setting to test answers, there is a related question: Do patients believe when responding to a test that they may gain from appearing more seriously disturbed? Within the settings of our research it was the norm that patients exhibiting psychotic behaviors were met with restrictions from privileges most patients seek out (e.g., freedom to move out of the hospital for passes). In such circumstances, it is a reasonable working assumption that the evidence of psychotic thinking occur in spite of patients' wishes to be perceived as "normal." None of the patients in our samples stood to profit for legal reasons or to gain monetary compensation from being considered pathological. While they were assured that no untoward consequences outside of treatment considerations would follow, all worked within a treatment milieu in which bizarre behavior or speech was regarded as a symptom.

PROJECTIVE AND NONPROJECTIVE USES OF THE RORSCHACH

Much of the heat of the controversy over the Rorschach arises from the "projective hypothesis"—the hypothesis that the subject projects onto ambiguous stimulus elements that reflect his preoccupations, conflicts, and defenses that are less visible in more structured situations. Many of the inferences from the Rorschach response, however, do not in fact depend on the projective hypothesis. One can instead assume that the Rorschach responses, like other behaviors, represent some consistent properties of the subject's perceiving, thinking, and communicating that tell us something about how he or she will behave in other settings. The preference for a relatively unstructured setting arises from the assumption that much of day-to-day behavior, and especially pathological distortions of behavior, arise in relatively ambiguous circumstances rather than in well-structured settings (see Wachtel, 1973). A subject's responses in a situation where there are no well-practiced or clearly perceived cues to "appropriate" behavior may possibly reflect some of the individual's tendencies to perceive other ambiguous situations in everyday life. The scoring of the Rorschach explored in this chapter and in earlier chapters attempts to look systematically at aspects of responding that can be linked theoretically and/or empirically to pathology or personality with the assumption of continuity of behaviors in different settings.

A number of systematic studies of a variety of indexes of disordered thinking have been reported. Many of the original formulations of types of responses reflecting thought disorder were developed by Rapaport, Gill, and Schafer in their classic (1946) and now revised (1968) work on diagnostic testing. A wide variety of indexes of different aspects of schizophrenic disorganization are detailed by Weiner (1966). A highly detailed and extensive scoring system extending and refining that of Rapaport and colleagues and integrating other concepts has been devised by Holt (1956, 1963, 1977; Holt and Havel, 1960), and we have utilized components of this scoring system in earlier chapters.

Previous general scoring systems of the Rorschach have tended to support the use of the Rorschach as an index of disordered thinking. Watkins and Stauffacher (1952) reported the use of the delta index, one of the first general systems, for assessing the protocols of schizophrenics and other pathological groups. The delta index weights different manifestations of disordered thinking (many derived from Rapaport and others) according to an *a priori* judgment of the degree of pathological implications on a five-point scale. The combined delta index did show discrimination among different patient groups. Powers and Hamlin (1955) used the scale to discriminate normal subjects (college students) from neurotics (outpatients), and in turn neurotics from psychotics (inpatients). Johnston and Holzman (1979) have reported a revision of this system with results discriminating schizophrenics from other patients.

The question of using the Rorschach to differentiate the various diagnoses within schizophrenia (e.g., catatonic, paranoid) was investigated by Bower, Testin, and Roberts (1960). Diverse elements were employed: form, content, and measures of "thought process." Bower and colleagues found that *within schizophrenics*, different manifestations of disordered thinking, perception, and choice of content appeared in different diagnostic subgroups and that several factors were needed to account for the various indexes of thought disorder.

One of the questions raised by these two approaches is whether disordered thinking is a single- or multidimensional construct. For the most part, these general scoring systems have considered pathology as a single dimension.

PERSPECTIVE AND RORSCHACH RESPONSES

The capacity to maintain perspective, or recognize when one's responses deviate from broad consensual standards of appropriateness, can be examined from a number of facets of the Rorschach response. One of the most basic approaches to a Rorschach response is to gauge the form accuracy of the percept. "Form accuracy" implies that areas that elicit the percept for the subject can elicit similar responses in others. "Poor" form accuracy implies that the percept cannot be readily shared by others, and often involves a private, idiosyncratic experience.

A second aspect of maintaining adequate perspective is the ability to establish boundaries between percepts, a topic already discussed in Chapter 9. Blurred, fused boundaries may be seen as an extreme in the loss of perspective of the other in one's own thinking.

Another aspect of thought-disordered responses on the Rorschach that is less emphasized in the literature is the adequacy of the patient's communication of the response to the examiner. Problems in perspective can manifest themselves in the breakdown of intelligibility of the communication. In a somewhat different way, they can become manifest in the *elaboration* of responses in an idiosyncratic fashion, which allows the patient's unique and unshared chain of associations to dominate the response.

VERBALIZATION OF DISORDERED THINKING

Much of the attention paid to scoring the Rorschach has focused on the properties of the inkblot or content of the response, such as location, determinants (color, form, etc.), barrier properties, and the like. Aspects that have received less attention have been the quality of communication and source of associations. Some of these aspects have been described by Rapaport and colleagues and utilized by Watkins and Stauffacher (1952) and Holt (1956, 1977; Holt and Havel, 1960).

The quality of the subject's verbalization in communicating his response has been classified by Rapaport into various categories, such as "peculiar," "queer," and, if quasi-logic is employed, "autistic logic." These categories form, in a general way, an ascending scale of disturbance in their varbalization. Peculiar verbalizations include unusual or inappropriate use of words, "mild" neologism (e.g., "the bird aspect of it made it look like it had wings"). Peculiar verbalizations can occur in normal or neurotic protocols (e.g., highly obsessive patients), but are assumed to be more frequent in more disturbed patients. Queer verbalizations are more severe indications of the subject's inadequate grasp of social conventions of speech. In comparison to a peculiar verbalization, "queer" verbalizations are more likely to be labeled as pathological and would not occur in casual conversation. Autistic logic, according to Rapaport and colleagues, represents a more severe disruption of the thinking process. While peculiar and queer verbalizations represent the end-products of illogical thinking, autistic logic, an even more pathological response, is the process of quasi-logical thinking presented in its clearest form. Such responses often include words that suggesting attempts to be "logical," for example, "therefore"; "because"; "it is necessary"; "it must be." An example of such autistic logic might be: "This is winter." "What made it look like winter?" "Well, because it's blue and this is December, so it had to be winter."

For our comprehensive measure of positive thought disorder from the Rorschach, we rated each response for its level of communication distortion, or "Deviant Thought Quality." Disruptions of thought quality occur as a function of how well or poorly the subject explains and reasons about his responses in describing them. Disturbed thought quality is potentially unrelated to where the response is seen on the card, the content of the response, or the adequacy of the form of the area chosen for the percept, but disturbed thought quality is likely to occur in the presence of "formal" aspects of thinking disorder, such as fabulized combinations or contaminations. Vague, confused, and fluid responses also represent a disruption of communication and thus are relevant to deviant thought quality. Our system for scoring the Rorschach for "deviant thought quality" is described at greater length in a detailed manual (Quinlan, Harrow and Carlson, 1973). This manual also describes our system for assessing two other characteristics of verbalizing the Rorschach responses: *overspecificity* and *affective elaboration.*

OVERSPECIFICITY

One aspect of Rapaport's system of evaluating Rorschach responses is based on the concept of "loss of distance." If the subject begins to respond to the percept as if it were real, then he has lost "distance" from the fact that it is an inkblot, e.g., Card V—"It's a bat—I'm frightened, take it away." To describe inappropriate "distance" from the test situation, Rapaport, Gill, and Schafer (1946) describe two types of Rorschach responses: *fabulization* and *confabulation.*

Two aspects of "loss of distance" appear to be scored within fabulizations and confabulations, an ideational element and an affective one. In the ideational elaboration, the percept may take on an air of reality or be elaborated in details that are beyond anything that can be justified from the inkblot. An example was given by the patient quoted at the beginning: "a shark and my boss [?], actually only the shark-prints are there, it has eaten my boss." A human figure could only be vaguely perceived. The elaboration of that figure as his boss, and that the boss had been eaten by the shark clearly originated within the subject's own private associations, without sufficient perspective on the lack of public verifiability of the percept. Self-references are scored on this scale, especially when they are not supported by specific details; for example, "That's the bear-skin rug in my daughter's den." This aspect has been labeled by us as *overspecificity* (OS) since, in general, the responses elaborate associations that are too specific to be justified solely by the stimulus properties of the inkblot. Three levels of overspecificity were detailed. Level 1 (mild) refers to moderate elaboration or embellishment of the response. This level is not necessarily pathognomic, and in this case may appear because the subject wants to add interest; for example, "That's the skull of a cow in the Mojave desert"; ("Why Mojave desert?"): "Oh, I just named a desert I knew." Level 2 (moderate) involves associations that are beyond simple embellishment, often reflecting particular concerns, at the expense of the reality of the stimulus. At this level, in contrast to level 3 (severe), the objective aspects of the blot are usually not distorted; an example of a level 2 response is: a cat skin, mangy, and decaying (where the subject or patient can point to details suggesting the elaboration). In level 3 (severe), the description of the responses is dominated by elements that are not present on the card. Often these are highly idiosyncratic responses that could only be perceived by the subject. An example of level 3 was given on card IX: "This is the triumph of evil over good." (Upper part = witches, lower part = babies). Level 3 approximates the full confabulation response described by Rapaport and others.

AFFECT ELABORATION

Affect elaboration includes another aspect of Rapaport's scores for fabulation and confabulation. Affect elaboration can occur in two ways, as an elaboration of affective properties of the figures perceived (e.g., "a sad clown") or as the affective reaction of the subject to the response (e.g., "a bat, oooh it's scary, makes me want to throw it away"). While in some sense the attribution of affect is an overly specific elaboration, the special role of affect in psychopathology suggested that it would be profitable to score separately for specifically affective elaborations. In another sense, affect cannot be proven or disproved; it is not a part of the "public" response. Scores in this scale range in three levels paralleling the scoring for overspecificity: mild, moderate, and severe.

A low level of affective elaboration (AE-1) can be seen in responses such as: "two people in love"; "two angry bugs fighting each other"; "a bat, the color makes me dreary." More severe examples would be: "A raging monster; his eyes are red with anger, his mouth is open and yelling"; "A miserable sick, depressed person; tears coming down here, really sad." At the most extreme level, the affect becomes the dominant features: "Cancer-dark-death-despair-gloom" (from a patient whose mother recently died from cancer); Card IX—"Love! The pink is sheer joy, the green the feeling of springtime and love, the orange the flowers of love. It's all so lovely it makes me want to sing."

PATIENTS

The patients we studied using our system of evaluating Rorschach responses to assess issues concerning thought disorders included a sample of 171 consecutive admissions to the inpatient unit of Yale-New Haven Hospital (Almond, 1971; also see Chapter 2). The sample included patients with the following diagnoses: Schizophrenia (undifferentiated, paranoid, catatonic, acute)—48; latent schizophrenia (borderline, pseudoneurotic)—35; personality or character disorders (e.g., sociopathy, obsessive-compulsive personality disorder)—38; neurotic depression—19; psychotic depression (excluding manic-depressive psychosis)—19; and miscellaneous other diagnoses (seizure disorder, anorexia nervosa, manic depressive disorder, other neuroses)—12.

Since the group of "mixed diagnoses" was heterogeneous with respect to the levels of expected thought disorder and no subgroup was large enough for statistical comparisons (all $n \leq 6$), these subjects were not used in the across-diagnosis comparisons. We compared the neurotic and psychotic depressed patients (19 of each); there were no significant differences, so we combined these groups for across-diagnosis comparisons, giving a group of 38 depressed patients.

SUBJECT CHARACTERISTICS

The median age of the total sample was 23 years. There was a significant difference in age between the schizophrenic group (median age = 20.5 years) and the nonschizophrenic groups (median age = 33 years). However, when two-way analyses of variance (age by diagnosis) were performed for the three scales, no significant effects for age or interactions of age with diagnosis were found. This suggests that age was not a significant factor in accounting for the differences in the diagnostic groups.

The sample included 98 females and 73 males. When two-way analyses of variance (sex by diagnosis) were performed on the scores, no significant effects for sex and no significant interactions of sex by diagnosis were found. Using the WAIS Information Scale as an index of intelligence (Wechsler, 1958), there were no significant differences in intelligence among the diagnostic groups (F [3,155] = 1.34,ns).

RORSCHACH TESTING

Within the first ten days of hospitalization, each patient was administered the Rorschach by one of the authors (DQ), or a trained assistant, using the method outlined by Rapaport and colleagues (Rapaport, Gill, and Schafer, 1946; Allison, Blatt, and Zimet, 1968). We included the additional provision that the examiner encourage the patient to give at least two but no more than three responses per card. (Mean number of responses = 22.64, SD = 7.07). (For this phase of our research, Mrs. Kathleen Carlson was a valuable collaborator, especially in relation to her administering the protocols and scoring the data.)

SCORING

Each protocol was scored by one of two scorers using our detailed manual, which is available from Microfiche Publications (Quinlan, Harrow, and Carlson, 1973). All protocols were scored by someone other than the administrator of the test to eliminate the use of cues outside of the written protocol. Reliabilities were at satisfactory levels (TQ, $r_{(18)}$ = .79; OS, $r_{(18)}$ = .92; and AE, $r_{(18)}$ = .90: all $P < .01$).

VERBALIZATIONS AND DIAGNOSIS

A one-way analysis of variance of the verbalization scores across the four diagnostic groups was computed using an index for each major score. The index was obtained by dividing the total weighted score by the number of responses, and then multiplying by 100. The means and analysis of variance appear in Table 15.1. It is clear that affect elaboration (AE) occurs at a much lower rate than deviant thought quality (TQ) and overspecificity (OS).

Examination of the results reveals that the thought quality measure significantly discriminated the schizophrenics from every other group. Schizophrenics had an average score that was more than 1½ times higher than the closest group, the latent schizophrenics. On overspecificity, the schizophrenic group was significantly higher than character disorders and depressed patients, while latent schizophrenics or borderline patients were higher than depressed patients. The results for affect elaboration are quite different from those for the other two scores. On this variable, character disorders had the highest score, while schizophrenics had the next to lowest score. Only the character disorders-depressive difference was significant.

The results support earlier data we have presented in this book, and in separate reports (Quinlan, Harrow, Tucker, and Carlson, 1972;

TABLE 15.1
Verbalization Scores: TQ, OS, AE by Diagnoses, Means and Analysis of Variance

Score Diagnostic Group		N	TQ Index	OS Index	AE Index
Schizophrenic	(S)	48	113.65	90.35	13.29
Latent schizophrenia	(L)	35	73.69	71.69	15.89
Personality or character disorder	(C)	38	63.34	59.95	20.32
Depression	(D)	38	45.34	43.32	5.55
MS			3095.26	2101.78	426.95
F (3,155)			11.84***	7.94***	3.41*
Significant differences[a]			S-L**, S-C**, S-D**	S-C**, S-D**, L-D*	C-D**

*P < .05

**P < .01.

***P < .001.

[a]Newman-Keuls test for *a posteriori* comparisons.

Tucker, Quinlan, and Harrow, 1972), indicating that the quality of the patient's verbalizations on the Rorschach responses does present important diagnostic information. Whether viewed from the standpoint of communication of logical and coherent content (deviant thought quality), or from the viewpoint of elaborating from personalized or idiosyncratic associations (overspecificity), the verbalization scores differentiated among diagnostic groups in ways that are plausible and potentially useful. Affect elaborations were low in that group with a presumed affective (depressive) disturbance, but the depressive disturbance was associated with a lowering of all aspects of verbalization scoring. Affect elaboration is clearly a different kind of elaboration from overspecificity.

Given encouraging results on the comparisons across diagnosis, we asked the question: How do verbalization scores relate to other signs of disordered thinking? To do so, we first performed a factor analysis of a larger set of Rorschach scores including those representing other features of loss of perspective and some that are used as indicators of personality traits.

FACTOR ANALYSIS

The question of the utility of the Rorschach in understanding the nature of thinking disorder and pathology in general can better be understood if the relationships of the various Rorschach indices to each other are explored. Factor analysis suggests itself as a procedure for assessing whether there is a unitary dimension of thought disorder, with each of the scores that are indicative of thinking disorder falling on a single factor, or whether two or more factors will better describe different facets of thought disorder.

A major question that can be addressed by factor analysis is whether scores indicative of *mild* levels of thinking disorder are on the same dimension or dimensions as scores reflecting more severe levels of disordered thinking (Harrow and Quinlan, 1977). Specifically, the implication of such procedures as the delta index (Watkins and Stauffacher, 1952; Johnston and Holzman, 1979) and the TQ, OS, and AE scorings, among others, is that mild deviations are of the same order as major deviations, so that a record with many mildly disordered responses is rated as equally disordered as one with a few responses with major deviance.

A third use of factor analysis is to provide a set of weighted combination scores that allow comparison of Rorschach dimensions with other measures of pathology, personality, and diagnosis. In order to have broad representation of Rorschach variables, scores were included that have traditionally been only partially related to descriptions of pathology, and more frequently used as measures of personality factors, e.g., human movement and color on the Rorschach.

The new scores included were:

1. deviant thought quality;
2. affect elaboration; and
3. overspecificity.

Other Rorschach scores included in this analysis were:

4. *Form accuracy:* the degree to which the subjects response matches the configuration of the blot. Two levels of accuracy were used, corresponding to unusually poor or unusually good accuracy (very poor, very sharp) as described by Rapaport, Schafer, and Gill (1946). In addition, a third category (vague or amorphous form) was included for responses where the percept could assume any vague or indefinite form (e.g., smoke, fire, islands). Form accuracy has been found to be lower in schizophrenia (see Weiner, 1966), and comprises a major component of "developmental level" scoring systems (Friedman, 1953; Phillips, Kaden, and Waldman, 1959).
5. *Fabulized combinations:* two percepts combined into one on the basis of contiguity in an arbitrary, impossible, or otherwise unjustified way (but with the distinctiveness of the component parts maintained, e.g., a bear with a chicken's head).
6. *Contamination response:* two percepts fused together, with the distinctiveness of the two percepts not maintained. (See Chapter 9 for further analysis of Rorschach responses involving fabulized combinations and/or contaminations.)
7. *Drive mainifestations:* these scores are based on a system developed by Robert Holt (Holt and Havel, 1960; Holt, 1963, 1970). Two levels of drive manifestation were scored: primitive and socialized. Chapter 6 presents detailed findings based on this construct.

The following scores were not predicted to relate necessarily to psychopathology but were included as measures potentially linked to personality characteristics which should be analyzed in relation to thought disorder:

8. Combinations: two or more areas of the blot related in a reasonable fashion.
9. Movement: *human* movement only was scored, following the suggestion of Rapaport and colleagues (1946).
10. Color: three types of color response were scored: form-dominated color (FC), color responses with form-related elements (CF), and pure color responses (C). These responses were weighted, respectively, 0.5, 1.0 and 1.5.
11. Responses: (R): the number of responses varied sufficiently and thus was included, even though the range of R was restricted by administration procedures to two or three per card.
12. Barrier and Penetration: responses emphasizing firm, protected boundaries or broken or penetrable boundaries were scored according to the Fisher-Cleveland system (1968).

Factor analyses were computed using the principal-axis solution, entering the simple frequencies of scores for mild deviation separately from the weighted sums of scores for major deviations. (For example, TQ 1 was entered as a frequency, and the weighted sum of TQ 2–4 also was used.) Separate scores for each type of color response and for two levels of drive domination of responses were employed.

By a number of criteria, it appeared that three was the appropriate number of factors. In the unrotated solution, three factors had eigenvalues greater than 1.0. Introducing a fourth factor did not influence the loadings after rotation of the first three in any major way, and the fourth factor had only two variables with loadings higher than .40.

The resulting varimax (analytic) rotation is presented in Table 15.2. The factors are presented in descending order of variance accounted for. Together, three factors accounted for 46 percent of the total variance.

The three factors could be described as follows:

1. Factor I had a high loadings (> .400) for most of the variables that could be considered more *severe* indicators of thought disorder: severe scores for thought quality, overspecificity, affective elaboration, contaminations, fabulized combinations, and primitive (*but not socialized*) drive content. For descriptive purposes, this factor was labeled "ideational disturbance."
2. Factor II had high loadings for number of responses, barrier and penetration, combinations, and for mild levels of deviant thought quality, overspecificity, very sharp form accuracy, and socialized-

drive content. The label assigned to it, "productive richness—mild deviance," was chosen because this factor seemed to be so strongly related to the amount the subject responded to the card and nonextreme elaborations of the responses. Its appearance in that factor structure suggests that high productivity is associated with mild deviance, and this factor is a relatively independent aspect of the Rorschach within the population and procedures used.

3. Factor III had high loadings for amorphous form, pure color, mild affect elaboration, and very poor form. The factor appeared to combine both diffuse perception and scores directly or indirectly related to forms of affective responses, and hence was labeled "affective/perceptual diffusion."

The results of the factor analysis may bear on issues of whether or

TABLE 15.2
Factor Analysis of Rorschach Variables:
Three-Factor Varimax Rotation, $N = 171$

		Loadings	
		Factor II	
		Productive	Factor III
	Factor I	Richness/	Affective/
	Ideational	Mild	Perceptual
Variable	Disturbance	Disturbance	Diffusion
Deviant thought quality: Mild	−.093	.652	.285
Severe	.807	.144	.297
Overspecificity: Mild	.028	.647	.351
Severe	.842	.241	.207
Affective elaboration: Mild	.184	.093	.567
Severe	.554	−.059	.041
Form accuracy: Amorphous	.008	.003	.776
Very Poor (−)	.353	.151	.422
Very Good (+)	−.245	.526	.144
Color: Form color (FC)	.068	.285	.115
Color form (CF)	.239	.074	.196
Pure color (C)	.078	−.066	.695
Contaminations	.800	−.078	.093
Fabulized combinations	.720	−.040	.025
Barrier	.078	.619	−.105
Penetration	.394	.448	−.052
Movement	.384	.361	−.280
Drive: Socialized	.383	.486	.102
Primitive	.672	.193	.050
Combinations	.059	.567	−.202
Number of responses	.130	.639	.365

not mild deviance is a possible sign of severe thought pathology. It could be inferred from the correlations and the composition of the first factor in the factor analysis that hospitalized psychiatric patients with mild cognitive deviance do not necessarily show a greater frequency of severe positive thought disorder than do other hospitalized psychiatric patients.

The first factor also suggests that diverse aspects of the Rorschach responses indicating major pathology tend to occur in the same record, if not on the same response. For example, fabulized combinations and contaminations are mutually exclusive scores for the same response, yet they load highly on the ideational-disturbance factor.

The number of responses had high loadings on the second factor. The loading of number of responses on the other factors was low enough to suggest that productivity is not a major element of those dimensions. The occurrence of high loadings for mild indices of disturbance on this factor along with more positive signs of conceptual and perceptual activity, such as good form or combinations, leaves open the possibility of this factor tapping richness of mental activity with mildly deviant responses sometimes occurring.

The third factor is an interesting one. The high loadings of amorphous form, pure color, and mild affective elaboration suggest the vague diffuse quality of responses. Previous descriptions of pure color responses have suggested they indicate labile affective response (see Rapaport et al., 1946; Shapiro, 1977; Blatt and Feirstein, 1977).

The appearance of mild affect elaboration (but not severe) on this third factor begins to suggest why the affect elaboration score reported above is only mildly related to other verbalization scores: the mild and more frequent occurrences of AE-1 scores are on a different factor compared to the mild scores for OS and TQ. It is only the more blatant evidence of AE (a rating of 2 or 3) that relates to other signs of ideational disturbance.

The interpretation of the factors thus far has been an "internal" analysis of Rorschach scores. Further support for the interpretation of factors was sought by comparing Rorschach factors to diagnoses and other key measures that are methodologically independent.

Factor scores and diagnosis

Factor scores for each subject on each of the three factors were computed. The factor score is a variable obtained as a weighted combination of each of the variables entered into the factor solution.

The weights are related to the loading of each variable and the standard deviation of the variable.

A one-way analysis of variance was conducted across the four major diagnostic groups: schizophrenic, latent schizophrenic, character disorder, and neurotic and psychotic depressed patients. The results are presented in Table 15.3. The analysis of variance indicated a very sharp variation across diagnostic groups for Factor I: Ideational Disturbance (F [3,155] = 10.22; $P < .001$). A *posteriori* comparisons (Newman-Keuls; Winer, 1962) indicated that schizophrenic patients were more pathological than patients with personality disorders and depression ($P < .01$). Depressed patients were also significantly lower on this factor than latent schizophrenics ($P < .05$). The analysis of variance for Factor II approached significance, F (3,155) = 2.18 ($P < .10$). Depressives tended to be lower on productive richness—mild deviance than schizophrenics ($t = 2.33$, $P < .05$), and personality disorders ($t = 2.18$, $P < .05$). The ANOVA on Factor III, affective/perceptual diffusion, was not significant, F (3,155) = 1.90 ($P < .13$), but this was the only factor that tended to differentiate schizophrenics from latent schizophrenics ($t = 2.09$; $P < .05$ on an *a priori* basis). Schizophrenics showed a trend to be high and latent schizophrenics to be low on this factor, with other patients in the middle.

Two variables, deviant thought quality and contaminations sum (see Chapter 9), significantly discriminate schizophrenics from all other diagnostic groups, so that the factor scores do not improve interdiagnostic discrimination. Factor I, however, does constitute a general "positive thought disorder" factor of Rorschach scores, while Factor II and III capture other facets of Rorschach scores that are worth further examination.

Relation of factor scores to other major aspects of psychopathology

The factor scores for each patient were assessed in relation to a number of key measures of psychopathology and to select personality variables. Subsequent to admission, the psychiatrist responsible for each patient's treatment completed a set of forms including a scale for bizarre speech and behavior, histrionic behavior, paranoid thinking, and depressed mood. Satisfactory reliability has been established for these scales, and they have been utilized successfully in a number of studies (Quinlan, Harrow, Tucker, and Carlson, 1972; Harrow, Tucker, and Shield, 1972; Shanfield, Tucker, Harrow, and Detre, 1970). Length of hospitalization was obtained as a rough index of short-term outcome.

TABLE 15.3
One-Way Analysis of Variance of Factor Scores[1] by Diagnostic Groups

Diagnoses: Variable	Schizophrenia (N = 48) Mean SD		Latent Schizophrenia (N = 35) Mean SD		Personality Disorder (N = 38) Mean SD		Depression (N = 38) Mean SD		F: df = 3,155
Factor I	0.46	1.10	0.15	1.06	-0.12	0.82	-0.62	0.52	10.22[2]
Factor II	0.12	0.95	0.06	1.06	0.13	1.02	-0.37	0.95	2.18[3]
Factor III	0.30	1.30	-0.22	0.70	-0.01	1.01	-0.06	0.77	1.90[4]

[1] Scores are "factor scores," mean = 0, standard deviation = 1.00.
[2] $p < .001$.
[3] $p < .10$.
[4] $p < .13$.

During the early weeks of hospitalization, patients completed a battery of psychological instruments that included measures of introversion-extroversion (Eysenck, 1959), the Zung Depression Scale (Zung, 1965), and the MMPI.

Factor scores were related, significantly, to a number of clinical ratings, and to other psychopathology scores assessed independently; the results obtained in this area are presented in Table 15.4. The pattern of correlations supports the interpretation of the factors as measures of disordered thinking, productivity, and affective lability.

The first factor, *ideational disturbance*, correlated significantly ($P < .05$ or better) in the positive direction with: longer length of hospitalization; bizarre speech and behavior; paranoid thinking; and the Schizophrenia,

TABLE 15.4
Correlations of Rorschach Factor Scores
with Other Variables (df = *169*)

Variable	Factor 1 Ideational Disturbance	Factor 2 Productive Richness/ Mild Disturbance	Factor 3 Affective/ Perceptual Diffusion
Days in hospital	.25**	.02	.16
Therapist rating:			
Histrionics	.14	.03	.20*
Depressed mood	−.16*	−.07	−.20*
Paranoid thinking	.25**	.00	.06
Bizarre speech & behavior	.30***	−.04	.13
Medications: Any medication	.12	−.03	−.08
Phenothiazines	.28**	−.08	.01
Tricyclics	−.22**	−.03	−.18*
Personality scales:			
Extraversion/introversion			
(Maudsley)	.06	.08	.34***
Zung SDS (depression)	.13	−.20*	−.12
MMPI: *K*	−.17	.09	.01
PA (*K* corrected)	.33***	−.03	.03
PT (*K* corrected)	.20*	−.05	−.05
SC (*K* corrected)	.37***	.01	.06
MA (*K* corrected)	.32***	.03	.25**
SI	.04	−.17	−.20*
Sex	−.13	−.15	.09
WAIS information	.22*	.21*	.06

*$P < .05$.
**$P < .01$.
***$P < .001$.

Paranoia, Psychaesthenia, and Hypomania scales of the MMPI (*K* corrected). Scores on ideational disturbance were significantly higher for patients on phenothiazines, lower for patients on tricyclics, and lower for patients rated for depressed mood. A moderate but significant positive correlation with WAIS information was found with Factor I, and a moderate significant negative correlation with age was found. This coincides with the general trend for schizophrenics to have earlier hospitalizations than depressed patients. Thus, there is a relatively mild but significant confounding of type of pathology with age.

Factor II, *productive richness—mild deviance,* was negatively correlated with the score on the Zung self-rating depression scale, and was moderately positively related to WAIS Information, an index of intelligence (*P* < .05).

Factor III, *affective/perceptual diffusion,* was significantly positively correlated with extroversion on the Maudsley Scale, with the MMPI Hypomania Scale, and with clinical ratings of histrionic behavior. It also was significantly negatively correlated with rated depressed mood, social introversion, and the use of tricyclic medication. Thus, it appears that this factor assesses some form of affect and aspects of social interaction, including several aspects of maniclike behavior.

IMPLICATIONS OF THE FACTOR ANALYSIS

A single factor, ideational disturbance, accounted for a substantial proportion of the variance. It had loadings on almost all of the scores related to severe positive thought disorder. Scores on this factor differentiated acute schizophrenic patients from other groups of patients. The factor scores for the ideational disruption factor correlated with several independently derived variables measuring aspects of disordered thinking. The results suggest that many different types of disturbed thinking can be found in the same patients. Thus, during the acute stages, the same patients show a variety of different aspects of positive thought disorder, and also in many cases, the same severely thought-disordered verbalizations by a patient reflect psychopathology on a number of scores. Some of the verbalizations for a given response are *simultaneously* deviant in terms of conventional social standards, suggest difficulty in boundaries, are loose, have personalized and affective elements, are overinclusive, are illogical, and so on.

This may help to explain why different theorists look at disordered speech and come up with different generalizations about it. They could each be looking at a different dimension of the same disordered speech (some are looking at it to see if it is "loose," some are studying it for illogical aspects, and some are studying whether it is overinclusive). Most of the different investigators are correct in noting a difference between schizophrenics and nonschizophrenics on the particular aspect they are studying, since the speech of acute schizophrenics shows disturbance of many dimensions simultaneously, and the generalizations about the type of thought disorder involved may depend on which aspect or dimension one studies.

The findings on the second factor, productive richness—mild deviance suggest that depressed patients tend to see fewer percepts and/or say less. The findings allow for the possibility that productivity is a useful diagnostic cue. Most important, more blatant forms of thought disorder are relatively independent of response productivity.

The third factor that emerged, affective perceptual diffusion, was somewhat unexpected. The appearance of pure color responses along with moderate levels of affective elaboration tends to lend some support for the traditional interpretation of pure color responses as indicative of affect lability (e.g., Rapaport et al., 1946; Shapiro, 1977). The relationships to extroversion and hypomania are conceptually consistent.

The data also help answer the question posed in the introduction as to whether mild forms of each type of positive thought disorder are closely tied in with more severe levels of the same type of disordered thinking. The data support the separation of different levels of thought disorder. The ideational disturbance factor that emerged contained only the more severe levels of positive thought disorder. The mild levels of disturbance did not distinguish schizophrenics from nonschizophrenic patients, in contrast to highly significant results at the more severe levels. The overall results suggest that for some purposes the mild and severe levels can be separated, and that while it is possible that there may be some commonality in the processes or underlying factors involved in producing both of them, *additional* underlying factors are involved in the appearance of the more severe levels.

The results support other research of ours indicating that *mild* degrees of disordered thinking are not schizophrenic features (Harrow and Quinlan, 1977). It would appear that mild forms of positive thought disorder are found in many types of acutely disturbed patients, including nonschizophrenics. As we have noted in several other chapters, it is only at the more severe levels of each type of thought disorder that the indices distinguish schizophrenic from nonschizophrenic patients during the acute stage. The data also suggest that, in practical clinical situations, if one attempts to differentiate acutely disturbed schizophrenics from other acutely disturbed psychiatric patients, the more severe levels of thought disorder might be separated and included as separate indices.

This aspect of the factor analysis carries implications concerning general scoring systems for assessing positive thought disorder. Since mild levels of thought disturbance have different implications from those of the severe levels, heavier weightings of severely pathological responses will be the main contributor to their successful discrimination of groups with varying levels of pathology.

The correlations of the third factor with extroversion, hypomania, and histrionic behavior are low but are statistically significant, and in a direction consistent with the interpretation of this factor. The fact that "classical" schizophrenics are high on this factor and latent schizophrenics are low is, in retrospect, a plausible description of one of the differences between these two groups of patients: they are differentiated from each other by the occurrence of a flagrant psychotic episode in the acute schizophrenics and an absense of an overt break in the latent schizophrenics.

We should also note that Factor I, ideational disturbance, has many similarities (e.g., contaminations) with two factors found by Efron and Piotrowski on their Long-Term Prognostic Index (1966). These same two factors were also the ones that correlated significantly with a rating of long-term outcome in psychiatric inpatients. A similar long-term outcome study including a large number of patients given the Rorschach is currently being conducted by the authors.

Impaired perspective and Rorschach scores

Examination of the Rorschach responses of the patients whose scores load highly on Factor I suggest that these deviant responses could be influenced by a breakdown of perspective. Poor form accuracy, major deviance of thought quality, highly overspecific responses, and boundary-disturbance scores could be a product of impaired perspective. The different loadings of primitive and socialized drive are also consistent. The primitive-drive response lacks the usual shaping and meeting that more socialized-drive expressions entail; the shock value of blatant drive representations violates the expectations of day-to-day functioning based on what is appropriate.

The emergence of a clear factor of ideational disturbance from Rorschach responses is consistent with the assumption that, with reduced cues as to the appropriate mode of responding, more disturbed patients will show a more impaired ability to take the perspective of a general other in shaping their responses.

16

Overview on Disordered Thinking and Schizophrenia

OVERALL GOALS AND THE ROLE OF EMPIRICAL RESEARCH ON THOUGHT DISORDER IN SCHIZOPHRENIA

In summarizing some of the key aspects of our research so that we can draw some conclusions about the nature of disordered thinking and the major disorders in which it occurs, such as schizophrenia, we will outline a few of our tentative conclusions.

To begin, we might note that there are a number of important issues that need to be dealt with: not only whether schizophrenics have disordered thinking, but also what type of disordered thinking, under what circumstances, what its longitudinal course is and how permanent it is, is there a particular kind of content or problem area specific to the schizophrenic patient's disturbed thinking, is disordered thinking unique to schizophrenia or is it also found in nonschizophrenics, does it fit along a continuum with mildly disturbed types of thinking found in normals, how prominent and important is disordered thinking in schizophrenia, and what kinds of factors might influence or lead to it?

When the field is able to answer these questions more completely, it will have advanced a good distance toward solving the major riddles about disordered thinking in schizophrenia, and will perhaps have moved in the direction of better understanding the riddle of what schizophrenia is all about. In other words, it is our belief that by acquiring knowledge about cognitive dysfunctioning in schizophrenia, one will get a better picture of the disorder and answer some of the major theoretical questions about it.

Most of the above questions, which we will discuss briefly below, have been examined in greater detail in earlier chapters. However, there are several that we have not covered in detail in this book.

RELEVANT ISSUES CONCERNING DISORDERED THINKING

1. Are All Types of "Thought Disorders" Proposed by Various Clinicians and Theorists as Schizophrenic Phenomenon Really of Importance?

The evidence provided by others and the evidence presented here indicate that many types of thought disorders are not important. We did find clear evidence for certain types of disordered thinking in schizophrenia. However, many types of disordered cognition that have been discussed at length by clinicians and theorists appear to be less important when examined closely at different phases of disorder, including the acute phase, phases of partial-remission, and the more chronic phases. Some of the earlier research on schizophrenic cognition is based on using comparison groups of normals as the main controls. In these cases, the patient's being schizophrenic is confounded with being a patient, and with being acutely disturbed and hospitalized. Differences found between schizophrenics and normals using this type of experimental design may be a consequence of any of these factors, since they are all confounded. As a result, some promising leads about aspects of cognition that are seen as important to schizophrenia become less salient when comparisons are made between schizophrenics and acutely disturbed nonschizophrenic patients. Our research leads to the following conclusions:

a. Some types of thinking that are often considered of major theoretical importance are not prominent in early stages of the disorder, although it is quite possible that they play a more important role in the later schizophrenic picture. One such type is concrete thinking, or the inability to abstract successfully, which shows some impairment in early schizophrenics, but is not a dominant factor at that phase of disorder. We have discussed research on this type of disordered thinking, which might be viewed as a deficit symptom or a negative symptom, in Chapter 7. In general, our research has indicated that various types of thought pathology that might be viewed as negative symptoms, and especially impoverished thinking, are not prominent at the early acute stages except in select patients, and are more prominent in a number of chronic schizophrenics.

b. Other types of thinking hypothesized as important in schizophrenia by a number of investigators are prominent at the early acute stages. It is questionable, however, how long they persist and how much these early, seemingly prominent, types of thought pathology are influenced by very acute disturbance, acute psychopathology, and disorganization. One such aspect is conceptual overinclusion, which seems to be influenced by overt disorganization and to be most prominent in the active stages of schizophrenia. Our research in this area was discussed in Chapter 10. Other aspects, such as boundary problems, also seem to be heavily influenced by acute disturbance and acute psychopathology, although some types of boundary problems may persist in a subgroup of schizophrenics. Boundary problems were discussed in Chapter 9. Another type of cognitive disturbance that has been written about extensively in the last twenty five years by Payne and other investigators (Payne, 1966) is what we have labeled "behavioral overinclusion," While this aspect is often quite high in acutely disturbed schizophrenics, it is not high at all in *chronic* schizophrenics and our evidence suggests that it is even less prominent in chronic patients than it is in normals. Our research and that of others suggest that behavioral overinclusion is partly a function of excessive behavioral output, or overproductivity.

c. Still other types of cognition that have been discussed at length by clinicians and theorists are prominent in many schizophrenics at early acute stages of the disorder, but are influenced by overall disturbance, and also are common in many disturbed *nonschizophrenics*. These types also seem to diminish after patients emerge from the acute or active stage of the disorder. One such type that fits under this category is stimulus overinclusion, or certain types of disorders in selective attention, that we found to be common in acutely disturbed nonschizophrenics. We have presented our research on stimulus overinclusion and disordered attention in Chapter 12. Depersonalization is another feature that many have hypothesized as important in schizophrenia. Our evidence suggests that depersonalization is extremely common in acute schizophrenic states. However, we have also found evidence indicating that it is quite common in many other types of disturbed patients, and heavily influenced by acute psychopathology, dysphoric affect, and overall disturbance. We have discussed depersonalization in Chapter 11.

Our results on the emergence of primitive-drive-dominated thinking have also shown that this feature is not uniformly positive for acute schizophrenics. In addition, we have found many types of acutely disturbed *non*schizophrenics who show severe problems concerning this type of thinking, including a number of patients with sociopathic or rule-breaking difficulties. Our research in this area was discussed in Chapter 6. One can see by the above research that not all types of disordered thinking that others have theorized as prominent in schizophrenia are actually of importance throughout the course of the disorder.

2. Is positive thought disorder unique to schizophrenia?

This question is one that still arises frequently among clinicians and therefore, the answer deserves considerable emphasis. As we have indicated in Chapter 4, and will discuss again later in this chapter, our research indicates that disordered thinking is not unique to schizophrenia. Some older formulations of positive types of thought pathology as uniform for schizophrenia, and exclusive to it, are imprecise, and should be revised. Many of the older observations are based on dramatic examples of severely thought-disordered schizophrenics, some studied during the acute phase and others studied during the chronic phase. They do not involve detailed examinations of large samples of severely thought-disordered manic patients, and also samples of psychotic nonschizophrenics, some of whom also show severe positive thought disorder.

Thus, some clinicians have believed that reliance on disordered thinking is a certain way to distinguish schizophrenics from nonschizophrenics. Our research suggests that this is not the case. However, during active stages of disorder, analysis of the presence and level of potential thought pathology is still a valuable clue to the presence of severe disorganization and possible psychosis, particularly schizophrenic or manic psychosis.

At our current stage of knowledge the concept of schizophrenia is a disjunctive one, a category that depends on a combination of features. Disordered thinking has been one of these signs, and along with other major features such as nondepressive delusions and hallucinations, it ranks as one of the better ones. Until our understanding of psychosis is advanced further and better criteria for schizophrenia are developed, disordered thinking can still be used as one possible sign of this disorder, although our research suggests that it is not an infallible one.

3. Does Thought Disorder Fit on a Continuum with Normal Thinking?

Several aspects of our evidence suggest that positive thought disorder, such as bizarre thinking, is not a discrete phenomenon, but that it lies on a continuum that extends all the way from normal thinking to mildly strange thinking and extends on the continuum to severe bizarre thinking. Among other aspects of our results this includes data reported in Chapter 4 using several different types of test instruments, indicating that: (a) mild levels of disordered thinking are extremely common in many acutely disturbed nonschizophrenics patients, and can be found in some normals; and (b) as one moves further out on the possible continuum, more severe levels of disordered thinking are frequent in (but still not exclusive to) overt schizophrenics and manic patients in active stages of their disorder.

As we have noted in Chapter 15, the factor-analytic data suggest that a factor with high loadings for variables that reflect severe levels of positive thought disorder separated schizophrenic from nonschizophrenic patients. A second factor with high loadings for variables reflecting mild levels of thought disorder did not separate schizophrenics from personality disorders. Fitting in with these results, we have constructed our more recent indices of bizarre-idiosyncratic thinking, a composite measure of positive thought disorder, to give considerably greater weight to responses involving severe positive thought disorder than to responses involving mild deviance or cognitive slips (see the manual included as the appendix to this book). It is our belief that normal thinking, mild levels of thought disorder, and severe levels of thought disorder may be placed on a continuum, with *some* of the underlying processes involved in mild and severe thought disorder being the same. However, additional underlying factors may be involved in responses at the extreme end of the continuum (severe levels of thought disorder).

Earlier, we have discussed the issue of mild versus severe levels of thought disorder, and of whether severe positive thought disorder lies on a continuum with normal thinking. As we have noted, without clear knowledge of the underlying factors involved, it is difficult to resolve with certainty questions about whether there is a "true" continuum in this area. Thus, the issue of disordered thinking in psychopathology as a possible continuum cannot be determined at present with any finality.

In general, formulations about whether a feature does or does not fit along a continuum are often difficult to resolve and one of the issues is what is the underlying continuum (e.g., normality versus severe pathology). Currently, either alternative (continuum or discrete phenomenon) is possible. It seems most probable, however, that severe positive thought disorder fits on the opposite end of a continuum with normal thinking.

We have also noted elsewhere that our evidence about thought disorder in schizophrenics, as compared to that found in other disorders, suggests that there is no unique "thought disorder" exclusive to overt schizophrenia. Our data indicate that the severe positive thought disorder found in schizophrenics includes many of the factors present in the severe positive thought disorder that can be found in some nonschizophrenic patients.

4. During a schizophrenic's active psychotic episode, is all thinking and behavior strange or bizarre?

As we have discussed earlier, even during an acute psychotic episode, not all of the schizophrenic's behavior is strange. The particular situation the schizophrenic faces at the moment is extremely important. The overt appearance of positive thought disorder depends on the type of stimuli present and on the opportunity for disordered thinking to show itself in the schizophrenic's verbalizations. It seems that in more ambiguous, socially oriented situations, disordered schizophrenic thinking is more likely to appear. Thought pathology is less likely to appear in structured situations, although even in structured situations, disordered thinking frequently appears as long as the patient's *response* is not strictly limited or forced into a tight structure. This can be seen most clearly in our research using the Proverbs test, using a test of social comprehension, and using the Object Sorting test. In contrast, the opportunity for deviant schizophrenic verbalizations to appear is diminished when a carefully structured response is presented to the patient or when he is given the opportunity to select a response in a multiple-choice situation, or when a stereotyped response is demanded. In situations where nonstereotyped responses are demanded, bizarre behavior or positive types of thought disorder are much more likely to appear. The presentation of unstructured stimuli is also of value if one wishes to assess idiosyncratic behavior. Some theorists, however, have focused exclusively on the value of unstructured stimuli and have underemphasized the importance of establishing situations that do not lend themselves to stereotyped, overpracticed, or over-learned responses.

5. Is Disordered Thinking a Permanent Characteristic of Schizophrenia?

One of the goals of our follow-up research program is to help answer this question, and we discussed some of our early results in this area in Chapter 5. After a series of follow-ups over a five-year period we have found some schizophrenics who were continuously thought disordered. This does not appear to be the case for all schizophrenics, and probably not even for the majority of early, young schizophrenics. The old notion that "once crazy, always crazy" has not been supported in a certain number of the schizophrenic patients we studied. On the whole, schizophrenics do show severe disordered thinking during the acute phase and during active chronic phases. In addition, for a certain percentage of schizophrenics some thought pathology may be a permanent part of their thinking. Thus, severe thought disorder may be continuous for a subgroup of schizophrenics. At the same time our overall results suggest that if bizarre-idiosyncratic thinking is more characteristic of schizophrenics during the nonpsychotic phase, this only applies to a subgroup of schizophrenic patients.

Clinicians and theorists should be speaking of *active* and *inactive* phases of schizophrenia for some early, young patients. Considered along this dimension, for some early schizophrenics the disorder is a phasic one. One possibity we have thought about is that schizophrenia could be a phasic disorder for some during the early stages, and could later become more continual for a certain number of schizophrenics in the chronic stages. Holzman, in a recent paper, has also emphasized the phasic nature of cognitive dysfunctioning in schizophrenia, noting that the structures for adaptive thinking and perceiving are not obliterated (Holzman, 1978). Aspects of our data showing the phasic quality of thought disorder also could fit ideas advanced by Zubin and Spring (1977) about vulnerability, although other aspects of our data suggest the persistence of some level of delusional activity in a number of schizophrenics, and suggest vulnerability to a more sustained disorder (Harrow and Silverstein, 1977; Silverstein and Harrow, 1981). In addition, other aspects of our follow-up research indicate that the great majority of schizophrenics show difficulties in other areas of adjustment, with only a small percentage of schizophrenics showing very favorable outcomes (Harrow, Grinker, Silverstein, and Holzman, 1978).

6. Is the Schizophrenic's Disordered Speech and Thinking Influenced by His Specific Concerns and Preoccupations?

Our research on intermingling, which is discussed in Chapter 5, indicates that material from the schizophrenic's particular concerns and preoccupations can often be found in his disordered speech and thinking. These data would indicate that the schizophrenic's concerns and preoccupations often do play some role in his bizarre verbalizations. Our data suggest, however, that these concerns are not enough to account for the whole picture. Other results of ours on a large number of preoccupied nonschizophrenics suggest that preoccupation and concern are not sufficient by themselves to lead to disordered schizophrenic thinking. Thus, research on groups of other disturbed nonschizophrenic patients has indicated that considerable preoccupation and concerns are also common among many of these patients. Aspects of their concerns and preoccupations sometimes appear among nonschizophrenics' responses to test material without the same degree of severe bizarre verbalizations.

If excessive preoccupation is the only factor responsible for bizarre verbalizations and thinking, one would expect some bizarreness in disturbed nonschizophrenics since they also show considerable preoccupation and tend to personalize in responses to test material. We have suggested, however, that because of other basic differences between schizophrenics and nonschizophrenics, when nonschizophrenics become acutely disturbed, they show personal content in their responses to test material (or personalize) but do not become bizarre. In contrast, when schizophrenics become acutely disturbed, they personalize and allow the emergence of this personal material to occur in a poorly controlled fashion, and this makes them look strange and/or bizarre. Thus, the emergence of schizophrenics' concerns and preoccupations plays a role in their bizarre speech, but since nonschizophrenics also personalize without showing as much bizarreness, an important factor is an impairment for schizophrenics in other mechanisms that under normal circumstances would prevent them from becoming bizarre.

We have proposed that impaired perspective about the social inappropriateness of their own thinking is one such mechanism that may play a role in the tendency of schizophrenic and thought-disordered patients to allow their personalized thinking to enter into their overt responses, making their speech seem strange. In contrast, many disturbed nonschizophrenic and non-thought-disordered patients may show some tendency to personalize but will not allow their personal concerns totally to dominate their speech or to make them look strange. We have provided some evidence suggesting that this is because of their better perspective about what type of speech would lead to their appearing inappropriate or bizarre to others. Some of our views on impaired perspective have been discussed in Chapters 3 and 5, and we have included further discussion later in this chapter. Elsewhere, in a recent report, we have presented data indicating that when nonpsychotic patients intermingled personal material into their speech, they did it more subtly and less directly than schizophrenics. When these nonpsychotic patients intermingled, they did so in a manner that was less likely to disrupt the external topic, and less likely to make them appear strange (Harrow, Lanin-Kettering, Prosen, and Miller, 1983). Consistent with this interpretation is the finding that thought-disordered and psychotic patients showed fewer metacognitive remarks to correct their overpersonalized and strange verbalizations, which suggests they have less awareness that their speech is inappropriate.

7. Does Disordered Schizophrenic Speech Show Content Reflecting a Universal Schizophrenic Theme or Does the Content Material Represent an Individual "Complex" or Concern for Each Patient?

Our research studying the particular content area that may appear in disordered speech has explored whether there is one universal schizophrenic conflict or schizophrenic problem that is reflected in their speech pathology. If there was one uniform problem area that appeared, it could fit some theories about a core schizophrenic conflict. Our studies have indicated that there is not one particular content area or one universal schizophrenic theme that appears in their disordered verbalizations. In our research using a free-verbalization technique, we found that the signs of disturbed verbalizations covered a wide number of different content areas, with these areas often being specific to each patient's particular, individual, major concerns.

In addition, as we have noted in Chapter 5, although most schizophrenics' particular concerns appeared in their disordered speech, there have been other schizophrenics whom we studied whose thought disordered verbalizations did not reflect, at least overtly, a particular concern of theirs. Whether these patients' thought-disordered utterances really do have some underlying conflicts or content areas from which they are derived is still an open question. As of the present, however, we do not have clear evidence that all disordered schizophrenic speech reflects particular conflicts, concerns, or other personal material.

Recently, using other techniques, we have conducted further exploration of the content area that might be related to disordered schizophrenic verbalizations. This research involved the interviewing of patients about their specific disordered verbalizations in response to proverbs and comprehension questions (see the research on intermingling discussed in Chapter 5). Using this technique, we found further evidence that for those schizophrenics who intermingled personal material into their responses, the particular type of content areas involved covered a wide range of issues and was apparently individual to each patient. Thus, we have data derived by means of several techniques that suggest that the problem areas indicated by the content of schizophrenics' verbalizations cover a number of different areas, rather than reflecting a universal schizophrenic theme.

Since the disordered verbalizations of the schizophrenic patients we studied do not reflect a universal schizophrenic theme, another issue in this area arises. This second issue concerns whether the content material in an individual schizophrenic's idiosyncratic verbalizations represents one central "complex" or area of concern for that patient, as opposed to representing a variety of topics and concerns for that schizophrenic. Data in this area have some bearing on older theories about schizophrenic patients having one disturbed central "complex" or problem area, with preoccupation over this central problem area dominating their lives and leading to emotional disturbance and disordered thinking.

Our results on the question of whether a schizophrenic's idiosyncratic verbalizations center on one central "complex" or on a variety of topics indicate a lack of uniformity. Overall, however, our data indicate that the disordered speech of most of the schizophrenics we studied seemed to show evidence of personal material from two or more areas of their experience, rather than from one central "complex" (Harrow and Prosen, 1979). Only a few of the individual schizophrenic patients we studied showed intermingling of personal material from only one problem area. The tendency for material from several different areas to appear in a patient's idiosyncratic verbalizations suggests that the important factor is the personal tendency of the schizophrenic to intermingle material from a variety of problem areas into his verbalizations during active phases of disorder, rather than the idiosyncratic behavior arising as a result of the magnitude of one central problem area.

8. Are Schizophrenics' Idiosyncratic Verbalizations Influenced by a General Impairment in Social Knowledge and Understanding of Social Conventions?

An important issue is whether the schizophrenic's idiosyncratic and odd thinking and behavior are influenced by a general lack of knowledge or understanding of what behavior is expected of him in the type of social situation he faces. Thus, it has been proposed by some that the schizophrenic's bizarre thinking and strange behavior are a consequence of his never having learned what types of behaviors are appropriate, and/or an absence of knowledge of social conventions. This possibility is enhanced by the research, which has suggested the prominence of idiosyncratic verbalizations and the analyses indicating that idiosyncratic verbalizations are deviant or odd in respect to conventional social norms. In addition, as we have observed in Chapter 5 and at several points in this and other chapters, our research has suggested that impaired perspective about what types of behaviors are appropriate for a particular situation is one major factor in the schizophrenic's bizarre thinking and behavior.

Our research, however, does not support the thesis that strange schizophrenic behavior is a consequence of a general lack of knowledge of social rules. Data we have collected on a number of samples, using several techniques, suggest that at least in the acute stage, schizophrenics do not show a greater impairment or more severe deficits on tests of social comprehension than they do on tests assessing other areas requiring complex cognitive decisions. It is always, of course, possible that there could be select deficits in very special social areas. Even here, however, less formal data of ours do not support this formulation. We would propose that schizophrenics do have such social knowledge, although there may be a problem in using this knowledge effectively in relation to judgments about their own behavior.

Thus, a number of areas of our research exploring impaired perspective suggest that schizophrenics' major difficulties are not a consequence of their never having learned what types of social behavior are appropriate or of never having learned social conventions. Data on this point include the following:

1. Despite the impaired perspective about their own responses by schizophrenics and by thought-disordered patients, they have better

perspective about others' responses and thus seem able to mobilize their judgments about social conventions adequately in judging others' behavior.

2. Even during their acute psychotic episodes, many schizophrenics seem to be able, sporadically to make adequate judgments about their own behavior in some situations.

3. Evidence about schizophrenics' premorbid status suggests that before their first psychotic break and before they came to the hospital, most of them were not behaving grossly inappropriately. Thus, one could presume that at that point, before their disorder began to become manifest, their perspective was either adequate or close to adequate. Exceptions occur in some patients with poor premorbid histories, but usually not in terms of grossly inappropriate behavior.

4. Our data indicate that for many schizophrenics their socially inappropriate behavior diminishes after a few weeks in the hospital during partial recovery, and they also show less bizarre thinking and behavior at follow-up. This indicates that most early-phase schizophrenic difficulties are temporary or sporadic concerning either the possession or the effective use of knowledge about what is socially appropriate.

Overall, it is our view that when the schizophrenic is socially inappropriate, it is not typically due to his or her never having acquired such consensual knowledge about what types of behaviors are socially appropriate. Rather, we would emphasize such factors as not using this knowledge effectively in certain types of situations.

9. Is a Disorder in Stimulus or Information Processing the Key Mechanism Producing Disordered Schizophrenic Thinking?

The issue of whether impaired stimulus or information processing is a key mechanism responsible for disordered schizophrenic thinking is a question that cannot be answered easily, in part because of the complexity of information processing. During the early stages of perception a variety of processes are involved, and there are a number of different possible ways in which faulty information processing can occur. These include possible difficulties associated with the sensory registers or very short term memory; difficulties in selective attention or "filtering"; difficulties in ability to process relevant information quickly enough through the limited capacity of short-term memory; possible quicker decay of memory traces; various possible difficulties in coding material, or in organizing material into larger units in short-term memory; various possible problems in search and retrieval processes in short-term memory; and various possible problems in other steps involved in information processing. Thus, the initial stages of information and stimulus processing involve a number of complicated steps, many occurring at very rapid speeds, and most of which are poorly understood at present. Increasingly sophisticated research in this overall area is beginning to make some progress, but it has also become apparent that the processes involved are much more complicated than was originally believed.

In view of this complexity, with many processes involved, it is difficult to study all or even most of them to rule out a possible disorder at one or several steps of information processing. Thus far our research has focused on select aspects of stimulus and information processing: This has included: (a) research on a possible impairment in selective attention; (b) research on kinesthetic figural after-effects to evaluate with *this* technique hypotheses about stimulus reduction in schizophrenics; and also (c) research on field dependence. The research has produced mixed results with a number of negative findings.

One example of our negative findings in areas that had initially seemed promising can be seen in our research studying potential stimulus reduction in schizophrenia. The kinesthetic figural after-effects (*KFA*) has been one of the standard techniques used in the past to evaluate hypotheses about stimulus reduction. Our most recent results in this area have been negative and have even suggested that the use of techniques such as the *KFA* to get at stimulus reduction may present major difficulties (Kuster, Harrow, and Tucker, 1975). While our results have questioned the *KFA* as a technique to get at the phenomenon, it is still possible that the concept of stimulus reduction could be an important one, but must be evaluated by other methods. This is currently being done by investigators such as M. Buchsbaum and others using evoked potentials for this research.

Aberrant Perceptual Experiences and a Disorder in Selective Attention in Schizophrenia

Among the most interesting hypotheses in the area of stimulus and information processing are formulations about the importance of aberrant perceptual experiences involving an impairment in selective attention. Such disorders of selective attention have been accepted by some as the key background factor leading to thought disorder and other aspects of the schizophrenic disorder. Our major research efforts in the area of stimulus and information processing, summarized in Chapter 12, have focused on the potential importance of a disorder in selective attention. The model for the types of aberrant perceptual experiences involved in such attentional disorders have been outlined in detail by J. Chapman and McGhie (Chapman, 1966; McGhie and Chapman, 1961). Their vivid descriptions of the types of disorders in selective attention that they feel are prominent in schizophrenia have been very influential in the literature on schizophrenic psychopathology. We have labeled these types of aberrant perceptual experiences that they describe, which are characterized by the schizophrenic's tendency to be distracted by or to focus unnecessarily on a wide range of irrelevant stimuli, as "stimulus overinclusion."

We described in Chapter 12 a series of three large studies of selective attention or stimulus overinclusion that we conducted, using as stimulus material the type of first-hand statements J. Chapman and McGhie have reported directly from their schizophrenic patients. Our results from all three experiments were either mixed or negative on the formulations in this area. Thus, the results from these three studies indicated that disorders of selective attention, or stimulus overinclusion, are found in many, but not all, schizophrenics. Most important, however, they are common in disturbed nonschizophrenic patients, and cut across the usual diagnostic lines. Such impairments in selective attention can also be found in some normals, especially during periods of anxiety and disturbance for them. Our research, then, suggests that an impairment in selective attention is not a necessary condition for schizophrenia (some schizophrenics do not have it), not is it a sufficient condition for schizophrenia (many nonschizophrenics have it).

How does one come to understand the frequency of disorders in selective attention in nonschizophrenic patients and in normals? We have proposed in Chapter 12 that such attentional disorders may arise from several different sources. We have suggested that the attentional and perceptual systems can be disrupted by any of a number of different factors. Variables associated with schizophrenic disorders are one of them. However, anxiety, acute distress, and other variables can also be included among the other factors that can disrupt attention. Anxiety and a high level of disruption can be found in most acute schizophrenics. They can also be found in many other types of disturbed people with psychopathology, and they occur periodically in normals, some of whom experience disruption in their attentional processes at such times.

If schizophrenia is viewed as a centrally based disorder, when there is an impairment in control mechanisms one might expect a disruption in the regulation of external and internal stimuli. With such a central cognitive impairment, some attentional and perceptual mechanisms might be disrupted, as well as mechanisms involved in other non-perceptual functions. This disruption of perceptual processes would not be uniform for all schizophrenics. It would vary according to the particular individual and would not be a core factor in producing schizophrenic psychopathology. Seen this way, the smooth regulation of attention could be disrupted by several factors, including the underlying factors associated with schizophrenia, as well as by anxiety and general disturbance in nonschizophrenics.

We presented in Chapter 12 a model downplaying the importance of an impairment in selective attention as a central etiologic agent in schizophrenia. This model was, in part, designed to deal with our data indicating that many nonschizophrenics have similar difficulties in this area. Our evidence in this area is incomplete, and there are still other possible means by which an impairment in selective attention could play a role in schizophrenia. It would seem important, however, that theories advocating the centrality of an impairment in selective attention deal with the negative evidence that research such as ours and others have found.

Currently, there are a large number of formulations about pathology in different aspects of stimulus and information processing, and especially about a disorder in selective attention as being a central factor in schizophrenia. Thus far, our research has produced some positive results on aspects of thinking that are disordered in schizophrenia and are not closely related to stimulus processing, and we have produced some negative findings on select hypotheses related to selective attention. We would propose that impairments in stimulus and information processing are important phenomena that can be found in many different types of people. We have suggested, however, that other aspects of cognition are more central to the schizophrenic disorder, and if information processing is an important influence on disordered thinking, then the relationship here is not as simple and uniform as some have hypothesized. Our view is that while formulations on selective attention cannot be ruled out and there are still some promising leads in this and other areas related to information processing, the burden of proof is on those who believe in the formulations.

10. Do Any Specific Types of Subgroups of Schizophrenics Show More Thought Disorder?

The question of whether to subcategorize schizophrenics into smaller, more homogeneous, subgroups of patients has been a center of interest since the original formulations about the concept of dementia praecox by Kraepelin, which united a group of disorders that many had viewed as separate illnesses. Since the renaming of this concept as "schizophrenia" in the early part of this century by Bleuler (1950), with the belief that it may represent a group of disorders, there has been a continual search for appropriate ways to subdivide schizophrenia into more homogeneous groupings. Over the years there have been various formulations about differences in the frequency and severity of thought disorder between different subgroups of schizophrenics, with the three most widely discussed systems of subcategorizing this disorder being the process-reactive dimension, paranoid versus nonparanoid schizo-phrenia, and acute versus chronic schizophrenia.

Process Versus Reactive Schizophrenia

Our analysis of potential differences in the frequency and severity of thought disorder between process and reactive schizophrenics using the Phillips Scale of premorbid social-sexual competence to assess this dimension (Phillips, 1953) has been discussed extensively in relation to positive types of thought disorder in Chapter 4. In Chapter 7, we discussed our results for the process-reactive dimension on one type of defect state or negative cognitive symptom, namely concrete thinking.

In relation to positive types of thought disorder, during the very early acute stages of schizophrenia we found a minor tendency for process schizophrenics to show more disordered thinking than reactive schizophrenics. This tendency was not a strong one, and was not even close to significant for most of our samples. Overall, our results on process versus reactive schizophrenics at the acute phase were inconclusive for positive thought disorder.

We also analyzed the results from the process-reactive dimension for the schizophrenic sample we followed up, in terms of both potential thought pathology and functioning, and adjustment, during the post-hospital phase. Our results did not show strong differences between the process and reactive schizophrenics concerning the extent of positive thought disorder at follow-up.

Rather surprisingly, despite the hypotheses by many theorists about a very strong link between the process-reactive dimension and later outcome (Garmezy, 1970), we did not find powerful differences in overall functioning and adjustment at follow-up between the process and reactive schizophrenics (as assessed by the Phillips Scale). There were a number of nonsignificant relationships, as well as some significant and near-significant relationships between the process-reactive dimension and outcome for our sample of young, early schizophrenics at follow-up. Our overall results indicated, however, that when early, young schizophrenics are studied, and the influence of chronicity and marital status is reduced, the relationship between the process-reactive dimension and subsequent outcome is not as powerful as some theorists have assumed (Westermeyer and Harrow, 1980; In press).

Paranoid Versus Nonparanoid Schizophrenia

Another way of subcategorizing schizophrenic patients that has long been of considerable interest to workers in the field is the paranoid-nonparanoid dimension (Ritzler and Smith, 1976). Some theorists have proposed that paranoid schizophrenics may constitute a different type of disorder with a more benign clinical course, and a large number of other theorists have discussed differences between paranoid and nonparanoid schizophrenics (Kendler and Davis, 1981; Kendler and Tsuang, 1981; Magaro, 1981; Meissner, 1981). While our follow-up studies have not found strong differences in positive thought disorder between process and reactive schizophrenics after the acute phase, we have in contrast found differences in paranoid versus nonparanoid schizophrenics. Paranoid schizophrenics, who have been hypothesized to have a more favorable posthospital course, tended to show less positive thought disorder than nonparanoid schizophrenics when we studied our follow-up results. These differences were near significant with some of our samples, and did achieve statistical significance with other samples of ours. In contrast to expectations, the paranoid schizophrenics did not show significantly better posthospital functioning and adjustment (e.g., work functioning, social adjustment, etc.) than the nonparanoid schizophrenics at the first follow-up. Thus, our first follow-up did not show differences between paranoid and nonparanoid schizophrenics in overall adjustment, but did find evidence of better cognitive functioning for the paranoid schizophrenics.

Acute Versus Chronic Schizophrenia

We have subcategorized schizophrenics according to whether they are acute as opposed to chronic schizophrenics, and studied potential differences between those groups in cognitive disorders, and in other areas. Our analysis of chronic schizophrenics has included studies of four different samples of multiyear, hospitalized, chronic schizophrenics, who have spent many successive years on the "back wards" of state hospitals. The research with these patients, some of which is outlined briefly below, is discussed in greater detail in Chapters 5 and 7.

Recently, several theorists have proposed that many of these chronic schizophrenics may be "burned out," with a preponderance of deficit or negative symptoms. The suggestion is that they no longer show any positive cognitive symptoms. Contrary to this suggestion, our more recent detailed analysis has shown very severe positive cognitive symptoms in a large number of these chronic schizophrenics, when we studied them more closely. Since acute schizophrenics also show severe positive thought pathology, at this point our results on whether the acute or chronic schizophrenics show more positive thought disorder are mixed, with both of these types of samples showing severe levels.

Our analysis of negative cognitive symptoms in our multiyear, chronic schizophrenic samples and our comparison of these samples with samples of early acute schizophrenics have produced results that are in accord with theoretical expectations. The multiyear, hospitalized, chronic schizophrenics, considered as a group, showed severe levels of deficit symptoms, significantly more than the early acute schizophrenics. Thus, the chronic schizophrenics had severe levels of intellectual deficit, they were extremely concrete, and a number showed some evidence of impoverished thinking.

Some or many of these negative symptoms may be associated with the general course of schizophrenic deterioration for these chronic groups, with this course not being uniform for all schizophrenics. If this is the case, then these chronic schizophrenics may be a select group, with some or many of them once having shown a clinical picture similar to the acute young schizophrenics we have studied. Thus, they may represent some of the same types of patients as the acute schizophrenics, but they are being studied at a later stage of the same disorder. In this possibility, however, the multiyear, chronic schizophrenics would be a selective sample; that is, they would represent the subsample of schizophrenics once showing an early acute picture, but from among this larger group they would represent those patients who were destined to show considerable deficits and negative symptoms later in the course of their disorder, and to spend many years continuously hospitalized in state institutions.

Another possibility, discussed in Chapter 7, is that some of these chronic, multiyear schizophrenics with severe deficits never performed at a much higher level and always showed signs of inadequate cognitive functioning, even prior to the onset of their disorder. According to this possibility, among those people who have acute schizophrenic breaks, those with lower levels of cognitive and other skills, and with poorer integrative ability, are less likely to show resilience in terms of a partial recovery from their schizophrenic breaks. In turn, these patients are more likely to wind up as long-term chronic schizophrenics than are acute schizophrenics with higher initial ability levels and better integrative skills.

We have proposed that each of the above possibilities accounts for a portion of the long-term chronically institutionalized schizophrenic sample with severe deficits and negative symptoms. Thus, some of these chronic schizophrenics may originally have been acute schizophrenics whose functioning has shown considerable deterioration, and others may be schizophrenics with initial low levels of functioning who are only showing slight or no declines in functioning during the chronic stage.

We should note that while we have reviewed three of the traditional ways to subcategorize schizophrenics, there are other possible methods. These include methods based on the longitudinal course of their clinical picture, such as a separate analysis of those schizophrenics with continuous positive or negative thought disorder over time. We are currently studying these possibilities within the framework of a longitudinal research design.

POSITIVE THOUGHT DISORDER: THE CONSTRUCT OF BIZARRE IDIOSYNCRATIC THINKING, FACTORS THAT MAY INFLUENCE IT, AND HOW IMPORTANT IS IT IN SCHIZOPHRENIA?

1. Positive Thought Disorder and Bizarre Idiosyncratic Thinking: The Constructs and Their Potential Usefulness

We have discussed our research on a number of different types of thought pathology, with these including both positive symptoms and select types of negative or deficit symptoms, such as concrete thinking. A greater part of our efforts has centered on positive types of thought disorder. We feel that the most promising leads in our investigations of various types of positive symptoms have arisen from our studies involving the construct of bizarre-idiosyncratic thinking, which encompasses almost all of the major features that would be considered as "positive thought disorder," and in this way could unite a large body of seemingly diverse studies. Some of our research on bizarre-idiosyncratic thinking is reported in earlier chapters. In these earlier chapters, and in other individual papers we have reported, we assembled evidence supporting the idea that seemingly different types of positive thought disorder can profitably be included in a single construct, such as bizarre-idiosyncratic thinking.

In analyzing the construct of bizarre-idiosyncratic thinking, the question arises: Since the constructs of positive thought disorder and bizarre-idiosyncratic thinking are broad constructs, can these broad constructs be used to generate research on factors that may influence positive thought disorder or may even produce it? There are various ways to study the individual types of bizarre-idiosyncratic thinking as well as the broader overall construct. In terms of the *individual* kinds of bizarre-idiosyncratic thinking, in earlier chapters we outlined aspects of our research studying some of the different types, such as loose associations (Chapter 8), primitive-drive-dominated thinking (Chapter 6), boundary disturbance (Chapter 9), and conceptual overinclusion (Chapter 10).

In terms of the broader overall concepts, one of the assumptions that the broader concepts of positive thought disorder and bizarre-idio-syncratic thinking carry with them involves an expectation that, in general, the different individual types of bizarre-idiosyncratic thinking will appear in the same patients. The factor-analytic research we conducted (Chapter 15) provides some support for this assumption.

Another assumption is that some of the same rules will apply to, and some of the same factors will influence and increase the levels of, various seemingly different types of bizarre-idiosyncratic thinking, such as loose associations, conceptual overinclusion, poor logic, and the like. We have found evidence indicating that this is the case. Thus, while there are also specific considerations that may be individual to each type, the major factors we have discussed as influencing positive thought disorder seem to be able to play a role in almost all of the different, individual types of bizarre-idiosyncratic thinking.

For instance, a factor such as the influence of the acute phase of disturbance, with its consequent increase in a patient's disorganization and lower levels of cognitive efficiency, seems simultaneously to effect almost all of the various specific types of bizarre-idiosyncratic thinking that have been of interest to investigators. Our evidence indicates that acute disturbance in a schizophrenic increases the prospects of loose associations, conceptual overinclusion, poor logic, and so on. Likewise, as time passes and patients begin to emerge from the acute phase, one can expect some reduction or decrease in overall bizarre-idiosyncratic thinking, and generally in *each* of the individual types of bizarre-idiosyncratic thinking.

There are various other types of evidence that suggest that the construct of bizarre-idiosyncratic thinking can be useful. The current trend by many to classify thought disorder into two broad types— positive and negative thought disorder—fits into this scheme. Fish, for example, defined the term "positive formal thought disorder" in terms of "unusual" thoughts (Fish, 1962, p.25). While we have equated Fish's concept of positive thought disorder (based on "unusual" thoughts) with our construct of bizarre-idiosyncratic thinking, at present we are not dealing with a fixed *entity*, but rather with a seemingly useful *construct* to categorize, label, and study one major type of thought pathology.

2. Positive Thought Disorder and Bizarre Idiosyncratic Thinking: Factors That May Influence It

In addition to our discussion of bizarre-idiosyncratic thinking in earlier chapters, we also have proposed various different factors that we believe influence positive thought disorder, with some of them also having some influence on other types of positive symptoms such as delusions, and possibly hallucinations.

Overall, we have proposed a model in which disordered thinking is not a consequence of one factor, but of several factors, often interacting with each other. We believe that some of these factors cut across the thought pathology and psychosis found in schizophrenia and in some other types of severe disorders. Among these factors may be impaired perspective, intermingling, the types of confusion-disorganization that can arise in the acute phases of a severe psychotic disorder, a focus on their own private ideas by select psychotic patients, and probably additional factors that are not completely understood at present. Other factors that play a role may be more specific to certain patient groups, such as a disorder in the rate of thinking that can be found in manic patients.

Although we have not discussed brain damage in this book, observations of occasional clearly brain-damaged nonschizophrenics who show thought disorder lead one to the belief that select types of cerebral damage and/or chemical imbalances in the central nervous system (e.g., toxic psychosis patients) can be a contributor. Research by G. Tucker, and by others (e.g., Tucker, Campion, and Silberfarb, 1975; Rochford, Detre, Tucker, and Harrow, 1970) provides some formal evidence that brain damage is also a factor that can interfere with cognitive processes and increase the possibility of thought pathology.

Some or all of these factors, especially *in combination*, seem to be able to interact with each other and lead to more severe levels of disordered thinking. This is particularly evident in the acute phase of schizophrenia when the increased confusion and disorganization associated with the acute phase of disorder interacts with the schizophrenic's poor perspective and inappropriate intermingling of aspects of his inner life into his external world behavior. This complex of factors increases the acute upset and the consequent confusion-disorganization, with this resulting in even poorer perspective and inappropriate intermingling, which can increase the level of acute upset and lead to further confusion-disorganization, and so on. This *combination* can produce some of the more flagrant and dramatic examples of disordered thinking seen in schizophrenics.

There are still many unknowns, and the extent of interaction between various mechanisms involved has not been explored. Even the potential interaction between intermingling and perspective raises some interesting questions. Thus, whether a press to intermingle personal concerns by an acutely upset patient will override adequate perspective and lead to poorer use of stored knowledge about social norms and social expectations, or whether poor perspective about social norms will lead to intermingling is still an issue. One possibility is that there is an interaction between perspective and intermingling, with some combination of the two occurring, and each influencing the other.

In Chapter 5 we reported our results and discussed in greater detail our research on several of these individual factors that can influence or are involved in positive thought disorder in schizophrenia, and that can play a role in the production of bizarre-idiosyncratic thinking. These various factors are *not* parallel to each other and do not operate at the same stage or level of the cognitive process.

Thus, one factor discussed in Chapter 5, the acute disturbance, emotional intensity, and higher level of cognitive arousal found at the acute phase, can produce a disruption of hierarchical skills and of cognitive processes in general. One frequent result of this is dis-organization and disordered thinking.

At a different level of the cognitive process, intermingling involves interference with thought and speech. There is some derailing of goal-directed thinking via the emergence of a specific type of content related to various aspects of a patient's personal, and usually recent, ex-periences. The emergence of this task-irrelevant personal material into active thinking and speech can make the patient appear strange and idiosyncratic, and as such, should be viewed as a type of cognitive pathology. Personal material of this type, based on people's needs and concerns, is present as a background potential for disruption in both pathological and nonpathological individuals. It does not usually emerge overtly in blatant form for most people, however, except when they become disturbed. Other evidence of ours suggests that intermingling of personal material occurs for a variety of schizophrenics and nonschizophrenics during the periods of acute disturbance and emotional intensity found at the acute phase. The intermingling usually diminishes after the acute phase, with reductions in acute disturbance.

In contrast to the above factors, which interfere with or disrupt cognitive processes, impaired perspective about the appropriateness of one's own thinking and behavior can be viewed as an impairment in an aspect of thinking that serves as a higher-level cognitive mechanism, and is a component of routine, moment-by-moment thinking. Perspective, which is discussed at greater length in Chapter 5, is a term we have used to describe a person's effective selection from and use of his long-term stored knowledge about the range of responses and types of behavior that are socially appropriate for a particular situation. Routine perspective involves, on a moment-by-moment basis, a continual integration of long-term stored knowledge with other newer material as an influence to help guide behavior (or responses) in the situation. This background knowledge of shared social rules for behavior, along with a person's perception of what the immediate situation is, is thus used as a major factor in judgments about how one should speak and behave in a given situation.

One model of the patient's (and normal person's) behavior is that the person's ongoing behavior could be viewed as arising from moment-by-moment judgments and decisions based on the integration of:

1. The person's perception (based in part on his previous experience) of what the immediate situation or context facing the person is; with
2. the person's background long-term stored knowledge about the range of verbal and nonverbal behaviors that are socially appropriate and preferable for that type of situation.

According to this model, the total response or behavior of a person is based on the effective integration and use of stored knowledge with his or her appropriate perception of the immediate situation. Perspective, then, involves the effective selection and use of background stored knowledge about what is socially appropriate for a given situation. Viewed in this way, perspective has a major guiding role in thinking, or an executive control function, in terms of the continual planning and selecting of behavior, and decision making about how one will talk and behave in the world.

Perspective, then, concerns the relevance and effective use of long-term knowledge and experience as it interfaces with decisions about ongoing behavior, and is an important component of moment-to-moment cognitive acts. Because of the nature of its influence on thinking in terms of bringing preselected, relevant previous experience and societal norms to bear on the immediate situation, it also serves as an important cognitive control process and could be viewed as including metacognitive functions. Thus, perspective, based on background information acquired during one's experiences in childhood and adulthood, influences almost all of one's behavior and plays an integral role in thinking.

3. How Prominent and Important is Positive Thought Disorder in Schizophrenia?

Now that we have studied disordered thinking in schizophrenia from a number of viewpoints, some final discussion is in order on the implications of our research for questions about the potential importance of positive thought disorder in schizophrenia. Years ago many clinicians regarded disordered thinking as a primary symptom of schizophrenia, frequently in a rather noncritical manner. It would seem appropriate at this point to ask: Does our research support this older assumption? The answer is that it provides partial support, with considerable mixed results. Thus, in designing our overall research program to help clarify the potential importance of thought disorder, one of the central issues was: (1) is thought disorder *the* major symptom in schizophrenia? (2) is it, rather, one of *several* key symptoms in schizophrenia? or (3) is it a *minor* accompanying feature of schizophrenia that has little or no significance or importance?

In terms of evaluating whether thought disorder is a key symptom in schizophrenia, a number of aspects of our results that we have reported bear on this question. These include the following:

1. Data we have collected and reported earlier in this book and a large number of studies reported by other investigators suggest that positive thought disorders are key symptoms of the acute phase of schizophrenia, in that they are often present in flagrant form, along with several other symptoms, such as nondepressive delusions, hallucinations, disorganization, autism, and at times, paranoid ideation.

2. Our research and that of others has clearly indicated that thought disorder at the acute phase is not unique to schizophrenia (Harrow and Quinlan, 1977). Some nonschizophrenic patients from a variety of diagnostic groups also show signs of severe thought disorder, although it is more frequent and severe among schizophrenics.

3. Perhaps of most importance, the issue has arisen as to whether, at the acute phase, positive thought disorder is as frequent and severe in manic disorders and in other psychotic disorders as it is in schizophrenics. As we have noted in Chapter 4, our evidence, and that of Andreasen and others (Andreasen and Powers, 1974; Andreasen, 1979; Harrow, Grossman, Silverstein, and Meltzer, 1982), indicate that severe positive thought disorder at the acute phase is as frequent or at times more frequent in manic patients as it is in schizophrenics.

4. The issue of whether severe positive thought disorder is merely characteristic of all groups of psychotic patients, regardless of diagnosis, has not been studied fully, Early evidence of ours suggests that thought disorder is somewhat more frequent in other psychotic disorders, such as psychotic depressives, than in nonpsychotic patients. Our early evidence suggests, however, that these other psychotic groups show considerably less thought disorders than do schizophrenic and manic patient groups (Marengo and Harrow, 1985; Marengo, Harrow, McDonald, and Grinker, 1983). Thus, although some other psychotic patients show positive thought disorders, our evidence suggests that thought disorder is not just a feature that can be found in all psychotic patients.

5. The issue of whether positive thought disorder is a persistent characteristic of schizophrenic patients over time is an important one. Some traditional theories about schizophrenia assumed that thought disorder was a permanent characteristic of schizophrenia. The evidence we reported in Chapter 5 suggests that, at follow-up or at the posthospital phase, schizophrenics show either significantly or near significantly more thought disorder than patients who were not psychotic at the acute phase.

6. The data presented in Chapter 5 and other data we have collected indicate, however, that thought disorder is not a permanent characteristic for many early schizophrenics. Thus, it does not persist in many early schizophrenics. We have assessed this in schizophrenic groups using broadly based diagnostic systems, such as *DSM II*, and also using narrowly based diagnostic systems, such as *DSM III*. Some theorists feel that the newer diagnostic systems that employ a narrow concept of schizophrenia, such as *DSM III*, have separated out a "pure" group of schizophrenics. Our recent research, however,

indicates that even when one analyzes this "pure" group of *DSM III* schizophrenics. severe thought disorder does not persist for all or even most of these early schizophrenics, although a number of them show signs of psychosis which persists at reduced levels of intensity for years.

7. The data in Chapter 5 and other data of ours also indicate that when various different types of criteria for the diagnosis of schizophrenia are used, there is a subgroup of schizophrenics who show persistent thought pathology during early phases of their disorder. Thus, in both cases, with broadly defined groups of schizophrenics (*DSM II* schizophrenics) and narrowly defined schizophrenic groups (*DSM III* schizophrenics), a subgroup of these patients do show persistent thought pathology during the early phases of their disorder. The significant and near-significant differences between schizophrenic and nonschizophrenic patients at follow-up, in terms of more thought disorder for the schizophrenics, are accounted for in part by this subgroup of schizophrenics with persistent thought disorder.

8. The issue then arises of whether those schizophrenics who continue to show thought disorder at follow-up are a "sicker" group of schizophrenics, or are they the true or nuclear schizophrenics who are destined to show a downhill clinical course? At present we cannot provide a complete answer to this question, although we have begun to explore the issue (Harrow, Silverstein, and Marengo, 1983). There is no simple characteristic present at the premorbid or morbid phase of their disorder that neatly separates those schizophrenics who continue to show thought disorder at follow-up from those schizophrenics whose thought disorder remits during the posthospital phase. The thought-disordered schizophrenics do, however, show poorer outcomes and a large percentage show continued psychosis at the posthospital phase. This suggests a link between severe thought disorder and adjustment in other areas, especially continued psychosis, among early, young schizophrenics. We have begun to study this subgroup of thought-disordered schizophrenics at subsequent follow-ups to explore whether those schizophrenics with positive thought disorder at the posthospital phase are a subgroup of true or nuclear schizophrenics with a declining clinical course over time and very poor outcomes.

9. In terms of the original question about the role or importance of thought disorder in schizophrenia, our results clearly indicate that positive thought disorder is a key feature of schizophrenia during the acute phase of this disorder. Positive thought disorder is less important for many schizophrenics at follow-up, although it is still

prominent in a subgroup of these patients during the posthospital phase. Our evidence suggests that positive thought disorder plays a clear role in schizophrenia, and is one of several major features during acute and active phases of schizophrenia, rather than being the single or only key symptom in schizophrenia.

BIBLIOGRAPHY

Ackner, B. Depersonalization. II: Clinical syndromes. *Journal of Mental Science,* 1954, **100,** 854–872.

Adler, D. A. *Thought disorder in schizophrenia.* Unpublished doctoral thesis, Yale University School of Medicine, Department of Psychiatry, 1973.

Adler, D., & Harrow, M. *Manual for assessing components of idiosyncratic or bizarre responses.* ASIS/NAPS #02191. P. 1-20. New York: *Microfiche Publications,* 1973.

Adler, D., & Harrow M. Idiosyncratic thinking and personally overinvolved thinking in schizophrenic patients during partial recovery. *Comprehensive Psychiatry,* 1974, **15,** 57–67.

Allison, J., Blatt, S. J., & Zimet, C. *The interpretation of psychological tests.* New York: Harper & Row, 1968.

Almond, R. The therapeutic community. *Scientific American.* 1971, **224,** 34–42.

American Psychiatric Association, *Diagnostic and statistical manual of mental disorders (Third ed.).* Washington, D.C. American Psychiatric Association, 1980.

Andreason, N. Thought, language and communication disorders. II: Diagnostic significance. *Archives of General Psychiatry,* 1979 **36,** 1325–1330.

Andreason, N. Negative symptoms in schizophrenia. Definition and reliability. *Archives of General Psychiatry,* 1982, **39,** 784–788.

Andreason, N., & Powers, P. Overinclusive thinking in mania and schizophrenia. *British Journal of Psychiatry,* 1974, **125,** 452–456.

Andreason, N., & Powers, P. Creativity and psychosis: An examination of conceptual style. *Archives of General Psychiatry,* 1975, **32,** 70–73.

Angrist, B., Rotrosen, J., & Gershon, S. Differential effects of neuroleptics on negative versus positive symptoms in schizophrenia. *Psychopharmacology*, 1980, **72**, 17–19.

Arieti, S. *The interpretation of schizophrenia* (2nd ed.). New York: Basic Books, 1974. (a)

Arieti, S. An overview of schizophrenia from a predominantly psychological approach. *American Journal of Psychiatry*, 1974, **131**, 241–249. (b)

Asarnow, R. F., Steffy, R. A., MacCrimmon, D. J., & Cleghorn, J. M. An attentional assessment of foster children at risk for schizophrenia. In L.C. Wynne, R. L. Cromwell, & S. Matthysse (Eds.), *The nature of schizophrenia: New approaches to research and treatment.* New York: John Wiley, 1978.

Astrachan, B.M., Harrow, M., Adler, D., Brauer, L., Schwartz, A., Schwartz, C., & Tucker, G.J. A checklist for the diagnosis of schizophrenia. *British Journal of Psychiatry*, 1972, **121**, 529–539.

Astrachan, B. M., Harrow, M., Becker, R. E., Schwartz, A. H., & Miller, J. C. The unled patient group as a therapeutic tool. *International Journal of Group Psychotherapy*, 1967, 17, 178–191.

Astrup, K., & Noreik, K. *Functional psychoses: Diagnostic and prognostic models.* Springfield, Ill.: Charles C. Thomas, 1966.

Bartko, J. J., Strauss, J. S., & Carpenter, W. T. The diagnosis and understanding of schizophrenia. Part II: Expanded perspectives for describing and comparing schizophrenic patients. *Schizophrenia Bulletin*, 1974, **11**, 50–60.

Bateson, G., Jackson, D. D., Haley, J., & Weakland, J. Toward a theory of schizophrenia. *Behavioral Science*, 1956, **1**, 251–264,

Beck, A. T. *Depression: clinical, experimental and theoretical aspects.* New York: Hoeber, 1967.

Beck, A. T., Ward, C. H., Mendelson, M., Moch, J., & Erbaugh, J. An inventory for measuring depression. *Archives of General Psychiatry*, 1961 **4**, 561–571.

Beers, C. *A mind that found itself: an autobiography.* New York: Longmans Green, 1908.

Bellak, L. A multiple factor psychosomatic theory of schizophrenia. *Psychiatric Quarterly*, 1949, **23**, 783–795.

Bellak, L. The schizophrenic syndrome: A further elaboration of the unified theory of schizophrenia. In L. Bellak (Ed.), *Schizophrenia: A review of the syndrome.* New York: Grune & Stratton, 1966.

Bellak, L. & Loeb, L. (Eds.) *The schizophrenic syndrome.* New York: Grune & Stratton, 1968.

Bendig, A. W. The development of a short form of the Manifest Anxiety Scale. *Journal of Psychology.* 1956, **20**, 384.

Benjamin, J. D. A method for distinguishing and evaluating formal thinking disorders in schizophrenia. In J. S. Kasanin (Ed.),*Language and thought in schizophrenia.* New York: W.W. Norton, 1944.

Bergler, E., & Eidelberg, L. Der mechanismus der depersonalisation. *Zeitschrift für Psychoanal.*, 1935, **21**, 258–285.

Blacker, K.H., Jones, R., Stone, G., & Pfefferbaum, D. Chronic users of LSD: The "acid heads." *American Journal of Psychiatry*, 1968, **125**, 341–351.

Blatt, S. J. *Object representation in psychosis.* Paper presented to the American Psychological Association, Washington, D.C., August 1971.

Blatt, S. J., & Feirstein, A. Cardiac response and personality organization. *Journal of Consulting and Clinical Psychology*, 1977, **45**, 115–123.

Blatt, S. J., & Ritzler, B. Thought disorder and boundary disturbance in psychosis. *Journal of Consulting and Clinical Psychology*, 1974, **42**, 370–381.

Blatt, S. J., & Wild, C. *Schizophrenia: A developmental analysis.* New York: Academic Press, 1976.

Bleuler, E. *Dementia praecox or the group of schizophrenias.* New York: International Universities Press, 1911 (English translation: 1950).

Bower, A., Testin, R., & Roberts, A. Rorschach diagnosis by a systematic combining of content, thought process, and determinant scales. *Genetic Psychology Monographs*, 1960, **62**, 165–172.

Bowers, M. B., Jr. *Retreat from sanity.* New York: Human Sciences Press, 1974.

Bowers, M. B., Jr. & Freedman, D. X. "Psychedelic" experiences in acute psychosis. *Archives of General Psychiatry* 1966, **15**, 240–258

Braff, D. L. & Beck, A. T. Thinking disorder in depression. *Archives of General Psychiatry.* 1974, **31**, 456–459.

Braff, D. L., & Sacuzzo, D. P. Information processing dysfunction in paranoid schizophrenia: A two-factor deficit. *American Journal of Psychiatry*, 1981, **138**, 1051–1056.

Brattemo, C. E. Interpretations of proverbs in schizophrenic patients: Further studies. *Acta Psychologica* (Amsterdam), 1962, **20**, 254–263.

Brauer, R., Harrow, M., & Tucker, G.J. Depersonalization phenomena in psychiatric patients. *The British Journal of Psychiatry*, 1970, **117**, 509–515.

Brenneis, B. Features of the manifest dream in schizophrenia. *Journal of Nervous and Mental Disease*, 1971, **153**, 81–91.

Brenner, C. *Textbook of psychoanalysis.* Garden City, NY: Doubleday, 1957.

Broen, W. *Schizophrenia, research and theory.* New York: Academic Press, 1968.

Broga, M. I., & Neufeld, R.W.J. Dimensions of thinking among process and reactive schizophrenics. *Psychological Record*, 1977, **27**, 265–277.

Bromet, E., & Harrow, M. Behavioral overinclusion as a prognostic index in schizophrenic disorders. *Journal of Abnormal Psychology*, 1973, **83**, 345–349.

Bromet, E., Harrow, M., & Kasl, S. Premorbid functioning and outcome in schizophrenics and nonschizophrenics. *Archives of General Psychiatry*, 1974, **30**, 203–207.

Bromet, E., Harrow, M., & Tucker, G. Factors related to short-term prognosis in schizophrenia and depression. *Archives of General Psychiatry*, 1971, **25**, 148–154.

Brown, R. Schizophrenia, language and reality. *American Psychologist*, 1973, **28**, 395–403.

Buss, A. H., & Lang, P. Psychological deficit in schizophrenia. I. Affect, reinforcement, and concept attainment. *Journal of Abnormal Psychology*, 1965, **70**, 2–24.

Buss, A. H. & Buss, E. H. (Eds.) *Theories of schizophrenia.* New York: Atherton Press, 1972.

Callaway, E. Schizophrenia and interference. *Archives of General Psychiatry*, 1970, **22**, 193–208.

Callaway, E., & Naghdi, S. An information processing model for schizophrenia. *Archives of General Psychiatry*, 1982, **39**, 339–347.

Cameron, N. Schizophrenic thinking in a problem-solving situation. *Journal of Mental Science*, 1939, **85**, 1012–1035.

Cameron, N. Experimental analysis of schizophrenic thinking. In J.S. Kasanin (Ed.), *Language and thought in schizophrenia.* New York: Norton, 1944.

Cameron, N. *The psychology of behavior disorders.* Boston: Houghton-Mifflin, 1947.

Cameron, N. *Personality development and psychopathology.* Boston: Houghton-Mifflin, 1963.

Cameron, N., & Margaret, A. *Behavior pathology.* Boston: Houghton-Mifflin, 1951.

Cancro, R. Abstraction on proverbs in process-reactive schizophrenia. *Journal of Consulting and Clinical Psychology,* 1969, **33,** 267–270.

Carlson, K., Quinlan, D., Tucker, G.J., & Harrow, M. Body disturbance and sexual elaboration factors in figure drawings of schizophrenic patients. *Journal of Personality Assessment,* 1973 **37,** 56–63.

Carlson, K., Tucker, G.J., Harrow, M., & Quinlan, D. Body image and mental illness: A study of the human figure drawings of psychiatric patients. In I. Jakab (Ed.), *Conscious and unconscious expressive art.* Basel, New York: Karger 1971.

Carson, R. Proverb interpretation in acutely schizophrenic patients. *Journal of Nervous and Mental Diseases,* 1962, **135,** 556–564.

Carpenter, W. T., Strauss, J. T. & Bartko, J. J. The diagnosis of schizophrenia. Part I: Use of signs and symptoms for the identification of schizophrenic patients. *Schizophrenia Bulletin,* 1974, **11,** 37–49.

Chaika, E. Thought disorder or speech disorder in schizophrenia? *Schizophrenia Bulletin,* 1982, **8,** 587–591.

Chapman, J. The early symptoms of schizophrenia. *British Journal of Psychiatry,* 1966, **112,** 225–251.

Chapman, L. Confusion of figurative and literal usages of words by schizophrenics and brain damaged patients. *Journal of Abnormal Psychology,* 1960, **60,** 412–416.

Chapman, L. A reinterpretation of some pathological disturbances in conceptual breadth. *Journal of Abnormal Psychology,* 1961, *62,* 514–519.

Chapman, L. J., & Chapman, J. P. *Disordered thinking in schizophrenia.* New York: Appleton-Century Crofts, 1973.

Chapman, L. J., Chapman, J. P., & Miller, G. A. A theory of verbal behavior in schizophrenia. *Progress in experimental personality research,* 1964, *1,* 49–77.

Cleveland, S. Body image changes associated with personality reorganization. *Journal of Consulting Psychology,* 1960, **24,** 256–261.

Cohen, B. Referent communication in schizophrenia In S. Schwartz (Ed.), *Cognition and language in schizophrenia.* Hillsdale, NJ: Erlbaum, 1978.

Cohen, B., Nachmani, G., & Rosenberg, S. Referent communication disturbances in acute schizophrenia. *Journal of Abnormal Psychology,* 1974, **83,** 1–13.

Colbert, J. & Harrow, M. Psychomotor retardation in depressive syndromes. *Journal of Nervous and Mental Disease.* 1967, **145,** 405–419.

Craig, W. J. Objective measures of thinking integrated with psychotic symptoms. *Psychological Reports,* 1965, **16,** 539–546.

Crowne, D. P. & Marlowe, D. *The approval motive.* New York: Wiley, 1964.

Deese, J. Thought into speech: Linguistic rules and psychological limitations in processing information determine how we put our ideas into words. *American Scientist,* 1978, **66,** 314–321.

Detre, T. P., & Jarecki, H. G. *Modern psychiatric treatment.* Philadelphia: J. B. Lippincott, 1971.

DeWolfe, A.S. Are there two kinds of thinking in process and reactive schizophrenics? *Journal of Abnormal Psychology,* 1974, **83,** 285–290.

Dixon, J. C. Depersonalization phenomena in a sample population of college students. *British Journal of Psychiatry,* 1963, **109,** 371–375.

Efron, H. Y., & Piotrowski, Z. A. A factor analytic study of the Rorschach Prognostic Index. *Journal of Projective Techniques and Personality Assessment,* 1966, **30,** 179–183.

Eliseo, T. S. Figurative and literal misinterpretation of words by process and reactive schizophrenics. *Psychological Reports,* 1963, **13,** 871–877.

Erlenmeyer-Kimling, L., & Cornblatt, B. Attentional measures in a study of children at high risk for schizophrenia. *Journal of Psychiatric Research,* 1978, **14,** 93–98.

Epstein, S. Overinclusive thinking in a schizophrenic and a control group. *Journal of Consulting Psychology,* 1953, **17,** 384–388.

Eysenck, H. J. The questionnaire measurement of neuroticism and extraversion. *Rivista di Psicologica,* 1956, **50,** 113–140.

Eysenck, H. J. *Manual of the Maudsley Personality Inventory.* London: University of London Press, 1959.

Federn, P. *Ego psychology and the psychoses.* New York: Basic Books, 1952.

Feffer, M. H., & Schnell, M. *Manual for the role taking test* (Document 9010). Washington, D.C.: American Documentation Institute, 1960.

Fenichel, O. *The psychoanalytic theory of neuroses.* New York: W. W. Norton, 1945.

Fierman, L. *Effective psychotherapy: The contributions of Hellmuth Kaiser.* New York: Free Press, 1965.

Fish, F.J. *Schizophrenia.* Bristol, UK: John Wright & Sons, Ltd., 1962.

Fisher, S. A further appraisal of the body image boundary concept. *Journal of Consulting and Clinical Psychology,* 1963, **27,** 62–74.

Fisher, S. Body image and psychopathology. *Archives of General Psychiatry,* 1964, **10, 519–529.**

Fisher, S. Body image and neurotic and schizophrenic patients. *Archives of General Psychiatry,* 1966, **15,** 90–101.

Fisher, S., & Cleveland, S. E. *Body image and personality.* New York: van Nostrand, 1958.

Fisher, S., & Cleveland, S. E. *Body image and personality* (2nd rev. ed.). New York: Dover, 1968.

Flavell, J. H. Metacognition and cognitive monitoring: A new area of cognitive developmental inquiry. *American Psychologist,* 1979, **34,** 906–911.

Foulds, G. A., Hope, K., McPherson, F. M., & Mayo, P. R. Cognitive disorder among the schizophrenias. I. The validity of some tests of thought-process disorder. *British Journal of Psychiatry,* 1967, **113,** 1361–1368.(a)

Foulds, G. A. , Hope, K., McPherson, F. M. , & Mayo, P. R. Cognitive disorder among the schizophrenias. II. Differences between the sub-categories. *British Journal of Psychiatry,* 1967, **113,** 1369–1374.(b)

Freedman, B. J. The subjective experience of perceptual and cognitive disturbances in schizophrenia. *Archives of General Psychiatry,* 1974, **30,** 333–340.

Freedman, B., & Chapman, L. Early subjective experience in schizophrenic episodes. *Journal of Abnormal Psychology,* 1973, **82,** 46–54.

Freud, S. *The ego and the id.* Trans. by J. Riviere. London: Hogarth Press, 1927 (1923).

Freud, S. *New introductory lectures on psychoanalysis.* New York: W.W. Norton, 1933.

Freud, S. *The interpretation of dreams.* New York: Avon Edition, Basic Books, 1965, (originally published: 1900).

Freud, S. *Inhibition, symptoms and anxiety.* Trans. by A. Strachey, Rev. ed. by J. Strachey. New York: Norton, 1977 (1926).

Friedman, A. S., Cowitz, B., Cohen, H. W. , et al. Syndromes and themes of psychotic depression. *Archives of General Psychiatry,* 1963, **9**, 504–509.

Friedman, H. Perceptual regression in schizophrenia: An hypothesis suggested by the Rorschach test. *Journal of Projective Techniques,* 1953, 17,171-185.

Galdston, I. On the etiology of depersonalization. *Journal of Nervous and Mental Disease,* 1947, **105**, 25–39.

Garmezy, N. Process and reactive schizophrenia: Some conceptions and issues. *Schizophrenia Bulletin,* 1970, **2**, 30–67.

Garmezy, N. Children at risk: The search for the antecedents of schizophrenia. Part II: Ongoing research programs, issues and intervention. *Schizophrenia Bulletin,* 1974, **1**, 55–125.

Garmezy, N. Attentional processes in adult schizophrenia and in children at risk. *Journal of Psychiatric Research,* 1978, **14**, 3–34.

Gathercole, C. E. A note on some tests of "overinclusive thinking." *British Journal of Medical Psychology,* 1965, **38**, 59–62.

Glass, G. & Bowers, M. B., Jr. Chronic psychosis associated with long-term psychotomimetic use. *Archives of General Psychiatry,* 1970, **23**, 97–103.

Goldstein, K. Methodological approach to the study of schizophrenic thought disorder. In J. S. Kasanin (Ed.), *Language and thought in schizophrenia.* New York: Norton, 1944.

Goldstein, K. Concerning the concreteness in schizophrenia. *Journal of Abnormal Psychology,* 1959, **59**, 146–148.

Goldstein, K. & Scheerer, M. Abstract and concrete behavior: Experimental study with special tests. *Psychological Monographs,* 1941, **53**, (2).

Goldstein, M., Rodnick, E.H., Jones, J.E., McPherson, S.R., & West, K.L. Familial precursors of schizophrenia spectrum disorders. In L.C. Wynne, R.L. Cromwell, & S. Matthysse (Eds.), *The nature of schizophrenia: New approaches to research and treatment.* New York: Wiley, 1978.

Goldstein, R. H., & Salzman, L. H. Proverb word counts as a measure of overinclusiveness in delusional schizophrenics. *Journal of Abnormal Psychology,* 1965, **70**, 244–250.

Gordon, R., Silverstein, M.L., & Harrow, M. Associative thinking in schizophrenia: A contextual approach. *Journal of Clinical Psychology,* 1982, 38, 684-696.

Gorham, D. R. Proverbs test for clinical and experimental use. *Psychological Reports,* Monograph Suppl. 1, 1956.

Gottschalk, L. A., & Gleser, G. C. *The measurement of psychological states through the content analysis of verbal behavior.* Berkeley and Los Angeles: University of California Press, 1969.

Grinker, R. R., Miller, J., Sabshin, M., Nunn, S., & Nunnally, J. *The phenomena of depressions.* New York: Hoeber, 1961.

Grossman, L., Harrow, M., Lazar, B., Kettering, R., Meltzer, H. & Lechert, J. Do thought disorders persist in manic patients? *Scientific Proceedings* of the 134th Annual Meeting of the American Psychiatric Association. Washington, D.C.: American Psychiatric Association, 1981.

Gruenberg, E. *The natural history of schizophrenia.* Boston: Little, Brown, 1974.

Gruenberg, E. M. From practice to theory: Community health services and the nature of psychoses. *The Lancet,* 1969, *1*(7597), 721–724.

Harrow, M., & Adler, D. *Are schizophrenics concrete?* presented at the 46th Annual Meeting of the Midwestern Psychological Association, Chicago, May 1974.

Harrow, M., Adler, D., & Hanf, E. Abstract and concrete thinking in schizophrenia during prechronic phases. *Archives of General Psychiatry,* 1974, **31,** 27–33.

Harrow, M., Bromet, E., & Quinlan, D. Predictors of posthospital adjustment in schizophrenia: Thought disorders and schizophrenic diagnosis. *Journal of Nervous and Mental Disease,* 1974, **158,** 25–36.

Harrow, M., Buckley-Marengo, J., Growe, G., & Grinker, R. R., Sr. Schizophrenic deterioration and concrete thinking. *Scientific Proceedings* of 132nd Annual Meeting of the American Psychiatric Association, 56–57. Washington, D.C.: American Psychiatric Association. 1979.

Harrow, M., & Ferrante, A. Locus of control in psychiatric patients. *Journal of Consulting and Clinical Psychology,* 1969, **33,** 582–589.

Harrow, M., Grinker, Sr., R. R., Holzman, P., & Kayton, L. Anhedonia and schizophrenia. *American Journal of Psychiatry,* 1977, 134, 794-797.

Harrow, M., Grinker, R. R., Sr., Silverstein, M. L., & Holzman, P. Is modern-day schizophrenic outcome still negative? *American Journal of Psychiatry,* 1978, **135** (10), 1156–1162.

Harrow, M., Grossman, L. S., Silverstein, M. L., & Meltzer, H.Y. Are manic patients thought disordered? *Scientific Proceedings* of the American Psychiatric Association. Washington, D.C.: American Psychiatric Association, 1980.

Harrow, M., Grossman, L.S., Silverstein, M.L., & Meltzer, H.Y. Thought pathology in manic and schizophrenic patients: At hospital admission and seven weeks later. *Archives of General Psychiatry,* 1982, **39,** 665–671.

Harrow, M., Grossman, L. S., Silverstein, M. L., Meltzer, H. Y., & Kettering, R. L. A longitudinal study of thought disorder in manic patients. *Archives of General Psychiatry,* in press.

Harrow, M., Harkavy, K., Bromet, E., & Tucker, G.J. A longitudinal study of schizophrenic thinking. *Archives of General Psychiatry,* 1973, **28,** 179–182.

Harrow, M., Himmelhoch J.M., Tucker, G.J., Hersh, J., & Quinlan, D. Over-inclusive thinking in acute schizophrenic patients. *Journal of Abnormal Psychology,* 1972, **79,** 161–168.

Harrow, M., Lanin-Kettering, I., Prosen, M., & Miller, J.G. Disordered thinking in schizophrenia: Intermingling and loss of set. *Schizophrenia Bulletin,* 1983, **9,** 354–367.

Harrow, M., Marengo, J., Pogue-Geile, M. & Pawelski, T. J. Schizophrenic deficits in intelligence and abstract thinking: Influence of aging and long-term institutionalization. In N. Miller (Ed.), *Schizophrenia, paranoia, and schizophreniform disorders in later life.* New York: Guilford Press, in press.

Harrow, M., & Miller, J. G. Schizophrenic thought disorders and impaired perspective. *Journal of Abnormal Psychology,* 1980, **89,** 717–727.

Harrow, M., & Prosen, M. Intermingling and disordered logic as influences on schizophrenic "thought disorders." *Archives of General Psychiatry*, 1978, **136:** 1213–1218.

Harrow, M., & Prosen, M. Schizophrenic thought disorders: bizarre associations and intermingling. *American Journal of Psychiatry*, 1979, **136**, 293–296.

Harrow, M., & Quinlan, D. M. Primary process thinking and schizophrenia. *Scientific Proceedings* of 126th Annual Meeting of the American Psychiatric Association, 226–227. Washington, D.C.: American Psychiatric Association, 1973.

Harrow, M., & Quinlan, D. M. Is disordered thinking unique to schizophrenia? *Archives of General Psychiatry*, 1977, **34**, 15–21.

Harrow, M., Quinlan, D., Wallington, S., & Pickett, L., Jr., Primitive drive-dominated thinking: Relationship to acute schizophrenia and sociopathy. *Journal of Personality Assessment,* 1976, **40**, 31–41.

Harrow, M., & Silverstein, M. L. Psychotic symptoms in schizophrenia after the acute phase. *Schizophrenia Bulletin,* 1977, **3,** 608–616.

Harrow, M., & Silverstein, M. L. Cognitive processes during the postacute phase of schizophrenia. In S. B. Sells & R. Crandall et al. (Eds.), *Human functioning in longitudinal perspective.* Baltimore: Wilkins, 1980.

Harrow, M., & Silverstein, M.L. The road to nosologic nirvana: A reply to M. Taylor. *Archives of General Psychiatry*, 1981, **38**, 1298–1299.

Harrow, M., Silverstein, M. L., & Marengo, J. Disordered thinking: Does it identify nuclear schizophrenia? *Archives of General Psychiatry*, 1983, 40, 765–771.

Harrow, M., Silverstein, M., Graef, R., Quinlan, D., & Lazar, B. *Disorders of attention and stimulus overinclusion in schizophrenia.* Presented at the 86th Annual Meeting of the American Psychological Association, Toronto, Canada, August 28–September 1, 1978.

Harrow, M., Tucker, G. J., & Adler, D. Concrete and idiosyncratic thinking in acute schizophrenic patients. *Archives of General Psychiatry*, 1972, **26, 433–439.

Harrow, M., Tucker, G. J., & Bromet E. Short-term prognosis of schizophrenic patients. In R. Cancro (Ed.), *The schizophrenic syndrome: An annual review.* New York: Bruner-Mazel, 1971.

Harrow, M., Tucker, G. J., Himmelhoch J., & Putnam, N. Schizophrenic "thought disorders" after the acute phase. *American Journal of Psychiatry*, 1972, **128,** 824–829.

Harrow, M., Tucker, G. J., & Shield, P. Stimulus overinclusion in schizophrenic disorders. *Archives of General Psychology*, 1972, **27,** 40–45.

Hasenfus, N. & Magaro, P. Creativity and schizohrenia: An equality of empirical constructs. *British Journal of Psychiatry*, 1976, **129**, 346–349.

Hawks, D. V. The clinical usefulness of some tests of overinclusive thinking in psychiatric patients. *British Journal of Social and Clinical Psychology*, 1964, **3,** 186–195.

Heaton, R. K., & Victor, R. G. Personality characteristics associated with psychedelic flashbacks in natural and experimental settings. *Journal of Abnormal Psychology*, 1976, **85,** 83–90.

Higgins, J. Process-reactive schizophrenia, recent developments. In R. Cancro (Ed.), *The schizophrenic syndrome: An annual review,* Vol 1. New York: Bruner-Mazel, 1971.

Himmelhoch, J., Harrow, M., Tucker, G. J., & Hersh, J. Manual for assessment of selected aspects of thinking: Object sorting test. New York: *Microfiche Publications,* ASIS/NAPS #02206, P. 1-25, 1973.

Hirsch, S. R., & Leff, J. P. *Abnormalities in parents of schizophrenics.* London: Oxford University Press, 1975.

Holt, R. R. Gauging primary and secondary process in Rorschach responses. *Journal of Projective Techniques,* 1956, **20,** 14–25.

Holt, R. R. *Manual for the scoring of primary process manifestations in Rorschach responses* (9th ed.). Unpublished manuscript, 1963.

Holt, R. R. *Manual for the scoring of primary process manifestations in Rorschach responses* (10th ed.). Unpublished manuscript, 1970.

Holt, R. R. A method for assessing primary process manifestations and their control in Rorschach responses. In M. A. Rickers-Ovsiankina (Ed.), *Rorschach psychology* (rev. ed.). Huntington, NY: Krieger, 1977.

Holt, R. R., & Havel, J. A method for assessing primary and secondary processes in Rorschach responses. *Journal of Projective Techniques,* 1956, **20,** 14–15.

Holt, R. R. & Havel, J. A method for assessing primary and secondary process in the Rorschach. In M. A. Rickers-Ovsiankina (Ed.), *Rorschach psychology.* New York: John Wiley & Sons, 1965.

Holtzman, W. H., Gorham, D. R., & Moran, L. J. A factor-analytic study of schizophrenic thought processes. Cited in Holtzman et al. *Inkblot perception and personality.* Austin: University of Texas Press, 1961.

Holtzman, W. H., Gorham, D. R. & Moran, L. J. A factor-analytic study of schizophrenic thought processes. *Journal of Abnormal Psychology,* 1964, 69, 355-364.

Holtzman, W. H., Thorpe, J. S., Swartz, J. D., & Herron, E. W. *Inkblot perception and personality.* Austin: University of Texas Press, 1961.

Holzman, P. S. Cognitive impairment and cognitive stability: Towards a theory of thought disorder. In G. Serban (Ed.), *Cognitive defects in the development of mental illness.* New York: Bruner-Mazel, 1978.

Holzman, P. S. & Rousey, C. Monitoring, activation, and disinhibition: Effects of white noise masking on spoken thought. *Journal of Abnormal Psychology,* 1970, **75,** 227–241.

Holzman, P. S., & Rousey, C. Disinhibition of communicated thought: Generality and role of cognitive style. *Journal of Abnormal Psychology,* 1971, **77,** 263–274.

Hughlings-Jackson, J. *Selected writings* (J. Taylor, Ed.). London: Hodeler & Stoughton, 1931.

Hunt, W. A., Jones, N. F. & Hunt, E. B. Reliability of clinical judgment as a function of clinical experience. *Journal of Clinical Psychology,* 1957, **13,** 377–378.

Jacobsen, E. Contributions to the metapsychology of cyclothymic depression. In P. Greenacre (Ed.), *Affective disorders: psychoanalytic contributions to their study.* New York: International Universities Press, 1953.

Jacobsen, E. *The self and the object world.* New York: International Universities Press, 1964.

Jefferson, G. Error correction as an interactional resource. *Language in Society,* 1974, **2,** 181–199.

Johnson, D. *Cognitive organization in paranoid and nonparanoid schizophrenia.* Doctoral dissertation, Yale University, 1980.

Johnson, D. R., & Quinlan, D. M. Fluid and rigid boundaries of paranoid and non-paranoid schizophrenics on a role-playing task. *Journal of Personality Assessment,* 1980, **44,** 523–531.

Johnston, M.H., & Holzman, P. S. *Assessing schizophrenic thinking* San Francisco: Jossey-Bass, 1979.

Jortner, S. An investigation of certain cognitive aspects of schizophrenia. *Journal of Projective Techniques and Personality Assessment,* 1966, **30,** 559–568.

Kantor, R. E., & Herron, W. G. *Reactive and process schizophrenia.* Palo Alto, CA: Science and Behavior Books, 1966.

Kaplan, B. *The inner world of mental illness.* New York: Harper & Row, 1964.

Keith, S. J., & Buchsbaum, S. NIMH activities: Workshop on factors related to premorbid adjustment. *Schizophrenia Bulletin,* 1978, **4,** 252–257.

Keith, S. J., Gunderson, J. G., Reifman, A., Buchsbaum, S., & Mosher, L. R. Special report: Schizophrenia 1976. *Schizophrenia Bulletin,* 1976, **2,** 510–565.

Kelly, D. H. W., & Walter, C. J. S. The relationship between clinical diagnosis and anxiety, assessed by forearm blood flow and other measurements. *British Journal of Psychiatry,* 1968, **114,** 611–626.

Kendler, K. S., & Davis, L. D. The genetics and biochemistry of paranoid schizophrenia and other paranoid psychoses. *Schizophrenia Bulletin,* 1981, **7,** 689–709.

Kendler, K. S. & Tsuang, M. T. Nosology of paranoid schizophrenia and other paranoid psychoses. *Schizophrenia Bulletin,* 1981, **7,** 594–610.

Khavari, K. A., Mabry, E., & Humes, M. Personality correlates of hallucinogenic use. *Journal of Abnormal Psychology,* 1977, **86,** 172-178.

Klein, D. F., & Davis, J. M. *Diagnosis and drug treatment of psychiatric disorders.* Baltimore: Williams & Wilkins, 1969.

Knight, R., Sherer, M., Putchat, C., & Carter, G. A picture integration task for measuring iconic memory in schizophrenics. *Journal of Abnormal Psychology,* 1978, **87,** 314–321.

Koh, S. D. Remembering of verbal materials by schizophrenic young adults. In S. Schwartz (Ed.), *Language and cognition in schizophrenia.* Hillsdale, NJ: Erlbaum, 1978.

Kornetsky, C., & Orzack, M. H. Physiological and behavioral correlates of attention dysfunction in schizophrenic patients. *Journal of Psychiatric Research,* 1978, **14,** 69–79.

Kraepelin, E. *Dementia praecox and paraphrenia* (Trans. R. M. Barclay). Edinburgh: Livingstone, 1950, (originally published in 1919).

Kris, E. *Psychoanalytic explorations in art.* New York: International Universities Press, 1952.

Kuster, G., Harrow, M., & Tucker, G. J. Kinesthetic figural aftereffects in acute schizophrenia: A style of processing stimuli? *Perceptual and Motor Skills,* 1975, 41, 451-458.

Kwawer, J. S., Lerner, H. D., Lerner, P. M., & Sugarman, A. (Eds.). *Borderline phenomena and the Rorschach test.* New York: International Universities Press, 1980.

Landis, B. Ego boundaries. *Psychological Issues,* 1970, **6** (Monograph 24).

Lang, P. J., & Buss, A. H. Psychological deficit in schizophrenia. II: Interference and activation. *Journal of Abnormal Psychology,* 1965, **70,** 77–106.

Lanin-Kettering, I. & Harrow, M. The though behind the words: A view of schizophrenic speech and thinking disorders. *Schizophrenia Bulletin,* In Press.

Lazar, B., & Harrow, M. Primitive drive dominated thinking. In R. Henley Woody (Ed.), *Encyclopedia of clinical assessment,* Volume 1. San Francisco: Jossey-Bass, 1980.

Lazare, A., Klerman, G.L., & Armor, D. Oral, obsessive, and hysterical personality patterns. *Archives of General Psychiatry,* 1966, **14,** 624–630.

Levitan, H. L. The depersonalizing process. *Psychoanalytic Quarterly*, 1969, **38**, 97–109.

Levitan, H. L. The depersonalizing process: The sense of reality and unreality. *Psychoanalytic Quarterly*, 1970, **39**, 449–470.

Lewis, A. Melancholia: A clinical survey of depressive states. *Journal of Mental Science*, 1934, *80*, 277–378.

Lewis, M. L. Rodnick, E. H., & Goldstein, M. J. Intrafamilial interactive behavior, parental communication deviance, and risk for schizophrenia. *Journal of Abnormal Psychology*, 1981, **90**, 448–457.

Lidz, T. *The origin and treatment of schizophrenic disorders.* New York: Basic Books, 1973.

Lidz, T., Cornelison, A., Fleck, S. & Terry, D. The intrafamilial environment of the schizophrenic patient: I. The father. *Psychiatry*, 1957, 20, 329-342.(a)

Lidz, T., Cornelison, A., Fleck, S. & Terry, D. The intrafamilial environment of the schizophrenic patient: II. Marital schism and marital skew. *American Journal of Psychiatry*, 1957, 114, 241-248. (b)

Lidz, T., Cornelison, A., Fleck, S. & Terry, D. The intrafamilial environment of the schizophrenic patient: IV. The transmission of irrationality. *Archives of General Psychiatry*, 1958, 79, 305-315.

Lidz, T., Fleck, S., Alanen, Y. O., & Cornelison, A. Schizophrenic patients and their siblings. *Psychiatry*, 1963, 26, 1-18.

Lidz, T., Fleck, S., & Cornelison, A. *Schizophrenia and the family.* New York: International Universities Press, 1965.

Liem, J. H. Effects of verbal communication of parents and children: A comparison of normal and schizophrenic families. *Journal of Consulting and Clinical Psychology*, 1974, **42**, 438–450.

Lloyd, D. N. Overinclusive thinking and delusions in schizophrenic patients: A critique. *Journal of Abnormal Psychology*, 1967, **72**, 451–453.

Lowe, C. M. *A study of the nature of guilt in psychopathology.* Unpublished doctoral dissertation, Ohio State University, 1961.

MacDonald, N. The other side: Living with schizophrenia. *Canadian Medical Association Journal*, 1960, **82**, 218–221.

Magaro, P. A. The paranoid and the schizophrenic: The case for distinct cognitive styles. *Schizophrenia Bulletin*, 1981, **7**, 632–661.

Maher, B. *Principles of psychopathology: an experimental approach.* New York: McGraw-Hill, 1966.

Maher, B. The language of schizophrenia: A review and interpretation. *British Journal of Psychiatry*, 1972, **120**, 3–17.

Maher, B. A., McKean, K., & McLaughlin, B. Studies in psychotic language. In P.J. Stone, D.C. Dunphy et al. (Eds.) *The general inquirer: A computer approach to content analysis.* Cambridge: MIT Press, 1966.

Mahler, M. *On human symbiosis and the vicissitudes of individuation. Vol. 1: Infantile psychoses.* New York: International Universities Press, 1968.

Marengo, J. B., & Harrow, M. *Abstract and concrete thinking in early schizophrenia: Previous assumptions and current realities.* Presented at the 51st Annual Meeting of the Midwestern Psychological Association. Chicago, May 1979.

Marengo, J. B. & Harrow, M. Thought disorder: A function of schizophrenia, mania, or psychosis? Journal of Nervous and Mental Disease, 1985, *173*.

Marengo, J., Harrow, M., Lanin-Kettering, I., & Wilson, A. A manual for scoring

idiosyncratic and bizarre responses to the proverbs and social comprehension test. In M. Harrow & D.M. Quinlan, *Disordered thinking and
schizophrenic psychopathology.* New York: Gardner Press, in press.

Marengo, J., Harrow, M., McDonald, C., & Grinker, R. The early course of
schizophrenic thought disorder. *Scientific Proceedings* of the 136th Annual
Meeting of the American Psychiatric Association. New York, April 30–
May 6, 1983.

Marengo, J., Harrow, M., & Rogers, C. *A manual for scoring abstract and concrete
responses to the proverbs test.* New York: *Microfiche Publications,* ASIS/
NAPS #03646. 1980.

Mayer-Gross, W. On depersonalization. *British Journal of Medical Psychology,*
1935, **15,** 103–122.

McGhie, A., & Chapman, J. Disorders of attention and perception in early
schizophrenia. *British Journal of Medical Psychology,* 1961, **34,** 103–116.

McGlothin, W. H., Arnold, D. & Freedman, D. X. Organicity measures following
repeated LSD ingestion. *Archives of General Psychiatry,* 1969, **21,** 704–
709.

McGlothin, W., Cohen, S., & McGlothin, M., Long-lasting effects of LSD on
normals. *Archives of General Psychiatry,* 1967, **17,** 521–578.

Meadow, A., Greenblatt, M., Funkenstein, D., et al. Relationship between
capacity for abstraction in schizophrenia and physiologic response to
autonomic drugs. *Journal of Nervous and Mental Diseases,* 1953, **118,** 332–
338.

Meadow, A., Greenblatt, M., Solomon, H., & Funkenstein, D. H. Looseness of
association and impairment in abstraction in schizophrenia. *Journal of
Nervous and Mental Disease,* 1953, **118,** 27–35.

Meissner, W. W. The schizophrenic and the paranoid process. *Schizophrenia
Bulletin,* 1981, **7,** 611–631.

Miller, J. G., Harrow, M., Lanin, I. B., & Neiditz, J. *The role of loss of perspective in
psychotic thinking.* Presented at the 1981 American Psychological Association Convention, Los Angeles, August 24–28, 1981.

Mishler, E. G., & Waxler, N. E. Decision process in psychiatric hospitalization:
Patients referred, accepted and admitted to a psychiatric hospital.
American Sociological Review, 1963, **28,** 576–587.

Mishler, E. G., & Waxler, N. E. *Family processes and schizophrenia: Theory and
selected experimental studies.* New York: Science House, 1968. (a)

Mishler, E. G., & Waxler, N. E. *Interaction in families: An experimental study of family
processes and schizophrenia.* New York: Wiley, 1968. (b)

Naditch, M. P. Acute adverse reactions to psychoactive drugs. *Journal of
Abnormal Psychology,* 1974, **83,** 394–403.

Naditch, M. P. Relation of motives for drug use and psychopathology in the
development of acute adverse reactions to psychoactive drugs. *Journal of
Abnormal Psychology,* 1975, **84,** 374–385.

Neale, J. M., & Crowell, R. L. Size estimation in schizophrenics as a function of
stimulus presentation time. *Journal of Abnormal Psychology,* 1968, **73,** 44–
48.

Nelson, J. C., & Bowers, M. B., Jr. Delusional unipolar depression: Description
and drug response. *Archives of General Psychiatry,* 1972, **26,** 546–552.

Neuchterlein, K. H. Reaction time and attention in schizophrenia: A critical
evaluation of the data and theories. *Schizophrenia Bulletin,* 1977, **3,** 373–
428.

Nunberg, H. *Allegemeine Neurosenlehre.* Bern and Berlin: H. Huber 1932.

Oberndorf, C. P. The role of anxiety in depersonalization. *International Journal of Psychoanalysis,* 1950, **31,** 1–5.

Oltmanns, T. F. & Neale, J. M. Abstraction and schizophrenia: Problems in psychological deficit research. In B. Maher (Ed.), *Progress in Experimental Personality Research,* Vol. 8. New York: Academic Press, 1978.

Oltmanns, T. F., Ohayon, J. & Neale, J. M. The effect of antipsychotic medication and diagnostic criteria on distractibility in schizophrenia. In L. C. Wynne, R. L. Cromwell, & S. Matthysse (Eds.), *The nature of schizophrenia: New approaches to research and treatment.* New York: John Wiley & Sons, 1978. Pp. 283-286.

Overall, J., & Gorham, D. The brief psychiatric rating scale. *Psychiatric Report,* 1962, **10,** 799–812.

Pavy, D. Verbal behavior in schizophrenia. *Psychological Bulletin,* 1968, 70, 164–178.

Pawelski, T. J., Harrow, M., Grinker, R. R., Sr., & Grossman, L. S. The construct of schizophrenia: Should a narrow or broad construct be used? In R. R. Grinker, Sr., & M. Harrow (Eds.), *A multidimensional approach to clinical research for schizophrenia.* Springfield, IL: Charles C. Thomas, in press.

Payne, R. W. An object-classification test as a measure of overinclusive thinking in schizophrenic patients. *British Journal of Social and Clinical Psychology,* 1960, **1,** 213–221.

Payne, R. W. The measurement and significance of overinclusive thinking and retardation in schizophrenic patients. In P. H. Hoch & J. Zubin (Eds.), *Psychopathology of schizophrenia.* New York: Grune & Stratton, 1966.

Payne, R. W. The long-term prognostic implications of overinclusive thinking in mental patients: A follow-up study using objective tests. *Proceedings of the IV World Congress of Psychiatry, Madrid, 1966,* New York: Excerpta Medica Foundation, 1968.

Payne, R. W. Disorders of thinking. In C. G. Costello (Ed.), *Symptoms of psychopathology: A handbook.* New York: Wiley, 1970.

Payne, R. W., Ancevich, S. S., & Laverty, S. G. Overinclusive thinking in symptom-free schizophrenics. *Canadian Psychiatric Association Journal,* 1963, **8,** 225–234.

Payne, R. W., & Caird, W. K. Reaction time, distractibility, and overinclusive thinking in psychotics. *Journal of Abnormal Psychology,* 1967, **72,** 112–121.

Payne, R. W., & Friedlander, D. A short battery of simple tests for measuring overinclusive thinking. *Journal of Mental Science,* 1962, **108,** 362–367.

Payne, R. W., Friedlander, D., Laverty, S. G., et al. Overinclusive thought in chronic schizophrenics and its response to "proketazine." *British Journal of Psychiatry,* 1963, **109,** 523–530.

Payne, R. W., Hawks, D. V., Friedlander, D., & Hart, S. D. The diagnostic significance of overinclusive thinking in an unselected psychiatric population. *British Journal of Psychiatry,* 1972, **120,** 173–182.

Payne, R. W., & Hewlett, J. H. G. Thought disorder in psychotic patients. In H. J. Eysenck (Ed.), *Experiments in personality.* London: Routledge & Kegan Paul, 1960.

Payne, R. W., Hochberg, A. C., & Hawks, D. V. Dichotic stimulation as a method of assessing disorder of attention in overinclusive schizophrenic patients. *Journal of Abnormal Psychology,* 1970, **76,** 185–193.

Payne, R. W., & Sloane, R. B. Can schizophrenia be defined? *Diseases of the Nervous System,* 1968, **29,** 113–117.

Phillips, J. E., Jacobsen, N., & Turner, W. J. Conceptual thinking in schizophrenics and their relatives. *British Journal of Psychiatry,* 1965, **111,** 823–
839.

Phillips, L. Case history data and prognosis in schizophrenia. *Journal of Nervous
and Mental Disease,* 1953, **117,** 515–525.

Phillips, L. Social competence, the process-reactive distinction, and the nature of
mental disorder. In P. H. Hoch & J. Zubin (Eds.), *Psychopathology of
schizophrenia.* New York: Grune & Stratton, 1966.

Phillips, L., Kaden, S., & Waldman, M. Rorschach indices of developmental
level. *Journal of Genetic Psychology,* 1959, **94,** 267–285.

Phillips L., & Zigler, E. Social competence: The action-thought parameter and
vicariousness in normal and pathological behaviors. *Journal of Abnormal
and Social Psychology,* 1961, **63,** 137–146.

Pishkin, V., & Bourne, L. E., Jr. Abstraction and the use of available information
by schizophrenic and normal individuals. *Journal of Abnormal Psychology,*
1981, **90,** 197–203.

Pishkin, V., Lovallo, W. R., Lenk, R. G., & Bourne, L. E., Jr. Schizophrenic
cognitive dysfunction: A deficit in rule transfer. *Journal of Clinical
Psychology,* 1977, **33,** 335–342.

Pogue-Geile, M., & Harrow, M. Negative and positive symptoms in schizophrenia and depression: A follow-up study. *Schizophrenia Bulletin,* 1984,
10, 371–387.

Pogue-Geile, M., Harrow, M. & Marengo, J. *The prognosis of schizophrenic
negative symptoms.* Presented at the 137th Annual Meeting of the
American Psychiatric Association, Los Angeles, CA, May 5-11, 1984.

Pogue-Geile, M. F. & Oltmans, T. F. Sentence perception and distractibility in
schizophrenic, manic and depressed patients. *Journal of Abnormal Psychology,* 1980, **89,** 115–124.

Powers, W. T., & Hamlin, R. M. Diagnosis of deviant verbalization on the
Rorschach. *Journal of Consulting Psychology,* 1955, **49,** 120–214.

Prosen, M., & Harrow, M. Do associative intrusions cause schizophrenia?
Scientific Proceedings of 129th Annual Meeting of the American Psychiatric Association, Washington, D.C., 1976.

Putterman, A. H., & Pollack, H. The developmental approach and process-
reactive schizophrenia: A review. *Schizophrenia Bulletin,* 1976, **2,** 198–
208.

Quinlan, D. M., & Harrow, M., Boundary disturbances in schizophrenia. *Journal
of Abnormal Psychology,* 1974, **83,** 533–541.

Quinlan, D., Harrow, M., & Carlson, K. *Manual for assessment of deviant responses
on the Rorschach.* New York: *Microfiche Publications,* ASIS/NAPS #02211,
P. 1-28, 1973.

Quinlan, D. M., Harrow, M., & Tucker, G. J. Schizophrenics and hallucinogenic
drug users: Differences in Rorschach boundary imagery. In *Proceedings,*
80th Annual Meeting of the American Psychological Association, 1972.

Quinlan, D. M., Harow, M., Tucker, G. J., & Carlson, K. Varieties of "disordered"
thinking on the Rorschach: Findings in schizophrenic and non-schizophrenic patients. *Journal of Abnormal Psychology,* 1972, **79,** 47–53.

Quinlan, D., Schultz, D., Davies, R., & Harrow, M. Overinclusion and transactional thinking on the object sorting test of schizophrenic and nonschizophrenic patients. *Journal of Personality Assessment,* 1978, **42,** 401–
408.

Rapaport, D., Gill, M. M., & Schafer, R. *Diagnostic psychological testing,* Vol. 2 Chicago: Year Book Publishers, 1946. (Rev. ed.), New York: International Universities Press, 1968.

Rattenbury, F. R., Silverstein, M. L. DeWolfe, A. S., Kaufman, C. F., & Harrow, M. Associative disturbance in schizophrenia, schizoaffective disorders, and major affective disorders: Comparisons between hospitalization and one-year follow-up. *Journal of Consulting and Clinical Psychology,* 1983, **51,** 621–623.

Redlich, F. C., & Freedman, D. X. *Theory and practice of psychiatry.* New York: Basic Books, 1966.

Reed, J. L. The Proverbs Test in schizophrenia. *British Journal of Psychiatry,* 1968, 114, 317-321.

Reed, J. L. Schizophrenic thought disorder: A review and hypothesis. *Comprehensive Psychiatry,* 1970, 11, 403-432.

Reich, W. *Character analysis.* New York: Orgone Institute Press, 1949.

Reilly, F. E., Harrow, M., & Tucker, G. J. Language and thought content in acute psychosis. *American Journal of Psychiatry,* 1973, **130,** 411–417.

Reilly, F., Harrow, M., Tucker, G. J., Quinlan, D. M., & Siegel, A. Looseness of associations in acute schizophrenia. *British Journal of Psychiatry,* 1975, **127,** 240–246.

Reilly, F., Quinlan, D. M., Harrow, M., & Tucker, G. J. Loose associations in the recovering schizophrenic. *Scientific Proceedings* of 128th Annual Meeting of the American Psychiatric Association. Washington, D.C.: American Psychiatric Association, 1975.

Rinkel, M. DeShon, H., & Hyde, R. Experimental schizophrenia-like symptoms. *American Journal of Psychiatry,* 1952, 108, 252-578.

Ritzler, B. A. & Smith, M. The problems of diagnostic criteria in the study of the paranoid subclassification of schizophrenia. *Schizophrenia Bulletin,* 1976, 2, 209-217.

Roberts, W. W. Normal and abnormal depersonalization. *Journal of Mental Science,* 1960, **66,** 478–493.

Rochester, S. R. Are language disorders in acute schizophrenia actually information processing problems? *Journal of Psychiatric Research,* 1978, **14,** 275–283.

Rochester, S. R., & Martin, J. R. *Crazy talk: A study of the discourse of schizophrenic speakers.* New York: Plenum Press, 1979.

Rochford, J. M., Detre, T., Tucker, G.J., & Harrow, M. Neuropsychological impairments in functional psychiatric disease. *Archives of General Psychiatry,* 1970, 22, 114-119.

Rodnick, E. H. & Garmezy, N. An experimental approach to the study of motivation in schizophrenia. In M. R. Jones (Ed.), *Nebraska symposium on motivation.* Lincoln, NB: University of Nebraska Press, 1957. Pp. 109-184.

Rosenthal, D., Wender, P.H., Kety, S., Schulsinger, F., Welnar, J., & Rieder, R. O. Parent-child relationships and psychopathological disorder in the child. *Archives of General Psychiatry,* 1975, **32,** 466–488.

Roth, M. The phobic-anxiety-depersonalization syndrome. *Proceedings of the Royal Society of Medicine,* 1960, **52,** 587–595.(a)

Roth, M., The phobic-anxiety-depersonalization syndrome and some general aetiological problems in psychiatry. *Journal of Neuropsychiatry,* 1960, **1,** 293–306. (b)

Roth, M. & Harper, M. Temporal lobe epilepsy and the phobic-anxiety-depersonalization syndrome, II. *Comprehensive Psychiatry,* 1962, **3**, 215–226.

Rotter, J. B. Generalized expectancies for external versus internal control of reinforcement. *Psychological Monographs,* 1966, 80, 1-28.

Saccuzzo, D. P., & Braff, D. Early information processing deficit in schizophrenia: New findings using schizophrenic subgroups and manic control subjects. *Archives of General Psychiatry,* 1981, **38**, 175–179.

Saltzman, L. Conceptual thinking in psychiatric patients. *Archives of General Psychiatry,* 1966, 14, 55-59.

Salzinger, K., Portnoy, S., Pisoni, D., & Feldman, P. The immediacy hypothesis and response-produced stimuli in schizophrenic speech. *Journal of Abnormal Psychology,* 1970, **76,** 258–264.

Schegloff, E., Jefferson, G., & Sachs, H. The preference for self-correction in the organization of repair in conversation. *Language,* 1977, **53**, 361–382.

Schilder, P. Selbstbewusstein und personlichkeit bewusstsein. Monograph from *Gesamgebiet der neurologie und psychiatrie,* 1914, 9.

Schilder, P. *Introduction to a psychoanalytic psychiatry.* Trans. by B. Glueck. New York and Washington, D.C.: Nervous and Mental Disease Publishing Company, 1928.

Schilder, P. *The image and appearance of the human body.* London: Kegan Paul, 1950.

Schneider, K. *Clinical psychopathology.* New York: Grune & Stratton, 1959.

Schwartz, D., Grinker, Sr., R. R., Harrow, M., & Holzman, P. Six clinical features of schizophrenia. *Journal of Nervous and Mental Disease,* 1978, 166, 831-833.

Searles, H. *Collected papers on schizophrenia and related subjects.* New York: International Universities Press, 1965.

Sedman, G. *An investigation of states of affect and alteration of consciousness as factors concerned in the etiology of depersonalization.* Doctoral dissertation, Sheffield University, 1968.

Sedman, G. Theories of depersonalization: A re-appraisal. *British Journal of Psychiatry,* 1970, **117,** 1–14.

Sedman, G. & Kenna, J. C. Depersonalization and mood changes in schizophrenia. *British Journal of Psychiatry,* 1963, 109, 669-673.

Shagass, C., & Bittle, R. Therapeutic effects of LSD: A follow-up study. *Journal of Nervous and Mental Psychology,* 1967, **144,** 471–478.

Shakow, D. *Adaptation in schizophrenia: The theory of segmental set.* New York: John Wiley & Sons, 1979.

Shanfield, S., Tucker, G.J., Harrow, M., & Detre, T. The schizophrenic patient and depressive symptomalogy. *The Journal of Nervous and Mental Diseases,* 1970, **151,** 203–210.

Shapiro, D. A perceptual understanding of the color response. In M. A. Rickers-Ovsiankina (Ed.), *Rorschach psychology* (rev. ed.). Huntington, NY: Krieger, 1977.

Shield, P., Harrow, M., & Tucker, G.J. Investigation of factors related to stimulus overinclusion. *Psychiatric Quarterly,* 1974, **48,** 109–116.

Shimkunas, A. M. Reciprocal shifts in schizophrenic thought processes. *Journal of Abnormal Psychology,* 1970, 76, 423-426.

Shimkunas, A. M. Conceptual deficit in schizophrenia: A reappraisal. *British Journal of Medical Psychology,* 1972, 45, 149-157.

Shimkunas, A. M., Gynther, M., & Smith, K. Abstracting ability of schizophrenics before and during phenothiazine therapy. *Archives of General Psychiatry,* 1966, 14, 79-83.

Shimkunas, A. M. Gynther, M. D., & Smith, K. Schizophrenic responses to the proverbs test: Abstract, concrete, or autistic? *Journal of Abnormal Psychology,* 1967, **72,** 128–133.

Shorvon, H. J. The depersonalization syndrome. *Proceedings of the Royal Society of Medicine,* 1945–46, **39,** 779–792.

Siegel, A., Harrow, M., Reilly, F., & Tucker, G.J. Loose associations and disordered speech patterns in chronic schizophrenia. *The Journal of Nervous and Mental Disease,* 1976, **162,** 105–112.

Siegel, A., Harrow, M., Reilly, F. E., & Tucker, G. J. Loose associations and disordered speech patterns in chronic schizophrenia. In R. Cancro (Ed.), *Annual review of the schizophrenic syndrome.* New York: Bruner/Mazel, 1978.

Siegel, A., Reilly, F. E., Harrow, M., & Tucker, G. J. Loose associations: Fact or fantasy. *Scientific Proceedings* of 126th Annual Meeting of the Psychiatric Association, Washington, D.C.: American Psychiatric Association, 1973.

Silverman, J. The problem of attention in research and theory in schizophrenia. *Psychological Review,* 1964, 71, 353-379.

Silverman, J. A paradigm for the study of altered states of consciousness. *British Journal of Psychiatry,* 1968, 114, 1201-1218.

Silverman, L., Lapkin, B., & Rosenbaum, I. Manifestations of primary thinking in schizophrenia. *Journal of Projective Techniques,* 1962, **26,** 117–127.

Silverstein, M. L., & Harrow, M. Schneiderian first-rank symptoms in schizophrenia. *Archives of General Psychiatry,* 1981, **38,** 288–293.

Silverstein, M., Warren, R. A., Harrow, M., Grinker, R. R., Sr., & Pawelski, T. M. Changes in diagnosis from *DSM II* to *DSM III. American Journal of Psychiatry,* 1982, **139,** (3), 366–368.

Sims-Knight, J. E., & Knight R. A. Nonlogical classification systems: A look at the underlying complexity of overinclusion in schizophrenics. *Journal of Clinical Psychology,* 1978, **34,** 857–865.

Singer, M. T., & Wynne, L. C. Thought disorder and family relations of schizophrenics: III. Methodology using projective techniques. *Archives of General Psychiatry,* 1965, **12,** 187–200. (a)

Singer, M. T., & Wynne, L. C. Thought disorder and family relations of schizophrenics. IV. Results and implications. *Archives of General Psychiatry,* 1965, **12,** 201–212. (b)

Singer, M. T., Wynne, L. C., & Toohey, M. L. Communication disorders and the families of schizophrenics. In L. C. Wynne, R. L. Cromwell, & S. Matthysse (Eds.), *The nature of schizophrenia: New approaches to research and treatment.* New York: Wiley, 1978.

Smart, R. G., & Jones, D. Illicit LSD users: Their personality characteristics and psychopathology. *Journal of Abnormal Psychology,* 1970, **75,** 286–292.

Sommer, R. & Osmond, H. Autobiographies of former mental patients. *Journal of Mental Science,* 1960, 106, 648–662.

Soskis, D. A., Harow, M., & Detre T. Long-term follow-up of schizophrenics admitted to a general hospital psychiatric ward. *The Psychiatric Quarterly,* 1969, **43,** 524–535.

Spitzer, R. Letter. *Archives of General Psychiatry,* 1981, **38,** 1299–1300.

Spohn, H. E. The case for reporting the drug status of patient subjects in experimental studies of schizophrenic psychopathology. *Journal of Abnormal Psychology,* 1973, **82,** 102–106.

Spring, B., Neuchterlein, K., Sugarman, J. & Matthysse, S. The "new look" in studies of schizophrenic attention and information processing. *Schizophrenia Bulletin*, 1977, **3**, 470–482.

Stephens, J.H. Long-term course and prognosis in schizophrenia. *Seminars in Psychiatry*, 1970, **2**, 464–485.

Stephens, J. Long-term prognosis and follow-up in schizophrenia. *Schizophrenia Bulletin*, 1978, **4**, 25–47.

Stephens, J. H. & Astrup, C. Prognosis in "process" and "nonprocess" schizophrenia. *American Journal of Psychiatry*, 1963, 119, 945-953.

Stoll, F., Harrow, M., & Rattenbury, F. R. Dimensions of delusions in schizophrenia. In R. R. Grinker, Sr., & M. Harrow (Eds.), *Multidimensional approach to clinical research in schizophrenia.* Springfield, IL: Charles C. Thomas, in press.

Storms, L. J., & Broen, W. E., Jr. A theory of schizophrenic behavioral disorganization. *Archives of General Psychiatry*, 1969, **20**, 129–144.

Storms, L. J., & Broen, W. E., Jr. Intrusion of schizophrenics' idiosyncratic associations into their conceptual performance. *Journal of Abnormal Psychology*, 1972, **79**, 280–284.

Strauss, J., & Carpenter, W. T., Jr. The prediction of outcome in schizophrenia: I. Characteristics of outcome. *Archives of General Psychiatry*, 1972, **27**, 739–746.

Strauss, J. S., & Carpenter, W. T. Prediction of outcome in schizophrenia: II. Relationships between predictor and outcome variables. *Archives of General Psychiatry*, 1974, **31**, 37–42.

Strauss, J. S., & Carpenter, W. T., & Bartko, J. J. The diagnosis and understanding of schizophrenia. Part III: Speculations on the processes that underlie schizophrenic symptoms and signs. *Schizophrenia Bulletin*, 1974, **11**, 61–69.

Strauss, J. S., Klorman, R., Kokes, R., & Sacksteder, J. Premorbid adjustment in schizophrenia: Concepts, measures and implications. Part I. The concept of premorbid adjustment. *Schizophrenia Bulletin*, 1977, **3**, 182–185.

Strauss, M. E. Behavior differences between acute and chronic schizophrenics: Course of psychosis, effects of institutionalization, or sampling biases? *Psychological Bulletin*, 1973, 79, 271-279.

Sullivan, H. S. *The interpersonal theory of psychiatry.* New York: Norton, 1953.

Tausk, V. On the origin of the "influencing machine" in schizophrenia (1919). In R. Fleiss (Ed.), *The psychoanalytic reader.* New York: International Universities Press, 1948.

Tucker, G. J., Campion, E. W., & Silberfarb, P.M. Sensorimotor functions and cognitive disturbance in psychiatric patients. *American Journal of Psychiatry*, 1975, 132, 17-21.

Tucker, G., Harrow, M., Detre, T., & Hoffman, B. Perceptual experiences in schizophrenic and nonschizophrenic patients. *Archives of General Psychiatry*, 1969, **20**, 159–166.

Tucker, G. J., Harrow M., & Quinlan, D. Depersonalization, dysphoria, and thought disturbance. *American Journal of Psychiatry*, 1973, **130**, 702–706.

Tucker, G. J., Quinlan, D., & Harrow M. Chronic hallucinogenic drug use and thought disturbance. *Archives of General Psychiatry*, 1972, **27**, 443–447.

Tutko, T. A., & Spence, J. T. The performance of process and reactive schizophrenics and brain-injured subjects on a conceptual task. *Journal of Abnormal and Social Psychology*, 1962, **65**, 387–394.

Vaillant, G. An historical review of the remitting schizophrenics. *Journal of Nervous and Mental Disease,* 1964, **138,** 48–56.

Vaillant, G. A 10-year follow-up of remitting schizophrenics. *Schizophrenia Bulletin,* 1978, **4,** 78–85.

Venables, P. H. Selectivity of attention, withdrawal and cortical activation. *Archives of General Psychiatry,* 1963, **9,** 74–78.

Venables, P. H. Input dysfunction in schizophrenia. In B. A. Maher (Ed.), *Progress in experimental personality research.* Vol. 1. New York: Academic Press, 1964. Pp. 1-47.

Venables, P., & O'Connor, N. A short scale for rating paranoid schizophrenia. *Journal of Mental Science,* 1959, **105,** 815–818.

Vigotsky, L. S. *Thought and language.* Edited and translated by E. Hanfman & G. Vakar. Cambridge, MA: MIT Press, 1962.

Von Domarus, E. The specific laws of logic in schizophrenia. In J. S. Kasanin (Ed.), *Language and thought in schizophrenia.* New York: Norton, 1944.

Wachtel, P. Psychodynamics, behavior therapy, and the implacable experimenter. *Journal of Abnormal Psychology,* 1973, **82,** 324–334.

Watkins, J. G., & Stauffacher, J. C. An index of pathological thinking in the Rorschach. *Journal of Projective Techniques,* 1952, **16,** 276–286.

Watson, C. G. Interrelationships of six overinclusion measures. *Journal of Consulting Psychology,* 1967, **31,** 517–520.

Watson, C. G. Abstract thinking deficit and autism in process and reactive schizophrenics. *Journal of Abnormal Psychology,* 1973, 82, 399-403.

Watson, C. G., Wold, J., & Kucala, T. A comparison of abstractive and nonabstractive deficits in schizophrenics and psychiatric controls. *Journal of Nervous and Mental Disease,* 1976, 163, 193-199.

Waxler, N. E. Parent and child effects on cognitive performance: An experimental approach to the etiological and responsive theories of schizophrenia. *Family Process,* 1974, **13,** 1–22.

Wechsler, D. *The measurement and appraisal of adult intelligence* (4th ed.). Baltimore: Williams & Wilkins, 1958.

Wechsler, D. *Wechsler Adult Intelligence Scale Manual.* New York: Psychological Corporation, 1955.

Weiner, I. B. *Psychodiagnosis in Schizophrenia,* New York: Wiley, 1966.

Welpton, D. Psychodynamics of chronic lysergic acid diethylamide use. *Journal of Nervous and Mental Disease,* 1968, **147,** 377–385.

Westermeyer, J. & Harrow, M. *The prediction of recovery in schizophrenia.* Presented at the 57th Annual Meeting of the Midwestern Psychological Association, St. Louis, MO, May 1-3, 1980.

Westermeyer, J. F., & Harrow, M. Prognosis and outcome using broad *(DSM II)* and narrow *(DSM III)* concepts of schizophrenia. *Schizophrenia Bulletin,* 1984, 10, 624–637.

Wild, C. *Adaptive regression in art students, teachers, and schizophrenics.* Doctoral dissertation, Yale University, 1962.

Wild, C. Disturbed styles of thinking. *Archives of General Psychiatry,* 1965, **13,** 464–470.

Wild, C. *Scoring transactional thought disorder on the Goldstein-Scherer Object Sorting Test: A revised manual.* Unpublished manuscript. Boston: Massachusetts Department of Mental Health, 1972.

Wild, C., Singer, M., Rosman, B., Ricci, J., & Lidz, T. Measuring disordered styles of thinking using the object sorting test on parents of schizophrenic patients. *Archives of General Psychiatry,* 1965, **13,** 471–476.

Winer, B. J. *Statistical principles in experimental design.* New York: McGraw-Hill, 1962.

Wing, J. K. Institutionalism in mental hospitals. *British Journal of Social and Clinical Psychology,* 1962, **1**, 38–51.

Wing, J. K., & Brown, G. W. *Institutionalism and schizophrenia.* London: Cambridge University Press, 1970.

Witkin, H. A., Lewis, H. B., Hertzman, M., Machover, K., Meissner, P., & Wapner, S. *Personality through perception.* New York: Harper, 1954.

Witkin, H. A., Dyk, R. B., Faterson, H., Goodenough, D. R., & Karp, S. A. *Psychological differentiation.* New York: Wiley, 1962.

Wright, D. M. Impairment in abstract conceptualization in schizophrenia. *Psychological Bulletin,* 1975, 82, 120–127.

Wynne, L. C., & Singer, M. T. Thought disorder and family relations of schizophrenics. I: A research strategy. *Archives of General Psychiatry,* 1963, **9**, 191–198. (a)

Wynne, L. C., & Singer, M. Thought disorder and family relations of schizophrenics. II: A classification of forms of thinking. *Archives of General Psychiatry,* 1963, **9**, 199–206. (b)

Wynne, L. C., Singer, M. T., Bartko, J. J., & Toohey, M. L. Schizophrenics and their families: Research on parental communication. In J. M. Tanner (Ed.), *Developments in psychiatric research.* London: Hodder and Stoughton, 1977.

Yates, A. J. Data-processing levels and thought disorder in schizophrenia. *Australian Journal of Psychology,* 1966, **18**, 103–117.

Zigler, E., & Phillips, L. Social competence and outcome in psychiatric disorders. *Journal of Abnormal Psychology,* 1961, **63**, 264–271.

Zigler, E., & Phillips, L. Social competence and the process-reactive distinction in psychopathology. *Journal of Abnormal Psychology,* 1962, **65**, 215–222.

Zubin, J., & Spring. B. Vulnerability—A new view of schizophrenia. *Journal of Abnormal Psychology,* 1977, **86**, 103–126.

Zucker, L. *Ego structure in paranoid schizophrenia.* Springfield, IL: Charles C. Thomas, 1958.

Zung, W. W. K. A self-rating depression scale. *Archives of General Psychiatry,* 1965, **12**, 63–70.

## PART VI

APPENDIX

The Assessment of Bizarre-Idiosyncratic Thinking: A Manual For Scoring Responses to Verbal Tests

Joanne Marengo
Martin Harrow
Ilene Lanin-Kettering
Arnold Wilson

Various approaches have been employed to assess severe thought pathology, or as it is most commonly called in the field, thought disorder. In the past, theoretical discussions of schizophrenia have explored the role of thought disorder through diagnostic and empirical work (Arieti, 1974; Bleuler, 1950; Cameron and Margaret, 1951; Kasanin, 1944). In turn, investigators have approached the question of assessing disordered thinking from a number of different viewpoints (Buss and Lang, 1965; Chapman and Chapman, 1973; Payne, 1970). Much of our own approach to studying thought pathology has revolved around the construct of bizarre-idiosyncratic speech and thinking (Harrow and Quinlan, 1977; Marengo & Harrow, 1983). A comprehensive assessment of bizarre-idiosyncratic thinking involves an evaluation of most of the major types of phenomena usually included under the term "formal positive thought disorder" (Andreasen, 1979a; Fish, 1962).

Since the concept of idiosyncratic thinking deals with a potentially important symptom of schizophrenic disturbance, we have focused on this feature as one major aspect of a long-term, multidisciplinary research project studying the course of psychosis and schizophrenic cognition (Chicago Follow-up Study, Michael Reese Medical Center,

Chicago, Illinois). One major thrust of this research program has been to address established beliefs and newer formulations regarding cognitive disturbances in schizophrenia. In this context, our studies of bizarre-idiosyncratic language have been primarily directed toward answering the following research questions: (1) Are bizarre-idiosyncratic verbalizations characteristic only of schizophrenia, or do other psychotic and nonpsychotic populations also demonstrate this behavior? (2) What changes in bizarre-idiosyncratic verbalizations occur over the course of the schizophrenic disorder? (3) Is the degree of bizarre-idiosyncratic language and thinking during the posthospital or "recovery" stage of schizophrenia an index of the severity of disturbance? (4) What is the association between disturbed language and thought and different stages of psychiatric illness (i.e., acute versus chronic conditions, early versus later phases of disorder)?

The purpose of the current manual is to describe our approach to defining and measuring bizarre-idiosyncratic speech and thought. The approach presented here focuses on assessing the frequency and severity of thought disorder. While more qualitative typologies exist, it is assumed that measuring degrees in the severity of disturbance, which relates to hypotheses regarding a continuum of disorder, will provide fruitful results.

The following manual outlines a system of scoring bizarre-idiosyncratic verbalizations from two short verbal tests. This system represents an extension of prior research efforts in this area. Some of the material from the current manual incorporates criteria developed by D. Adler that has been used successfully in previous research (Adler and Harrow, 1973, 1974; Harrow and Quinlan, 1977; Harrow, Tucker, and Adler, 1972). However, more specific criteria are now included for evaluating bizarre-idiosyncratic responses, and characteristic examples of bizarre-idiosyncratic verbalizations are offered as an aid to assessment. Analyses of disturbed language and thought, drawn from a variety of patient populations in various settings and contexts, have provided the framework for the current work.

THE DEFINITION AND CRITERIA OF BIZARRE-IDIOSYNCRATIC LANGUAGE

We have defined bizarre-idiosyncratic speech and behavior as that which is: (a) *unique to the particular subject;* (b) *deviant with respect to conventional social norms;* and (c) *frequently hard to understand or to empathize with.* While these three features are central to the concept, other less frequent characteristics are verbalizations that: (d) *may appear confused, contradictory, or illogical;* (e) *may involve sudden or unexpected contrasts;* and (f) *are usually inappropriate or unresourceful in relation to the task at hand.*

The first two of the above features are directly linked to social norms, though they are viewed from different vantage points: that of the individual and that of society. The last three characteristics listed in the definition may also appear as features of bizarre-idiosyncratic thinking, but they are features that are present some of the time, rather than being invariant.

It is surprisingly easy to spot bizarre-idiosyncratic statements since the manner of presentation or the ideas themselves impress the rater (including a naive rater) as unusual, strange, odd, or inappropriate. As the rater proceeds in gaining more experience in scoring numerous records, the empathic aspect is likely to emerge as one of the most significant signals for judging a response as bizarre and assigning an overall score.

The above definition provides us with a broad conceptualization of what are usually considered idiosyncratic statements. It is important to emphasize that bizarre or idiosyncratic qualities may be found in abstract and concrete as well as correct and incorrect responses, but they are analyzed and scored as a dimension separate from these other aspects of response behavior.

To illustrate, suppose the examiner presents the proverb:

Strike while the iron is hot.

And the subject responds with:

It could mean [pause] Hercules! [Could you say more?] I saw the movie Hercules. [Yes . . .] and it means don't iron over your hands and don't strike anybody before you cast the first stone.

Although a response may be scored as bizarre without meeting all of the above criteria, this particular response meets all of the criteria for bizarre-idiosyncratic thinking noted above (namely, a, b, c, d, e, and f). It represents a rather extreme but explicit example of disordered thinking. The investigator first wonders, "Hercules?—What is the relation of the response to the original proverb?" The response deviates in a very idiosyncratic way from the consensual norms for answering this question. Upon reflection one sees some of the possible reasons for the subject's interpretation in the suggestion of striking and violent action, with this leading to a response involving Hercules. In both this and other components of the response, it is not very easy for the observer to empathize with or understand the context from which the answer arose. In addition, the idea of ironing one's hands is unexpected with respect to what has preceded it, and unusual on its own account. The entire statement appears confused, and the line of thinking that has led to the response has resulted in an incorrect or unresourceful answer to the question.

PROCEDURE

The general assessment of bizarre-idiosyncratic thinking provides the basis for our scoring system. The procedure includes: (1) assessing subjects with two short verbal tests; and (2) assigning an overall score for the severity of bizarre-idiosyncratic thinking to each of the subject's responses. This procedure is outlined below. In addition, scoring criteria have been developed to characterize the subtypes of disordered thinking found in each response more specifically. Five categories and eleven subcategories of bizarre-idiosyncratic thinking have been defined and are included in Section I of the addendum. In Section 2 of the addendum, we have provided examples representing the range of overall and category scores for bizarre-idiosyncratic thinking. In Section 3 of the addendum, we have enclosed two scored protocols that may be used as a basis for scoring comparisons. We urge the researcher or clinician to review the scoring of the first few responses, rate the remainder of the responses on these protocols "blind," and then compare these ratings with ours before using this manual.

INSTRUMENTS AND ADMINISTRATION
OF TESTS

During the course of pilot work it became clear that test materials vary in their potential for eliciting idiosyncratic verbal behavior. Even for those patients whose speech would be labeled as odd by many, some types of verbal materials and tests do not readily elicit idiosyncratic responses. We have found that more open-ended procedures better lend themselves to eliciting this response behavior in those subjects with a potential for thought-disordered speech. Other tests prove cumbersome or unreliable. However, two verbal tests, the Gorham Proverbs Test (Gorham, 1956) and the Comprehension subtest of the WAIS (Wechsler, 1955; 1981), which are relatively short and easy to administer, were found to be good tools for evoking idiosyncratic verbal responses in those individuals with a potential for disordered thought.

The Proverbs Test

The Gorham Proverbs Test (clinical, free-answer set) consists of three parallel forms, each containing twelve proverbs. In our research, the multiple forms have been useful in the collection of longitudinal data over time from the same subject.

For purposes of standardizing subject assessment, directions for the proverbs test are read as follows:

I am going to read you some sayings. For example, the saying, "Large oaks from little acorns grow" could mean that great things may have small beginnings. Now, please tell me what each saying means rather than to just tell me more about it. Try to answer every one.

WAIS Comprehension Subtest

The Comprehension subtest of the Wechsler Adult Intelligence Scale, WAIS (Wechsler, 1955) or WAIS-R (Wechsler, 1981) consists of questions relating to social comprehension and judgment (e.g., Why does land in the city cost more than land in the country?). Twelve of these questions provide the materials for our evaluation of bizarre-idiosyncratic thinking (Questions 3–14).

The Comprehension subtest is introduced to the subject as instructed in the WAIS manual. Encouragement toward responding is sometimes needed in this test as well as in the proverbs test and is appropriate to utilize in the manner standardized by the Wechsler manual.

Recording the Data

It is essential that the verbalizations of the subject, as well as those of the examiner, be written down verbatim. The protocol also should include notations with reference to the behavior or affect stimulated by the test material or expressed during the course of testing. If it is impossible to record the verbalizations of an acutely disturbed patient, a transcribed tape recording may result in the most accurate test protocol. The examiner should inquire about all unclear or odd words or responses in a curious but nonintrusive manner, and these inquiries should be noted in parentheses. Since the object of these tasks is to obtain enough information to assess the various underlying processes that contribute to idiosyncratic responses, examiners must exercise judgment based on their own understanding of what has been said as the criteria for initiating inquiry.

Other Verbal Tests

Other comparable proverbs tests and other verbal tests have been employed in previous research (Benjamin, 1944). Recently, we also have used a verbal test (The Lanin-Berndt Communications Interview) involving a series of structured questions designed to tap several important dimensions of verbal behavior (Berndt, 1981). It is from our efforts to derive a scoring system for tests of this general type that the current manual was developed.

The Rorschach test and free-verbalization situations have also been useful in our assessments of bizarre-idiosyncratic thought (Quinlan et al., 1972; Quinlan and Harrow, 1974; Reilly et al., 1975). Both of these techniques show many valuable features. However, the Rorschach test takes longer to administer and is considerably more cumbersome to transcribe. The free-verbalization technique, while sensitive to eliciting bizarre-idiosyncratic behavior, also presented some problems in its standardization and transcription, and in obtaining reliability.

SCORING: THE OVERALL SCORE FOR BIZARRE-IDIOSYNCRATIC RESPONSES

The overall score for bizarre-idiosyncratic thinking is the first global evaluation of the record. It represents an assessment of each response from the point of view of its fit with the current verbal context and what is generally considered appropriate and understandable in our society. The extent to which a response as a whole is bizarre as well as the extent to which it meets the criteria of any or all of the specific types of bizarre-idiosyncratic thinking varies greatly. In the present scoring system, we evaluate degrees of bizarre-idiosyncratic thinking by assigning scores of

0, .5, 1, or 3, ranging from absent to severe bizarre-idiosyncratic thinking. Several examples of responses at each level of bizarre-idiosyncratic speech are provided here. A large number of other examples with the appropriate overall score for bizarre-idiosyncratic thinking are presented in Section 2 of the addendum.

Overall Score Values

0 = Idiosyncratic verbalizations are absent.

.5 = *Minimal bizarre qualities*. Verbalizations that contain some mildly strange material. The response is slightly "off" but in a social situation the verbalization is not strange enough to draw considerable attention. Mild cognitive slips would be scored here. Two examples of responses scored ".5" are presented below:

> Q: Why does land in the city cost more than land in the Country? A: Because land is scarce and people need land to build on. Soon it will be city all the way from New York to Florida—stretching and expanding, striving to survive.

> Q: Why should people pay taxes? A: Taxes are necessary. Obsessive takes help the government. I could give a whole thesis on it.

1 = *A definite idiosyncratic or bizarre response*. This type of response is noticeably unusual or strange, but usually still understandable. Most responses in which bizarre or idiosyncratic aspects are present will receive this rating. These responses would clearly be noticeable for their strangeness in a social situation. Two examples are presented below:

> Q: Why should we keep away from bad company? A: They produce an aura of ill-effect. [Q] They're not—you shouldn't be "subseeded" or deceited by people who are bad. They're just no good.

> Q: Rome was not built in a day. A: It's love, I think of it as love. I have to work towards love and love has to work towards me. And this has to gradually come.

3 = *A very severe bizarre response*. Such responses reflect a very serious deviation from consensual statements, may contain considerable confusion, and are very socially atypical. It is often hard to understand why that response was given to that particular question. This type of response is very rarely found

in normal population and is even infrequent among patients. Two examples are presented below:

> Q: When the cat's away the mice will play. A: Yeah. On the earth, up at the top, in the middle. XYZ. The end, the beginning of the end of the beginning.

> Q: One swallow doesn't make a summer. A: Boy, that's greedy as hell, man, that's real greedy. That's like pulling my actual backwards.

Total scores for the proverbs and comprehension tests range from 0 to 24. In assigning the overall score for potential bizarre-idiosyncratic thinking to each response, the rater is essentially assessing how strange or deviant the response is in relation to more conventional answers. In those cases where nonconventional answers are given, the rater is assessing how easy it is, at first glance, to understand the reason that a particular response was given or to empathize with the processes involved in arriving at the answer. Even responses that one can understand or empathize with may at times be scored, since they may show odd features or deviate from social convention in an unusual or unexpected manner. However, responses that deviate from the conventional answer and that are also difficult to understand are assigned even more severe ratings for bizarre-idiosyncratic thinking.

As outlined above, an overall score of 0 is assigned when the response is not bizarre or idiosyncratic in any way. An overall score of .5 is assigned when the response is slightly off, or contains cognitive slips that are not grossly deviant. In a social situation, this response would not really startle people or raise deep questions. This score is meant to capture slight deviations, some of which are expected to be found in normal records as well. An overall score of 1 is assigned to a response that is clearly idiosyncratic or bizarre. An overall score of 3 is assigned only to extremely unusual or very bizarre statements.

It should be noted that in scoring bizarre-idiosyncratic thinking, incorrect answers are not penalized, since lack of knowledge does not represent strangeness or bizarreness. However, incorrect answers in which it is difficult to understand why the particular incorrect answer was given, and incorrect answers that have no relationship at all to the question, will usually involve bizarre or strange thinking and be scored as such.

The *overall* score has emerged in our research as the most accurate estimate of bizarre-idiosyncratic thinking. It is based on a judgment of positive thought disorder in the response as a whole and is based both on the scorer's understanding of the definition of bizarre-idiosyncratic thinking as well as on the coherence and appropriateness of the response. The overall score is a qualitative assessment of the degree of idiosyncracy reflected in a response.

ESTABLISHING SUBJECT GROUPS BASED ON THE SEVERITY OF BIZARRE-IDIOSYNCRATIC THINKING

The Continuum Model

We believe that responses reflecting bizarre-idiosyncratic thinking can be placed on a continuum extending from very severe bizarre-idiosyncratic thinking to normal, socially consensual thinking, with considerably heavier weightings for very severely bizarre responses, as opposed to mildly bizarre responses, or mild cognitive slips. We have found that it also can be useful to have some system available to facilitate the placing of subjects into rough categories according to whether they show severe thought pathology, moderate levels of thought pathology, or no thought pathology. Accordingly, we assign subjects' total overall scores from the Proverbs and Comprehension tests to categories or levels reflecting various degrees of bizarre-idiosyncratic thinking.

In the system we have constructed, subjects' total overall scores have been categorized into a continuum of thought pathology. The five specific categories included in the current system are: (1) no bizarre-idiosyncratic thinking; (2) minimal to mild bizarre-idiosyncratic thinking; (3) moderate levels; (4) severe levels; and (5) very severe levels of bizarre-idiosyncratic thinking. The conversion levels presented in Table A.1 are used.

In terms of the degree of psychopathology reflected by the continuum of bizarre-idiosyncratic thinking, levels 1 and 2 of the Thought Disorder scale are representative of little or no pathological thinking and lie within the normal range. Level 3 (moderate level) reflects definite evidence of thought pathology or abnormal thinking. The number of patients at levels 4 and 5 provides an estimate of *severely* thought-disordered patients. The combined number of patients at levels 3, 4, and 5 gives the percentage of patients with definite signs of thought pathology or abnormal thinking.

The Composite Index of Bizarre-Idiosyncratic Thinking

A composite index of bizarre-idiosyncratic thinking also can be computed from both verbal tests, the Proverbs and the Comprehension tests, using the five levels of bizarre-idiosyncratic thinking described above. In this composite index, each subject is assigned to the highest (most severe) level into which he or she fits on either of the two tests. This composite index classifies subjects according to whether they show any pathological signs of bizarre-idiosyncratic thinking, given opportunities on two separate tests to show such behavior.

In our previous research we also have obtained measures of bizarre-idiosyncratic thinking from the Goldstein and Scheerer (1941, 1944) Object Sorting test and have categorized the scores from the Object Sorting test into the same five levels of bizarre-idiosyncratic thinking. We have combined the category scores or levels from the Object Sorting test with the parallel category scores or levels from the Proverbs and Comprehension tests to obtain a composite index of bizarre-idiosyncratic thinking.

This overall index is based on patient' scores from the three separate measures of thought disorder. For this overall index, each patient is assigned to one of the five categories or levels ranging from no bizarre-idiosyncratic thinking (level 1) to very severe cognitive disturbance (level 5) according to the most severe level attained on *any of the three tests*. This classification system categorizes patients according to whether they show any bizarre-idiosyncratic thinking, given three

TABLE A.1
Continuum of Bizarre-Idiosyncratic Thinking

Thought Disorder Group	Thought Disorder Scale	Thought Disorder Continuum	Proverb or Comprehension Test Total Score
No abnormal	1	Absent	0– .5
thinking	2	Mild	1–2.5
Abnormal thinking	3	Definite	3–6.5
Severe thought	4	Severe	7–11.5
disorder	5	Very Severe	12–36

separate opportunities to do so. The overall score encompasses a broad sample of patients' behavior and is more comprehensive than indexes that include only one or two tests.

Validity of the Subgroups Based on Severity of Bizarre-Idiosyncratic Thinking

The question arises as to the *validity* of the thought disorder groups we have established. The issue is partly centered on whether the cutoff points are useful in separating patients into groups that behave differently in distinct clinical or non-clinical areas and show differences in the severity of other types of psychopathology.

In a series of studies using the cutoff points to demarcate groups according to the 5 levels of thought disorder, we have found that the system described above has proved a useful means of delineating patients with more versus less severe cognitive pathology. We have found significant associations between the thought disorder *scale* (based on the composite index from the Proverbs test, the Comprehension test and the Object Sorting test), and other major psychopathology, such as delusions (Harrow, Silverstein and Marengo, 1983). In addition, we have found that there are significant relationships between the continuum of thought disorder severity (1-5 point scale) and the degree of dysfunction shown by schizophrenics in their overall adjustment (Harrow, Silverstein and Marengo, 1983; Marengo, 1983).

While we view the points of the thought disorder *scale* as lying on a continuum, we also have found the specific cut-off points that establish the thought disorder groups of value in other studies. When we have categorized patients into groups according to whether they have severe thought disorder, as opposed to signs of abnormal thinking, as opposed to little or no thought disorder on our composite index, we have found significant differences among the groups in various types of major psychopathology (Marengo & Harrow, 1983). This has occurred when we have contrasted schizophrenics with no or only mild thought disorder (thought disorder scale levels 1 and 2), with schizophrenics with signs of abnormal thinking (thought disorder scale levels 3), with schizophrenics with severe or very severe thought disorder (thought disorder scale levels 4 and 5). Thought disorder group differences have been found in concurrent assessments of work functioning, overall psychotic activity, and rehospitalization rates during posthospital phases of schizophrenia and depressive disorders (Marengo, 1983;

Marengo, Harrow & Silverstein, 1982). These data indicate some degree of validity for the cut-off points established and listed above.

In addition, the thought disorder scale and the thought disorder groups were predictive of the future functioning of patients when thought disorder was assessed at an early, posthospital phase of disorder (Pogue-Geile, Harrow & Marengo, 1984). The presence of severe thought disorder (thought disorder scale levels of 4 or 5) was a good prognostic indicator of future sustained functioning impairments in schizophrenia and the depressive disorders. Non-thought disordered patients and those showing abnormal thinking (but not severe thought disorder) evidenced a more benign or remitting subsequent course of psychosis and other functional impairments over the longitudinal course of disturbance (Marengo, 1983).

THE RELATION OF THIS SYSTEM OF EVALUATING BIZARRE-IDIOSYNCRATIC THINKING TO OTHER SYSTEMS OF THOUGHT PATHOLOGY ASSESSMENT

Rapaport, Gill, and Schafer (1968) System

We should note that in several ways the conceptual framework we employ to assess bizarre-idiosyncratic thinking is different from that used by Rapaport in his research studying disordered thinking, although the two systems are comparable in several respects. Our conceptual framework is closely tied to implicit conceptual norms that people have acquired over time about what is appropriate and what is deviant in a particular response situation. The framework used by Rapaport is based, in part, on assessing pathological verbalizations in terms of whether they involve too much distance or a loss of distance from the original stimuli, with such judgments based on implicit social norms (Rapaport, Gill, and Schafer, 1968). However, while there is some difference in the conceptual basis of the systems, in the actual practice of scoring disordered verbalizations, there is much similarity. The system we use involves assessing consensually deviant responses and behavior along dimensions of bizarre-idiosyncratic thinking that Rapaport might have labeled as "too much distance" or a "loss of distance" from the original stimuli.

JOHNSTON-HOLZMAN THOUGHT DISORDER
INDEX (1979)

The construct of bizarre-idiosyncratic thinking that we use and Johnston and Holzman's Thought Disorder Index also show similarity. In both systems, bizarre, strange, and deviant responses are assigned scores, and in both systems more severely deviant responses are given heavier or more pathological weighting. Johnston and Holzman's Thought Disorder Index has been used with the WAIS Comprehension scale and with other WAIS subtests, as well as with the Rorschach Test.

Our Proverbs test measures of bizarre-idiosyncratic thinking showed significant correlations ($r = .61$) with thought pathology as measured on Johnston and Holzman's Thought Disorder Index (1979) in a sample of young schizophrenics we studied during post-acute phases of disturbance.

During the course of previous research, we have employed the Rorschach and have constructed a manual to be used with it to assess bizarre-idiosyncratic thinking (Quinlan, Harrow, & Carlson, 1973). We have found these systems valuable. We tend, however, to favor the current verbal tests and system of assessment, since the Rorschach is more time-consuming in terms of administration, transcribing, and scoring.

THE RDC AND DSM III CRITERIA OF
THOUGHT DISORDER

The key components of bizarre-idiosyncratic thinking in the current system also can be helpful in assessing whether a patient has the type of formal thought disorder listed in major diagnostic systems such as the Research Diagnostic Criteria (RDC) and *DSM III* (Spitzer & Endicott, 1968; *DSM III*, 1980). Four of the five types of pathological speech and thinking outlined in the Research Diagnostic Criteria as constituting formal thought disorder (impaired understandibility of speech, loosening of association or derailment, illogical thinking, and neologisms) are viewed in the present system as components of bizarre-idiosyncratic thinking. Even the examples usually given for poverty of content of speech, which is included under "formal" thought disorder in the RDC, would be scored as bizarre-idiosyncratic thinking in the current system when they contain strange or idiosyncratic content.

Similarly, although *DSM III* is a little less optimistic about the concept of formal thought disorder, three of the specific types of thought pathology which, in effect, are substituted in *DSM III* for formal thought disorder (incoherence, marked loosening of associations, and markedly illogical thinking), are included in the present system. Again, many of the examples of the fourth type of thought pathology, marked poverty of content of speech, would be scored as bizarre-idiosyncratic thinking. It should be noted that these four types of thought pathology are included as symptoms that can be used in *DSM III* as partial criteria for a diagnosis of schizophrenia.

RELIABILITY AND VALIDITY

Evaluations of both reliability and validity of the current system of assessment have been based on normal subjects, and on outpatient and inpatient psychiatric groups. These assessments have taken place in a variety of settings and have included chronic and acute, psychotic and nonpsychotic, and medicated and unmedicated patient samples.

Reliability

Interrater reliability has been obtained for: (a) the overall system of assessing bizarre-idiosyncratic thinking using Proverbs and Comprehension tests; and (b) for the categories of bizarre-idiosyncratic thinking presented in the addendum. Interrater reliability estimates always have been high for the overall system and moderate to high for the specific categories of bizarre-idiosyncratic thinking. Four separate assessments of twenty patient records produced interrater reliabilities of $r = .93$, $r = .88$, $r = .67$, and $r = .91$ for total overall scores on the Proverb and Comprehension tests. Interrater reliabilities for each category of idiosyncratic thinking were as follows:

Category	Range of r
I. Linguistic Form and Structure	.82–.99
II. The Content of the Statement: The Ideas Expressed	.84–.99
III. Intermingling	.75–.85

IV. Relationship Between Response and Question   .73–.99
V. Behavior   .47–.98

In addition to interrater reliability, internal consistencies for the Proverbs test using Cronbach's Alpha produced a reliability of .85 for all possible combinations of item-by-item scores. Patients were also tested on two parallel forms of the Proverbs test administered successively in the same test session. Gorham's (1956) Proverbs Set 1 and Proverbs Set 3 were utilized. The correlation of subjects' overall scores for bizarre-idiosyncratic thinking between these two sets of proverbs was $r = .79$ (Harrow and Miller, 1980).

Comparisons of the total scores on Proverb and Comprehension tests for the same subjects have also been undertaken to determine whether a subject who obtains more pathological scores on one of these tests is likely to obtain more pathological scores on the other test. In a sample of eighteen nonmedicated inpatient, state-hospital subjects assessed with both tests during the first week of hospitalization, the reliability coefficient was $r = .74$ between Proverb and Comprehension total scores. A second sample of 104 medicated patients (63 schizophrenics and 41 nonschizophrenics) from a private and state hospital setting provided a reliability coefficient of $r = .53$ between Proverbs and Comprehension total scores. Significant correlations emerged for: (a) the total number of bizarre responses, $r = .57$; (b) the number of moderate and severe bizarre responses, $r = .55$; and (c) the frequency of severe bizarre responses, $r = .47$, between the Proverbs and Comprehension tests. This indicates that the bizarre-idiosyncratic thinking found was not peculiar to a specific test, and suggests that it is characteristic of a specific person in a variety of situations.

However, a significant difference emerged between the total scores derived from the two tests, $t (102) = 2.69$, $P<.01$. The Proverbs test elicited more severely bizarre responses than the Comprehension test when administered at the acute phase of patients' disorders. The Proverbs test appears to be more sensitive in terms of eliciting bizarre-idiosyncratic responses in acute patients who have a tendency toward bizarre thinking (Marengo, 1983). This appears to be a function of the differences in test stimuli and demand characteristics. The Proverbs test presents less familiar material to the patient, demanding more abstraction and more complex thinking. The subject cannot rely as much upon previous experience and socially stereotyped responses when responding to many of the proverbs.

Validity

In addition to the reliability studies, we have begun to conduct a number of studies to assess the validity of various aspects of the system. These have included longitudinal studies to assess empirically a) the relationship between bizarre-idiosyncratic speech and other aspects of psychopathology, and b) the level of bizarre-idiosyncratic thinking at different stages of patients' disorders.

Early results on various patient and normal samples have provided positive support for the validity of the construct of bizarre-idiosyncratic thinking, although such data obviously do not provide final evidence on validity. Our research on bizarre-idiosyncratic thinking with the Proverbs and Comprehension tests have indicated the following:

1. Schizophrenic and nonschizophrenic patients ($n = 85$) with a disturbance of associative processes on a word association test also manifested significantly more severe idiosyncratic thinking on the Comprehension test of the WAIS (Silverstein, Harrow, & Marengo, unpublished).

2. Bizarre-idiosyncratic thinking was positively correlated with linguistic errors on a structured communication task (Lanin-Kettering, 1983). Thought disorder as measured on the Proverbs test showed a significant association with an overall index of contextual coordination, $r = .48$, $p<.001$, and was also correlated with several component measures, including the ability to maintain topic, $r = .29$, $p<.03$, and to produce sentence-to-sentence coherence, $r = .43$, $p<.003$. Assessment included a sample of psychiatric and normal subjects.

3. Correlations of the Proverbs and Comprehension test total scores with our Object Sorting test measure of bizarre-idiosyncratic thinking were $r = .60$ and $r = .50$, respectively, in 50 psychiatric subjects we assessed at the acute inpatient phase.

4. A number of theories have been proposed concerning disturbed families and their possible role in their schizophrenic offsprings' disorders. Many of these theories are centered around concepts concerning communicative deviance in families of schizophrenics and other disordered patients. We have assessed the relationship between our measure of bizarre-idiosyncratic thinking and one of the measures of communicative deviance, that employed by Wild and Lidz, using the Object Sorting test (Wild, 1965, 1972). Bizarre idiosyncratic thinking on the Comprehension test, using an earlier version of the present scoring system (Adler and Harrow, 1973) showed a significant relationship ($r = .45$) with Wild and Lidz's measure of transactional

thinking, in a sample of 40 schizophrenic and nonschizophrenic patients we studied during the acute phase of disorder (Quinlan, Schultz, Davies and Harrow, 1978). In addition, the correlation between bizarre-idiosyncratic thinking as assessed on the Object Sorting test and Wild's measure of transactional thinking was $r = .67$ (Quinlan, Schultz, Davies and Harrow, 1978). These results suggest a strong relationship between our measure of bizarre-idiosyncratic thinking, or positive thought disorder, and measures of communicative deviance from family studies.

5. At the acute phase of disturbance, early schizophrenic patients showed significantly more severe bizarre-idiosyncratic thinking than other psychotic and nonpsychotic patient groups, indicating the tests' sensitivity to diagnostic factors. (Marengo & Harrow, 1983).

6. Differences existed in the severity of bizarre-idiosyncratic thinking over different stages of psychiatric disturbance. A decline in the severity of bizarre-idiosyncratic thinking was evident between acute-phase assessment and the stage of partial recovery (seven weeks after acute-phase assessment). This reduction was significantly associated with improvement in other aspects of the patients' clinical condition (Crittenden et al., 1980; Harrow, Marengo, & Lanin-Kettering, 1983).

7. In a longitudinal study we found significant schizophrenic-nonschizophrenic differences in bizarre-idiosyncratic thinking at the acute phase, and considerably smaller differences during posthospital periods of remission (Harrow and Silverstein, 1978; Marengo, Harrow, & McDonald, 1983).

8. Schizophrenics with severe thought pathology in post-acute phases of disorder also functioned significantly more poorly in other major areas of posthospital functioning (e.g., rehospitalization, work, social functioning) (Crittenden et al., 1980; Harrow, Silverstein, & Marengo, 1983).

9. Relatively high correlations between the composite score of bizarre-idiosyncratic thinking (derived from the Proverbs and Comprehension tests) and delusions, $r = .42$, have been used to support formulations about a general psychosis factor in schizophrenia (Harrow, Grossman, Silverstein, & Meltzer, 1982).

Thus, in these early studies the results from the Proverbs and Comprehension measures have generally fit in with common clinical observations and theories about bizarre-idiosyncratic thinking and positive thought disorder.

It should also be noted that in our assessments of nonpatient control samples, some normal subjects have manifested signs of abnormal thinking (Marengo and Harrow, 1983). We have also found that normal subjects demonstrate signs of severe bizarre-idiosyncratic thinking. Ten to fifteen percent of normal subjects showed levels 4 or 5 on the Comprehension or Proverbs test when one of these tests was used alone, and 10 percent showed severely disordered thinking on the overall index (Marengo and Harrow, 1983). The finding of some control subjects with severe levels of thought pathology should not be surprising, in view of various findings over the years of certain levels of psychopathology, and even severe psychopathology, in some "normals."

We should also point out that thought-disordered individuals show a great deal of normal speech. This attests to the phasic nature of thought disorder, even during periods of acute upset. Our measures assess the behavioral *potential* for bizarre-idiosyncratic thinking in spontaneous, open-ended speech situations.

Addendum to Manual for the Assessment of Bizarre-Idiosyncratic Thinking

SECTION 1. SPECIFIC CATEGORIES AND SUBCATEGORIES OF BIZARRE-IDIOSYNCRATIC THINKING

In addition to overall response scores for bizarre-idiosyncratic thinking, we have outlined a system for subsequent evaluations of each response focusing on criteria constructed to delineate specifically the anomalies of positive thought disorder. Five categories and eleven subcategories of bizarre-idiosyncratic thinking (based on both traditional and newer concepts of thought disorder) provide the criteria for evaluating components of bizarre-idiosyncratic verbalizations in greater detail. These major categories and subcategories represent various types of bizarre ideas, behavior, and language. They also provide one way of categorizing some of the different types of bizarre behavior one can find in responses to specific tasks, as well as in people's day-to-day behavior.

The presence of these components of disordered speech and language can be independently studied in light of different theoretical predictions, developments at different points in the unfolding of, or recovery from, a particular disorder, and in understanding differences among clinical populations. With bizarre-idiosyncratic thinking as a more general construct, these categorical evaluations provide the opportunity to study particular kinds of language disorders.

We have found these subtypes of bizarre-idiosyncratic verbalizations and behavior useful, and we do score them in our own research. *We should emphasize, however, that scoring or attending to these specific criteria is not absolutely necessary for attaining the overall score for bizarre-idiosyncratic thinking. One can utilize the overall system of assessment of bizarre-idiosyncratic thinking on the basis of the criteria outlined in the previous pages without attending to the detailed and specific subcategories noted in the following pages.* Interested readers might wish to study the system for categorizing bizarre-idiosyncratic thinking outlined below. We should again note, however, that even if one uses the following subcategories, the *initial overall rating of bizarre-idiosyncratic thinking should be made first, before scoring these individual subcategories.*

In terms of the specific components, we have used five basic categories to study both the subject's linguistic form (i.e., the manner in which ideas are communicated) and the content of the responses (i.e., the ideas themselves). In Section 2 of this addendum we have provided detailed examples of specific responses and how they should be scored within the five categories and eleven subcategories of bizarre-idiosyncratic responses. It should be noted that these categories are not exclusive and many responses will be scored for several types of component problems, particularly since problems in form and problems in content are often difficult to tease apart.

The Five Categories of Bizarre-Idiosyncratic Thinking

I. *Linguistic Form and Structure*: Here, the structure of language within the response is under scrutiny. A problem in this area implies that it is difficult to understand the subject's statement owing to *distortions in word use, grammatical form, or the linkage of words and phrases. A response also may be communicated poorly.* Questions are raised in terms of peculiarities in the individual's verbal style, the linguistic structure of the response, or gaps in communication that may interfere with the clear communication of meaning.

II. *The Content of the Statement: The Ideas Expressed*: Under primary consideration are the ideas presented within the response. This category pertains to peculiarities within a response such as *idiosyncratic reasoning, asocial attitudes, and disorganized or confused ideas.* Evaluations are made in terms of the ideas or attitudes the subject presents when viewed in terms of conventional attitudes, logical thought, or cogent explanations.

III. *What is Intermixed into the Response*: In this category the focus is on whether the response moves away from a consensual answer owing to a shift to loosely associated ideas or the subject's personal preoccupations. The twofold emphasis of this category is on: (1) the mixing or blending into the response of personal material from the subject's past or current experience, and (2) the extensive elaboration of a theme or idea, which does not fit neatly into the structure of the response, making it appear somewhat unusual. The question raised is: Are there any personal associations or tangential ideas that the subject is expressing as part of his response that detract from the quality of the verbalization?

IV. *The Relationship between Question and Response*: Here, the focus of evaluation is on *the ideas the subject presents in terms of how they relate to the question asked.* One considers whether the subject is able to address the task of interpretation, or answer a question. Is the subject inappropriately, or totally, focused on private, autistic associations or thoughts? Questions are raised regarding the relation between the ideas the subject presents and the question asked.

V. *Behavior*: Behavior is assessed in relation to conventional norms for conduct in a testing situation, including physical, affective, and verbal behavior. The question raised is: Is the subject's behavior deviant either in its extreme expression or in its incongruity and impropriety within the testing context?

A Suggested Step-By-Step Procedure for Evaluating the Categories of Bizarre-Idiosyncratic Thinking

The assignment of scores within these categories is determined using the criteria listed below. The extent to which a response meets each (or none) of the relevant category criteria is evaluated and the response is assigned a score of 0, .5, 1, or 3 for each category.

In assigning category and subcategory scores, it helps to:

a. Consider how the subject expresses his ideas. Is the response poorly structured, composed of vague elements, or obscured by idiosyncratic terminology? What is the subject's choice of words? Is there any unusual word usage or use of artificial, pedantic, or stilted language? Does the subject communicate his ideas in a reasonable fashion, or are there unexplained gaps or missing referents that make it very difficult to understand. If yes, then evaluate the response in terms of subcategory indicators and assign a score reflecting the degree of thought disorder in Category I.

b. Consider next the ideas presented. Does the subject's statement make any sense at all? If the response makes no sense, score a 3 in Category II. Does the reasoning deviate from rules of logic or social convention? Does the statement involve an odd meaning or outlook? If yes, then evaluate the extent and assign an appropriate score in Category II and in its appropriate subcategories.

c. Then consider the content of the response in terms of intermingling. After a smooth beginning (at times the initial thrust of the response may be partially or completely correct), does the subject's response then wander onto tangential or irrelevant topics? Does the response reflect intermingled personal material? If yes, then evaluate the extent to which this additional material causes the response to appear odd and assign scores to the appropriate subcategories and to Category III.

d. Now consider the relation of the responses to the question or proverb. Does the content of the response (at least initially) refer to the question asked (irrespective of whether it is correct or incorrect, concrete or abstract, and despite other aspects of bizarreness)? Is there any discernible association between the words or concepts of the question or proverb on the one hand, and the subject's statement on the other? Assign a score reflecting the distance of the response from the question or proverb in Category IV.

e. Finally, consider whether or not the patients' physical, affective, or verbal behavior deviates from conventional norms during the test situation. If it does, then evaluate the degree and assign a score of 0, .5, 1 or 3 in Category V.

Each of the five categories is scored on the scoring sheet. This score should be at least equal to or greater than the highest score on any of the component subcategories.

The scoring of the above five categories is based primarily upon the following eleven subcategories of disturbed language and thinking. These indicators have proven useful in orienting raters to the behavioral foundations of the five descriptive categories of idiosyncratic thinking. In addition, it is possible that some of these subcategories may be related to specific mechanisms involved in bizarre-idiosyncratic thinking. It is possible that some bizarre-idiosyncratic responses may be influenced by, or in part be a consequence of, confusion-disorganization, a tendency to intermingle personal concerns when thinking about neutral material, a disorder in logical reasoning, or attending to part rather than all of a question. However, while these eleven subtypes of bizarre-idiosyncratic thinking may be important, they do not represent an exhaustive list of all possible types of bizarre behavior and ideas, or all the possible dimensions with which one can look at these phenomena. There are a vast number of ways one can be strange and bizarre, and a vast number of ways one can deviate from social convention in a personal or idiosyncratic manner.

Eleven Subcategories of Bizarre-Idiosyncratic Verbalizations

CATEGORY I: LINGUISTIC FORM AND STRUCTURE
  1. Strange Verbalizations
      A. Single words used in an unusual or peculiar manner (which are, in the rater's best judgment not attributable to intellectual or cultural deficits).
      B. Mild or moderate cognitive slippage in regard to sentence structure, the expression of ideas, or the construction of new words (the new word is close in form to the correct word).
      C. Neologisms (a new word with *private* meaning). Real neologisms (involving a private meaning) are very unusual, and are scored a "3."
      D. Artificial, pedantic, or stilted language, inappropriate to the level of discourse in the testing situation.
  2. Lack of Shared Communication
      A. Responses that are not explicitly stated.
      B. Small gaps in communication, in which words are not explained or referents are unclear.
      C. Larger gaps in communication, in which phrases are not explained. Elements of private language may be apparent with unshared or unexplained concepts or ideas.
      D. Disorganized or poor linkage between consecutive words, phrases, or sentences within the response.
CATEGORY II: THE CONTENT OF THE STATEMENT
  3. Responses Involving Coherent but Odd Ideas
  4. Responses that are Deviant with Respect to Social Convention
  5. Peculiar or Idiosyncratic Reasoning or Logic
      A. Responses that are incorrect and illogical in terms of common knowledge about people, events, or the environment.
      B. Responses violating a logical paradigm, such as predicate logic.
      C. Self-contradictory responses or responses with confused logic.
      D. Responses with peculiar, autistic logic.

6. Confused or Disorganized Ideas
   A. Combinations of words put together in a manner that only dimly makes sense.
   B. Grammatically correct sentences that do not hold a logical thought.

CATEGORY III: INTERMIXING

7. The Overelaborated Response
   A. Irrelevant wandering within a partially correct or correct answer.
   B. Elaboration that is far too extensive, to the point where the original question is almost lost from sight.
8. Intermingling of Personal Concerns or Associations into the Response

CATEGORY IV: RELATIONSHIP BETWEEN QUESTION AND RESPONSE

9. Attending to Part Rather than Whole: associations or interpretations of a word or phrase that suggest that the subject's response is not based on the question as a conceptual whole, and that also make the response appear strange or idiosyncratic.
10. The Lack of a Relationship between the Subject's Statement and the Question Asked—almost as if a different question is being asked.

CATEGORY V: BEHAVIOR

11. Strange Behavior—including physical and affective behavior.

In scoring a response according to the list of major categories and subcategories outlined above, the subject's response is first analyzed and scored according to each of the eleven subcategories, and then assigned scores on the five major categories. The presence of one type of subcategory of bizarre-idiosyncratic thinking in a response (e.g., lack of shared communication) does not exclude the simultaneous presence of another type or subcategory from that same response (e.g., intermingling or an overelaborated response).

The categories listed above were constructed to focus on the distinct properties of a response that may contribute to an overall impression of unusual or odd verbal behavior. However, at times, although a category score is indicated (i.e., something unusual occurs in linguistic style, or in how a response is stated), the idiosyncracy is not attributable to any specific subcategory or behavioral indicator. In such instances, a category score for bizarre-idiosyncratic thinking is still justified, while the individual behavioral descriptors are left blank.

As we have indicated, we conceive of the categories and the subcategories that comprise them as a list of possible aspects of idiosyncratic thought and language that are not exhaustive. The overall response score is a general barometer of bizarre-idiosyncracy, and the categories and their foci are probes for the components of such verbal behavior. Thus, it is possible that any one response may be scored for overall bizarreness but may not fit neatly into any of the outlined categories or subcategories, with all of the categories and subcategories consequently rated as 0.

On the other hand, if a score of 1 is assigned for any of the five categories, an *overall* score of at least 1 is logically indicated, as the overall response or part of it is clearly bizarre or idiosyncratic. Although the overall score should be at least as great as that given in any individual category, the accumulation of category scores may, and often does, add up to more than the overall score.

As we have indicated, many responses will be scored in more than one category or subcategory. In a sample of hospitalized schizophrenic patients, for example, we found that of those responses scored for bizarre-idiosyncratic language and thought, approximately 50 percent were scored in one subcategory, 30 percent in two subcategories, and 20 percent in three or more subcategories. This ratio, however, may differ with varying populations.

SECTION 2. BEHAVIORAL INDICATORS AND SCORING EXAMPLES OF BIZARRE-IDIOSYNCRATIC RESPONSES

I. Linguistic Form and Structure

This category addresses the subject's verbal style, the particular way a response is worded, and the manner of communication. A problem in this category implies that it is difficult to understand what the subject means owing to: (a) alterations of language, or (b) gaps in verbal communication. We have listed below, in the left-hand column, some of the types of linguistic behaviors that may receive a score in this category. A typical range of scores is also listed below in the right-hand column for the various types of bizarre-idiosyncratic responses. While the ranges listed below may provide helpful guidelines, other more (or less) pathological scores can be assigned, depending on the severity of the particular bizarre responses.

This Category Includes

Peculiar Word Form or Use   *Points Typically Scored*
Using incorrect words   .5–1

Peculiar word alterations	.5–1
Unusual word combinations	.5–1
Neologisms	3
Pedantic-stilted language	.5–1

Lack of Shared Communication	
Vague, diffuse expressions	.5–3
Private language	1–3
Word play	.5–1
Verbal cognitive slips	.5–1
Disorganized linkage of ideas	.5–3
Phrase and word salads	3

Additional Scoring Guidelines

1. Raters should be cautioned against scoring unconventional modes of speech attributable to low intellect or to subcultural habits, if the subject has had little opportunity to learn about more conventional modes of expression.
2. To merit a score of 1 for this category, the damage done to the response must be at least moderately severe. Although rare, extremely severe slips in word use occasionally occur and in some cases might be sufficiently pathological to be assigned a score of 3.
3. Scores for slippage in regard to word structure and use are influenced by: (a) the subject's ability to correct stumbling or awkward grammar (reduces score usually .5 point); (b) the extent of pedantry; and (c) the damage done to the comprehensibility of the response.
4. Scores for vague, diffuse expressions resulting from some gap in communication are on a continuum of poorly explained responses. Scoring is influenced by: (a) the subject's further explication of any vague comments after inquiry (reduces score); (b) the extent of the demand for understanding placed on the rater (increases score); and (c) the amount of real or specific information given.
5. The rater must be particularly careful *not* to consider incorrect answers or concrete interpretations of proverbs as examples of scoreable responses in this category. *A problem in expression* implies that it is difficult to understand what the subject means because of (a) alterations of normal language usage, or (b) gaps in the communication of ideas.
6. Strange verbalizations occurring *after inquiry* merit a lower score.
7. The disorganized linkage of ideas includes responses in which the grammatical structure is very poor. In less serious forms of this phenomenon, dangling phrases, missing verbs, and missing con-

junctions typically contribute to a disorganized sentence structure. More serious forms impress the rater as lacking the foundation of an idea and are also scored in Category II.

8. Phrase and word salads are defined as words that are strung together in a meaningless fashion. Distinctions between a 1- and 3-point response are dependent upon the pervasiveness of the disorganization and the extent of incoherence.

II. The Content of the Statement, The Ideas Expressed

This category pertains to peculiarities within a response that reflect confusion in ideas, peculiar or idiosyncratic logic, and asocial attitudes (descriptions of behavior that most people would recognize as strange, unusual, or taboo in our society). More serious forms of bizarre responses fitting under this category impress the rater as lacking the foundation of an idea or organized explanation.

This Category Includes	*Points Typically Scored*
Coherent but Odd Ideas: Well-articulated thoughts that are counter to socially acceptable ideas and are not associated with current subcultural trends	.5–3
Responses that are deviant in respect to social convention: a. violations of conventional belief systems— unconventional ideas about the efficacy of various means of accomplishing certain ends.	.5–3
b. Violations of conventional values. c. Violations of conventional rules—legal regulations and formal norms.	
Peculiar or idiosyncratic reasoning: a. Responses that are incorrect and illogical in terms of common knowledge about people, events, or the environment.	1–3

Examples of Category I:* Linguistic Form and Structure	Subcategory Score	Notes on Subcategory Score	Overall Scores	Additional Notes
Peculiar Word Form or Use:				
THE WIFE IS THE KEY TO THE HOUSE "Huh! Doesn't make any *rhetorical sense* at all. Urr . . . it is rhetorical—no sense to me at all."	.5	Peculiar use of the word "rhetorical"; however, subject spontaneously makes correction, reducing score from 1 point to .5 point for this cognitive slip.	.5	
ROME WAS NOT BUILT IN A DAY "You should take your time. *Haste makes pace* as they say, or haste makes waste. You should never really work too fast."	.5	Because "Haste makes pace" is corrected, a score of 1 is reduced to .5.	.5	
A STREAM CANNOT RISE HIGHER THAN ITS COURSE "I guess it means the stream is conservative even if it rains it is not enough to overflow it. It's a *conservative stream* if it never rises above its peak—it never rises above what it really is."	.5	The word "conservative" is odd in this context.	.5	
BARKING DOGS SELDOM BITE "A dog with a bark normally, his bark is worse than his bite, *is badder, is better.*"	.5	This case shows idiosyncratic verbalization in relation to a loose use of words.	.5	
WHAT SHOULD YOU DO IF YOU'RE THE FIRST PERSON TO SEE SMOKE AND FIRE? "I'd go to the usher or person with an air of officialdom."	.5	Slightly pedantic	.5	Only slightly unusual

Continued

Examples of Category I:* Linguistic Form and Structure	Subcategory Score	Notes on Subcategory Score	Overall Scores	Additional Notes
Peculiar Word Form or Use:				
WHY ARE PEOPLE WHO ARE BORN DEAF USUALLY UNABLE TO TALK? "They can't hear vocal tones and it's difficult to form *verbage* because they can't hear others talking."	.5	Slight alteration of an existing word—we know what the subject intended to say.	.5	
A STREAM CANNOT RISE HIGHER THAN ITS SOURCE "A good seed grows a good plant. [Q] That means that if you have a good start you'll probably . . . it probably means that if you're full of shit then you're full of shit whether you like it or not."	.5	An inappropriate level of discourse is used. However, the original statement, giving another proverb, is correct and not bizarre.	.5	Receives a .5 rather than 1 because bizarreness is stimulated by inquiry.
DISCRETION IS THE BETTER PART OF VALOR "Pliant rectitude is a trait more appropriate for successful living than hotheadedness which is either stubborn or crusady."	1	Adds syllable to forcefit a word. Also responds at an inappropriate level of discourse.	1	Although the response involves an idea that accurately answers the question, the response is pedantic, and also fits other criteria for bizarre language.
DON'T JUDGE A BOOK BY ITS COVER "A facade of regal compliance bides an etiology of ire."	1	Very pedantic—too abstract—out of proportion with the task.	3	
WHY SHOULD WE KEEP AWAY FROM BAD COMPANY? "So you don't intoxicate yourself with poison."	1	"Intoxicate" is inappropriate here. The idea of "poison" also is idiosyncratic.	1	

	Score	Comment	Score	Comment
THE GRASS IS ALWAYS GREENER IN THE OTHER FELLOW'S YARD "Don't trouble trouble till trouble troubles you."	1	Word play spoils the response.	1	
DON'T SWAP HORSES WHEN CROSSING A STREAM "That's wish-bell. Double vision [Wish bell?] It's like walking across a person's eye and reflecting personality. It works on you, like dying and going to the spiritual world, but landing in the *Vella* world [Vella?]"	3	Neologisms are presented.	3	Also scored for confused idea, lack of shared communication, odd outlook, lack of relation to the proverb, and illogic.

Lack of Shared Communication:

	Score	Comment	Score	Comment
SPEECH IS THE PICTURE OF THE MIND "That's true."	.5	Subject comments without any attempt at clearly verbalized interpretation.	.5	Meets a criterion of bizarreness—is inappropriate for the task at hand.
WHERE THERE'S A WILL, THERE'S A WAY "You can't do everything though."	.5	The comment is on an implicit, unstated interpretation.	.5	
TO FIDDLE WHILE ROME BURNS "To amuse oneself when the avoidance of responsibility shouldn't be."	.5	The grammer is poor and disorganized. However, the rater is able to understand the meaning of the awkward verbalization.	.5	

Continued

Examples of Category I:* Linguistic Form and Structure	Subcategory Score	Notes on Subcategory Score	Overall Scores	Additional Notes
Lack of Shared Communication				
WHY DOES LAND IN THE CITY COST MORE THAN LAND IN THE COUNTRY? "Land in the city, it's more of a public concern to have a house in the city, so there are more taxes on it."	.5		.5	
WHEN THE CATS AWAY, THE MICE WILL PLAY "When law and order is out, the group under will slack off and tend to go away, instead of a set law that is restricting them will think more of them."	1	The last part of this response seems unconnected to the rest of the response.	1	
THE USED KEY IS ALWAYS BRIGHT "The right path, you'll know the right path."	3	The rater is impressed with a large amount of missing information.	3	Very difficult to empathize with—little idea of where response comes from.
ROME WAS NOT BUILT IN A DAY "Yeah. It means never. We're together, We're here together."	3		3	

*Although in a number of these examples, scores in other categories in addition to Category I are appropriate, only Category I scores will be noted and explained at this point.

b. Responses violating a logical paradigm,
   such as predicate logic.*   1–3

c. Self-contradictory responses with confused
   logic

Confused ideas   .5–3

Additional Scoring Guidelines

1. At times, the response to a question is so severely bizarre or odd that one cannot recognize why it would in any way be given as a response, since it seems to contain little material related to the original proverb or question. If it is hard to recognize it at all as a response to the original question it should be scored under Category IV, rather than Category II, unless the response is independently peculiar or strange.
2. Scores for peculiar or idiosyncratic reasoning or logic require an *explicit* statement involving faulty reasoning.
3. Scoring distinctions among the various types of idiosyncratic reasoning or logic are made on the basis of: (a) the deviance of reasoning from conventional or consensual thought, and (b) the type of illogic shown, with predicate logic considered as the most severe form and typically scored at the 3-point level.
4. If an illogical response comes after inquiry or encouragement, leniency in scoring is in order.
5. This category includes confused or jumbled communications and responses that show little evidence of a cogent idea. In some cases, disorganized sentence structure is apparent, and a score in Category I also is appropriate.

III. Intermixing Tendencies

This category assesses tendencies to mix or blend material into the response from the subject's past or current experience, or to extend or elaborate a seemingly neutral theme or idea, making the response appear strange. The result of the intermingling process is that relatively neutral proverb and comprehension items will show one or several

---

*Predicate logic is the establishment of equivalence between objects, things, ideas, etc. by focusing on the predicate rather than the identity of the equivalent. Thus, if:

  a. an angel is encircled by a halo;
  b. a cigar is encircled by a halo;
  c. an angel equals a cigar because both are encircled.

Examples of Category II: The Content of the Statement	Subcategory Score	Notes on Subcategory Score	Overall Score	Additional Notes
Coherent but Odd Ideas:				
WHY ARE CHILD LABOR LAWS NEEDED? "So the old can help the young. [Q] What's the question? [Repeat question] *It's a matter of distributing responsibility so the young don't have all the responsibility.*"	.5	Subject does not seem to be communicating what was originally intended.	.5	
WHY ARE PEOPLE WHO ARE BORN DEAF USUALLY UNABLE TO TALK? "Because they have nothing to talk about except that they are bored."	1		1	
ONE SWALLOW DOESN'T MAKE A SUMMER "Just because a bird says it's summer and acts like it's summer, it really isn't."	3	Strange ideation emerges in both the idea of birds verbally telling us that it is summer, and the "twist" that the birds are inaccurate and it really is not summer.	3	Clearly idiosyncratic with several odd ideas.
Deviant with Respect to Social Convention:				
IT'S BETTER TO BE HAPPY THAN WISE "Right. The retarded don't know how good they've got it."	.5	This response is considered deviant in terms of conventional beliefs.	1	Unusual with regard to outlook, and deviates from social convention.
IF YOU WERE LOST IN THE FOREST IN THE DAYTIME, HOW WOULD YOU FIND YOUR WAY OUT? "Jump on a tree."	1	Violates conventional beliefs about the efficacy of various means of accomplishing an end.	1	Also involves odd logic.

Item	Score	Comment
WHAT WOULD YOU DO IF WHILE IN THE MOVIES YOU WERE THE FIRST PERSON TO SEE SMOKE AND FIRE? "Just keep quiet. [Q] Just ignore it—think it's from the movie screen."	1	
WHAT WOULD YOU DO IF WHILE IN THE MOVIES YOU WERE THE FIRST TO SEE SMOKE AND FIRE? "I'd start picking up all the paper from the floor so it wouldn't burn."	3	This response would also fit under "odd outlook."
WHY ARE PEOPLE BORN DEAF USUALLY UNABLE TO TALK? "Because nobody wants to have anything to do with stupid people like that. They should all be put away in home."	1	
IF YOU WERE LOST IN THE FOREST IN THE DAYTIME, HOW WOULD YOU FIND YOUR WAY OUT? "I'd walk around in circles until I got dizzy and fell down asleep and dream about a passageway—wouldn't you?"	3	

Peculiar Reasoning or Logic:

Item	Score	Comment
ONE SWALLOW DOESN'T MAKE A SUMMER "Because two swallows make the summer more beautiful." A response that is illogical	.5	This response is also strange in terms of common knowledge about the environment.

Continued

Examples of Category II: The Content of the Statement	Subcategory Score	Notes on Subcategory Score	Overall Score	Additional Notes
Peculiar Reasoning or Logic:				
IF YOU WERE LOST IN THE FOREST IN THE DAYTIME, HOW WOULD YOU FIND YOUR WAY OUT? "First of all, I always know where the sun goes out and in; East and West. If I go into the forest I know where I go in, in relation to my house, so I can know where the closest way out is."	1		1	May also contain confusion of ideas ("in relation to my house"), although this is unclear from subject's presentation.
ONE SWALLOW DOESN'T MAKE A SUMMER "Summers are warm and it takes more than one summer to cool off."	1	An illogical response.	1	Also contains gaps in communication.
WHY SHOULD WE KEEP AWAY FROM BAD COMPANY? "Is that a question? Why is Jesus to me. It sounds like you are asking Jesus to me. Like asking Jesus the question—so it's none of my business. You know how he hung on the cross in like a Y. So he's 'why' to me. You'll have trouble with every 'why' question you ask me until I have this straightened out. That wasn't me talking—that was Peter the Apostle."	3	An example of predicate logic.	3	A severe type of bizarre response.
Confused Ideas:				
WHY DOES LAND IN THE CITY COST MORE THAN LAND IN THE COUNTRY? "Land in the city. It's more of a public concern to have a house in the city, so there are more taxes on it."	5		.5	

Proverb / Response		Description		Note
WHEN THE CAT'S AWAY THE MICE WILL PLAY "When law and order is out, the group under will slack off and tend to go away instead of a set law that is restricting them will think more of them."	1	After a reasonably coherent response, the subject makes a cognitive jump and ideas become difficult to decipher.	1	Also score in Category 1.
SHALLOW BROOKS ARE NOISY "Because they flood or make a sand."	1	Disorganized explanation.	1	Also scored in Category I ("make a sand").
DON'T COUNT YOUR CHICKENS UNTIL THEY'RE HATCHED "One chicken might go bad, and if it had twelve, but then only eleven, so don't count on it."	1		3	Difficult to empathize with—missing communication is also apparent (Category I).
DON'T CROSS YOUR BRIDGES TILL YOU COME TO THEM "Working continuously a person can only imagine."	3	Subject presents an incoherent thought.	3	A score in Category I is also appropriate here.
WHEN THE CAT'S AWAY THE MICE WILL PLAY "If something has to do with freedom to do with something you want to do. When they're gone you can do whatever it is. Do you want it another way? When something is injured or you have been injured then you aren't like you were catching mice."	3	An odd response that becomes more severely bizarre as the patient gives a strange overelaboration.	3	Also scored in Category III as a bizarre overelaborate response.
WHY ARE PEOPLE WHO ARE BORN DEAF USUALLY UNABLE TO TALK? "When you swallow in your throat like a key it comes out, but not a scissors. A robin, too, it means spring."	3	Rater is impressed by lack of organization and coherence in the response.	3	Verbalizations are generally confused and contradictory.

features. It may show an intermingling of fragments or parts of the patient's problems or concerns into the response, or the response will become extensively and needlessly elaborated. It will move away from the typical correct answer and shift into the direction of the subject's associations.

Some intermingling contains weak or mild evidence that the irrelevant material added might possibly be a consequence of personal concerns, and thus a case of intermingling. Unless there is moderate or strong evidence that the extra material is related to personal concerns, it is scored as an overelaborated response.

This Subcategory Includes	*Points Typically Scored*
Intermingling of personal themes	.5–3
Overelaboration on a theme not of a personal nature	.5–3
Irrelevant wandering from the task, not of a personal nature	.5–3
Extensive and unnecessary elaboration of a concept, not of a personal nature	1–3
Loose association of ideas	.5–3

Additional Scoring Guidelines

1. Intermingled material will usually be of a personal nature or contain affectively loaded words. The content may represent conflicts, wishes, concerns, attitudes or problems, that are inserted at the beginning, middle, or end of the response. As a criterion for scoring, the response would contain more than a casual personal reference— i.e., the intermingled material should make the response appear strange. Response-relevant personal examples that are appropriate *are not scored* for this category.
2. A score of 3 for intermingling applies to only the very obviously intermingled material that does not fit at all, and that makes the response seem extremely strange or bizarre (e.g., extensive anecdotes by the patient about himself or his own past or current experience).
3. If intermingling occurs after inquiry, leniency in scoring is called for (what is scored a 3 prior to inquiry is scored 1 postinquiry; 1-point responses are dropped to .5-point scores postinquiry).
4. *Do not score* story telling or explanations that, in response to inquiry, are clarifications of an appropriate response.
5. Scores of .5–1 for overelaborated responses and irrelevant wandering pertain to short transgressions—a phrase or one sentence—in

which the subject overattends to one aspect of the question or to one idea or thought. In this type of tangential wandering, although the subject is off the track, we can usually identify the association that governs the speech.

6. If the wandering is more extensive than a phrase or one sentence, 3 points are scored for the loss of distance. In these cases, the elaboration is so extensive that the original question is almost lost from sight.

IV. The Relationship between Question and Response

The emphasis in this category is on determining if the subject is able to address the task of interpreting the proverb or responding to a question.

This Category Includes	*Points Typically Scored*
Attending to a part of the question *rather than the whole*, making the response appear strange or idiosyncratic.	.5–3
Responses in which there is *no or very little trace of the original question.*	3

Additional Scoring Guidelines

1. At times, the individual partially interprets the proverb and then goes off on a loosely associated tangent. In these cases, the interpretative task has not been ignored, but the individual has overincluded tangential topics within the response. These bizarre responses should be scored under Category III.
2. Attending to a particular aspect of the proverb rather than understanding the proverb as a whole will be scored when there is a failure to interpret the stimulus material. That is, attention is given to a particular word or phrase only to the extent that the word or phrase dominates the entire response and leads the subject away from consensual responses.
3. A 3-point response in this category is characterized as so grossly bizarre that it is hard to match the response with the item given. It is hard to think of an extenuating circumstance or justification for these responses.
4. By contrast, a 1-point response contains a hint as to how the response is related to the proverb or question asked. However, even

Examples of Category III: Intermixing	Subcategory Score	Notes on Subcategory Score	Overall Score	Additional Notes
The Overelaborated Response				
IF YOU WERE LOST IN THE FOREST IN THE DAYTIME, HOW WOULD YOU GO ABOUT FINDING YOUR WAY OUT? "Go up to the main road if there was one, and if there wasn't, I wouldn't go back into the woods. There are swamps, poison oak, poison ivy, snakes, etc."	.5	The subject overattends to one aspect of the question.	1	
WHEN THE CATS AWAY THE MICE WILL PLAY "When something kind of happens, you know that you're doing something wrong, but if the authority is gone, then it's not wrong anymore. Thus, it's like taking advantage of it, the authority that's gone, and then you won't feel guilty about it, etc., etc."	1	If the subject extends his association to a couple of sentences or to a few associations, a 1-point score is appropriate.	1	This response contains some material that may be related to personal concerns (e.g., guilt) and is scored for intermingling.

A ROLLING STONE GATHERS NO MOSS

"That was a yesterday thing. If you keep yourself moving towards your goal whatever it may be and if you keep the goal in mind when you make decisions then you are most likely not to be led astray by feeling sorry for yourself, or greed or that type of thing. And if you just forget about your goals and values and give up hope and say the hell with everything, deteriorate, then you can get yourself in trouble."

3   Here the amount of extra material is extensive.

3   Also scored for intermingling.

The Intermingled Response

A STREAM CANNOT RISE HIGHER THAN ITS SOURCE

"A father is—no—a son is not greater than his father. I was talking about age not wisdom, but I'll say age."

.5   The answer is a personalized example of what the abstract, consensual answer depicts. It is slight intermingling.

.5   It is only mildly idiosyncratic.

THE USED KEY IS ALWAYS BRIGHT

"In the future, the key to my parent's house is a key for me to come there for anything at all. That's the way I want it."

1   The intermingling in this example is clear.

1   Although mildly off, the response remains fairly comprehensible.

DON'T SWAP HORSES IN THE MIDDLE OF A STREAM

"You shouldn't switch decisions or switch friendships with another just because he seems friendly—he might not be. May only be pretending. Stand your ground."

1   The first phrase and the last sentence are very close to the consensual answer. The middle part seems to be a topic that has personal meaning for the subject and makes the answer stray off the track in an inappropriate manner.

Continued

Examples of Category III: Intermixing

	Subcategory Score	Notes on Subcategory Score	Overall Score	Additional Notes
The Overelaborated Response				
WHY SHOULD WE KEEP AWAY FROM BAD COMPANY? "I've got a lot of friends that do a lot of dope. It's better to stay away from it so I can dry myself out. Misery loves company—that's a proverb. [Q: Can you say more?] Because they influence you like anybody else would."	1	In this example there is an overt reference to the self concerning a topic that is important to the patient. However, upon inquiry, the subject gives the consensual response, making it slightly less idiosyncratic.	1	
ROME WAS NOT BUILT IN A DAY "It's love. I think of it as love. I have to work towards love and love has to work towards me. And this has to gradually come."	1		1	
SHALLOW BROOKS ARE NOISY "There's a lot of rocks in shallow brooks. Sin and grief. [Q: Could you say some more?] The rocks kind of symbolize sin and grief."	1	"Sin and grief" look out of place in the answer and are not part of the consensual or typical response. They probably have a certain importance for the subject.	1	
A DROWNING MAN WILL CLUTCH AT A STRAW "Duh. Help! Is anyone going to save him? [Q: Could you say some more?] I could say I'm a drowning man right now. Anyone who asks for help. Ask and you shall receive. Seek and you shall find. It all has to do with Christ."	3	This answer is clearly affected by the subject's concern over his status and asking for help. This is a case of severe intermingling.	3	The response reflects a radical departure from the original question. While one can understand that the response has been influenced by both the original question and the subject's concerns, it is somewhat irrelevant, highly individualistic, and appears very strange.

with this clue, the response cannot be characterized as an appropriate interpretation.

V. Behavior

This category assesses behavior as it relates to conventional norms for conduct in a testing situation. A score in this category is attributed for behavior that is deviant either in its extreme expression, or in its incongruity and inappropriateness to the requirements of the situation. These requirements include both: (a) performance expectations associated with the formal testing procedures (e.g., responding with attention and verbalizations to the test questions), and (b) more general expectations associated with the interpersonal social context in which testing occurs.

This Subcategory Includes	*Points Typically Scored*
Physical behavior	
a. extremes in activity level	.5–3
b. behaviors showing loss of conventional social restraint	.5–3
c. exaggerated or unusual posture, mannerisms or gestures	.5–3
d. unusual modulation of pitch, speed volume or length of speech	.5–3
e. verbalizations showing loss of conventional social restraint	.5–3
f. nonsocial speech	.5–3
Affective behavior	
a. extremes in level of affective expression	.5–3
b. extreme lability of affect	.5–3
c. inappropriateness of affect in relation to situational context	.5–3

Additional Scoring Guidelines

1. In general, responses receiving higher ratings (1–3 points) in this category represent behaviors that would tend to appear idiosyncratic in a wide range of interpersonal contexts outside the formal testing situation.
2. Responses receiving minimal (.5) ratings tend to be those that, while unusual in the testing context, are less obtrusive and do not interfere as much with the subject's responding to the task.

Examples of Category IV:

The Relation between Question and Response	Subcategory Score	Notes on Subcategory Score	Overall Score	Additional Notes
Attention to limited part of the stimulus				
ONE SWALLOW DOESN'T MAKE A SUMMER "When you swallow something, it could be all right, but the next minute you could be coughing, and dreariness and all kinds of miserable things coming out of your throat."	1	The individual overincludes tangential themes associated to the most dominant meaning of the word "swallow."	1	We should note even when the word "swallow" is interpreted in terms of its alternate meaning, the response to it is still strange. Category II is also scored.
TOO MANY COOKS SPOIL THE BROTH "Too many killing people are around here."	1	This response is apparently not focused on the issues or questions raised by the proverb but rather is focused on issues associated to a phrase in the proverb.	1	
THE MORE COST THE MORE HONOR "The more the bad man cares, the worse he gets."	1	Although one can recognize pieces of the original proverb, the response fails to address the main theme of the question.	3	The examiner has little idea of where the response has come from.
DON'T SWAP (TRADE) HORSES WHEN CROSSING A STREAM "Horses run courses, there are racetracks all over the country."	1	Focus on the part (word "horse") rather than the whole, so that the proverb is interpreted in a strange and irrelevant manner	3	Also scored in Category I.

The Lack of a Relation between the Subject's Statement and the Question Asked:

WHY SHOULD WE KEEP AWAY FROM BAD COMPANY? "Say your prayers."	3	There is little trace of the original question; the examiner or scorer has only a vague hint of where the response has come from.	3	This type of response is very inappropriate and unresourceful to the task.
WHY SHOULD PEOPLE PAY TAXES "Show me the time to reason."	3	Again, it almost seems as if a different proverb or question is being answered.	3	
THE GRASS IS ALWAYS GREENER IN THE OTHER FELLOW'S YARD "There's a baby in my young man that calls me daddy."	3		3	Also scored in Categories I and II.
DON'T THROW GOOD MONEY AFTER BAD "Don't go to bed with your mother or your father if you want to go to sainthood."	3		3	Also scored in Category III.

Examples of Category V: Behavior	Subcategory Score	Notes on Subcategory Score	Overall Score	Additional Notes
BARKING DOGS SELDOM BITE "People who appear to be tough and abrasive many times on the inside are somewhat kind, considerate, compassionate and sad [subject begins to cry softly].	.5	The patient's personal concerns have overtly influenced her behavior, although this has occurred in a way that one can understand or empathize with.	.5	Also scored in Category III.
A STREAM CANNOT RISE HIGHER THAN ITS SOURCE "You can't go higher than your abilities." [Subject giggles for awhile.]	.5	Slightly inappropriate affect.	.5	
RICHES SERVE A WISE MAN BUT COMMAND A FOOL "You should always spend your money wisely, honey." [Grabs examiner's hand.]	1	Loss of conventional social restraint.	1	
WHY SHOULD WE KEEP AWAY FROM BAD COMPANY? "Darn you. Why did you ask me that?"	1		1	

IT NEVER RAINS BUT IT POURS "God's rule comes in huge storms." [Covers her head with her coat and giggles.]	1	Unusual behavior and affect.		Idiosyncratic; evokes a personal association of the individual's that is difficult to understand. Also scored in Category III.
THE WIFE IS THE KEY TO THE HOUSE "I'll agree with that." [sings, "A house is not a home without a wife."]	3		3	Also scored in Category I.
GOLD GOES IN ANY GATE EXCEPT HEAVEN'S "When you go in everything looks golden. Then comes the knock [subject knocks table]. Then who's there? [knocks again] Who's there?" [uses profane language.]	3	Inappropriate activities and speech.	3	Also scored in Categories I and IV.
WHAT SHOULD YOU DO IF WHILE IN THE MOVIES YOU WERE THE FIRST PERSON TO SEE SMOKE AND FIRE? "Report the fire [yells] FIRE! FIRE!" [runs around room wildly.]	3	Extreme activity level, grossly inappropriate affect and speech.	3	Not scored in any other category.

3. Behavior scored in this category must take place during administration of either the Proverb or Comprehension tests. The behavior, however, need not occur as part of the subject's response to specific test items (e.g., "Will you go out for a drink with me?").

SECTION 3. SCORING SHEETS AND PRACTICE PROTOCOLS

SUBJECT #1

Comprehension Subtest (Wais, 1955)

*3. *What is the thing to do if you find an envelope in the street that is sealed, and addressed, and has a new stamp?*

   Put it in the mailbox.

*4. *Why should we keep away from bad company?*

   You hit the nail on the head on what brought me into this place. I will say, there's people, and we pray for them but we must stay away from them.

*5. *What should you do if while in the movies you were the first person to see smoke and fire?*

   Try to put it out. That's what I do here. I tell them not to smoke. You don't holler help because you cause panic.

6. *Why should people pay taxes?*

   They have to, to help the other half live.

7. *What does this saying mean? "Strike while the iron is hot."*

   IDK. (Might mean?) If the iron was hot, I'd mess my shirt. If not, I'd burn my shirt. I'd have to test it first so I wouldn't be burnt. I don't want to be burnt.

8. *Why are child labor laws needed?*

   It's very important because of all our children going to college, there's such a vast amount of people. We need labor laws that will help them get a job—like myself.

9. *If you were lost in the forest in the daytime, how would you go about finding your way out?*

> I've been lost in the forest, kept going around in circles. The sun didn't shine, I was scared. Then this leg is shorter than the other. I found my way out.

10. *Why are people who are born deaf usually unable to talk?*

> Because they can't hear what you're saying—but that's not so they do talk to you eventually through Braille because I've driven with them. Handicapped people I drove for.

11. *Why does land in the city cost more than land in the country?*

> Because it's incorporated.

12. *Why does state require people to get a licence in order to get married?*

> It's mostly for the women's welfare. They have it binding so the women can protect the children's interest in case there's the mishap of a divorce—then they're protected.

13. *Saying mean? "Shallow brooks are noisy."*

> Somebody, you listen to them. It's the same melody all day long. (Melody?) If you listen to it rain it puts you to sleep.

14. *Saying mean? "One swallow doesn't make a summer."*

> I don't know.

Proverbs Test (Gorham, 1956)

PROVERBS TEST I   Name ___Subject #2___ Date _____

Circle One: TP_1 F_1 F_2 F_3 F_4 F_5

Directions: I am going to read you some sayings. For example, the saying: "Large oaks from little acorns grow" could mean that great things may have small beginnings. Now, I want you to tell me what the saying means rather than to just tell me more about it. Try to answer every one.

1. *Where there's a will, there's a way.*

> There's a way then. You just put your whole self in; you put a lot

Score Sheet for Bizarre-Idiosyncratic Responses

Subject ID _____ Subject #1 _____ Rater _____ Date: _____
                                                                    Administration

Setting: Reese ISPI Other _____ Proverbs Form 1 Form 2 Form 3
                                                                    Date: _____
TP1 TP2 F1 F2 F3 F4 F5   Comprehension (circle one)   Scoring
          (circle one)

Response Number	Overall Score	I. Linguistic Form and Structure			II. The Content of the Statement The Ideas Expressed				
		Peculiar word form or use	Lack of Shared Communicat.	Overall Category I.	Coherent but odd ideas	Deviant with respect to social convention	Illogic	Confused ideas	Overall Category II.
Prov. Comp	0,.5,1,3								
1	.5								
2	.5		.5	.5					
3 3	0								
4 4	0								
5 5	1				.5		1	.5	1
6 6	1								
7 7	1								
8 8	1								
9 9	3		3	3					
10 10	.5								
11 11	.5		.5	.5					
12 12	3	.5	1	1	1				1
13									
14									

CARD A: CARDS B-E:
Keypunch This   Keypunch These Rows Reading Across Left to Right
Column

Overall Sum	8.5	.5	3.5	4.0	0	0	1.0	2.5	3.5
Sum: 1 & 3pt. rsp.	7	0	3	3	0	0	1	2	3
# of 0's	4	11	8	7	12	12	11	9	8
# of .5's	3	1	1	2	0	0	0	1	1
# of 1's	4	0	3	3	0	0	1	2	3
# of 3's	1	0	0	0	0	0	0	0	0

# of Don't knows _____ 1

# of no Responses _____ 0

# of not scoreable _____ 0

Total Unrated _____ 1

Subject #1 (Continued)

| | III. Intermixing | | IV. Relationship Between Response and Question | | | V. Behavior |
Over Elaborated	Intermingled	Overall Category III.	Attention to limited part of stimulus	Lack of Relationship to stimulus material	Overall Category IV.	Overall Category V.
.5	1	1				
	.5	.5				
	1	1	.5		.5	
	.5	.5				
	1	1				
.5		.5				
				1	1	
3.0	2.5	5.0	2.5	0	2.5	1.0
2	1	3	2	0	2	0
8	8	5	9	12	9	10
2	3	4	1	0	1	2
2	1	3	2	0	2	0
0	0	0	0	0	0	0

Score Sheet for Bizarre-Idiosyncratic Responses

Subject ID _____ Subject #2 _____ Rater _____ Date: _____
Administration

Setting: Reese ISPI Other _____ Proverbs Form 1 Form 2 Form 3
Date: _____
Scoring

TP1 TP2 F1 F2 F3 F4 F5   Comprehension (circle one)
(circle one)

Response Number	Overall Score	I. Linguistic Form and Structure			II. The Content of the Statement — The Ideas Expressed				
		Peculiar word form or use	Lack of Shared Communicat.	Overall Category I.	Coherent but odd ideas	Deviant with respect to social convention	Illogic	Confused ideas	Overall Category II.
Prov. Comp	0,.5,1,3								
1									
2									
3	3	0							
4	4	1							
5	5	.5							
6	6	0							
7	7	1		1	1			1		1
8	8	.5		.5	.5				.5	.5
9	9	3		1	1				1	1
10	10	1							1	1
11	11	0								
12	12	.5	.5		.5					
	13	1		1	1					
	14	0								

CARD A:
Keypunch This Column

CARDS B-E:
Keypunch These Rows Reading Across Left to Right

Overall Sum	12	.5	5.0	5.0	1.5	0	1.0	.5	2.0
Sum: 1 & 3pt. rsp.	10	0	4	4	1	0	1	0	2
# of 0's	2	11	8	8	10	12	11	11	10
# of .5's	4	1	2	2	1	0	0	1	0
# of 1's	4	0	1	1	1	0	1	0	2
# of 3's	2	0	1	1	0	0	0	0	0

# of Don't knows   0

# of no Responses   0

# of not scoreable   0

Total Unrated   0

Subject #2 (Continued)

	III. Intermixing		IV. Relationship Between Response and Question			V. Behavior
Over Elaborated	Intermingled	Overall Category III.	Attention to limited part of stimulus	Lack of Relationship to stimulus material	Overall Category IV.	Overall Category V.
.5		.5				.5
1	.5	1	1		1	
1		1	1		1	
.5		.5	.5		.5	
	.5	.5				
	.5	.5				
	1	1				.5
1.0	4.0	4.5	.5	1.0	1.5	0
0	1	1	0	1	1	0
10	1	6	11	11	10	12
2	2	3	1	0	1	0
0	3	3	0	1	1	0
0	0	0	0	0	0	0

of fortitude in; if it's really what you want. You really go after it. I want a discharge, do you think I'll get it?

2. *Rome was not built in a day.*

   It wasn't. It takes time to build democracy, and a lot of churches and government, our whole being.

3. *When the cat's away the mice will play.*

   That's when momma isn't looking, the kids are doing what they want to.

4. *Barking dogs seldom bite.*

   They usually don't.

5. *A stream cannot rise higher than its source.*

   That's the truth. It can't rise higher because it's the same out of water. It can't raise any higher. If it rains enough, it might.

6. *Don't swap (trade) horses when crossing a stream.*

   Depends on the horses, I guess. Maybe you might have a wild horse. Maybe you might want to borrow the other person's horse that's tamer. I was almost killed on one, it took off on me.

7. *The used key is always bright.*

   Usually its dull, isn't it? It could be a key to a piano, too. It depends on what kind of key you're thinking of. It could be a thought. A key to a city. A key to anything, you know.

8. *Gold goes in at any gate except heaven's.*

   There's jewelry, there's platinum. They use it on your teeth for filling. There's gold in churches. There's gold in these mosque areas; like Lincoln's Tomb.

9. *One swallow (bird) doesn't make a summer.*

   It does make a summer, because they only come out in the summertime, in warm weather. A play on words, I have that any time I go for any driver's license.

10. *The wife is the key to the house.*

    She is because she is a doctor, a nurse, a psychologist. She keeps the family going. If she's upset then the children are too.

11. *Riches serve a wise man but command a fool.*

Yes. They do. Money goes where money is. It dominates the poor. We all struggle through that.

12. *Don't cast pearls before swine (pigs).*

That's like taking a good person, virtue unlimited, feasting them before a swine that just wants to make something little of you, swine shit. That's what happened to me. That's what brought me in here.

BLANK
Score Sheet for Bizarre-Idiosyncratic Responses

Subject ID _____ Rater _____ Date: _____
Administration

Setting: Reese ISPI Other _____ Proverbs Form 1 Form 2 Form 3

Date: _____
Scoring

TP1 TP2 F1 F2 F3 F4 F5   Comprehension (circle one)
(circle one)

Response Number	Overall Score	I. Linguistic Form and Structure				II. The Content of the Statement The Ideas Expressed			
		Peculiar word form or use	Lack of Shared Communicat.	Overall Category I.	Coherent but odd ideas	Deviant with respect to social convention	Illogic	Confused ideas	Overall Category II.
Prov. Comp	0,.5,1,3								
1									
2									
3	3								
4	4								
5	5								
6	6								
7	7								
8	8								
9	9								
10	10								
11	11								
12	12								
	13								
	14								

CARD A: CARDS B-E:
Keypunch This   Keypunch These Rows Reading Across Left to Right
Column

Overall
Sum

Sum: 1 &
3pt. rsp.

# of 0's

of .5's

of 1's

# of 3's

# of Don't
knows _____

# of no
Responses _____

# of not
scoreable _____

Total
Unrated

Blank Score Sheet (Continued)

	III. Intermixing		IV. Relationship Between Response and Question			V. Behavior
Over Elaborated	Intermingled	Overall Category III.	Attention to limited part of stimulus	Lack of Relationship to stimulus material	Overall Category IV.	Overall Category V.

Author Index

Subject Index

Affect, 7, 8
  blocking, 9
  blunted, 15
  inappropriate, 15
  labile, 15
Affective elaboration, 217, 334, 336
American Psychiatric Association, 33, 88
Amphetamines, 285, 297, 299, 303, 307
Analysis of Variance, 198
Anhedonia, 113
Anxiety, 277-279, 286, 291, 359
Association, 7, 8
  association links, 8
  "looseness," 13, 14, 45, 187-210

Beck Depression Inventory, 256
Bizarre-idiosyncratic thinking, 6, 12, 23, 24,
    44-78
  acute psychopathology influence, 115-117
  assessment of, 394-411
  categories and subcategories, 412-449
  chronic versus acute schizophrenics,
    108-111
  continuum hypothesis, 88

correlation among tests, 60, 61
definition and criteria, 45, 364-372
diagnostic indicators, 68, 88
dichotomy hypothesis, 88
family member differences, 317
frequency, 54
index of, 76
influences, 90-105
intermingling, 118-123
long-time study, 90-105
mild versus severe levels, 79-82
monitoring, 53
perspective, 53, 57
phase of partial recovery, 91-105
positive thought disorder, 364-372
process-reactive schizophrenia, 72-79
social context, 71
unique to schizophrenia, 83-85
Bizarre speech, 49-51
  definition, 49
  unique to schizophrenia, 83, 84
Boundaries, 212-235
  barrier, 218-221, 223, 224, 227-230, 337
  confabulation, 216-218, 330